Men's Health Concerns

SOURCEBOOK

SIXTH EDITION

Health Reference Series

Men's Health Concerns
SOURCEBOOK

SIXTH EDITION

Basic Consumer Health Information about Trends and Issues in Men's Health, Including Information about Gender-Specific Health Differences, the Leading Causes of Death in Men, Reproductive and Sexual Concerns, Male-Linked Genetic Disorders, Mental-Health Concerns, Alcohol and Drug Abuse, and Other Concerns of Special Significance to Men

Along with Information about the Screenings, Vaccinations, and Self-Examinations Recommended for Men, Guidelines for Nutrition, Physical Activity, Weight Control, and Other Lifestyle Choices That Affect Wellness, a Glossary of Related Terms, and a Directory of Resources for Further Help and Information

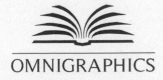

OMNIGRAPHICS

615 Griswold, Ste. 520, Detroit, MI 48226

Bibliographic Note
Because this page cannot legibly accommodate all the copyright notices, the Bibliographic Note portion of the Preface constitutes an extension of the copyright notice.

* * *

OMNIGRAPHICS
Angela L. Williams, *Managing Editor*
* * *

Copyright © 2019 Omnigraphics

ISBN 978-0-7808-1717-3
E-ISBN 978-0-7808-1718-0

Library of Congress Cataloging-in-Publication Data

Names: Omnigraphics, Inc., issuing body.

Title: Men's health concerns sourcebook: basic consumer health information about trends and issues in men's health, including information about sex-specific health differences, the leading causes of death in men, reproductive and sexual concerns, male-linked genetic disorders, mental-health concerns, alcohol and drug abuse, and other concerns of special significance to men; along with information about the screenings, vaccinations, and self-examinations recommended for men, guidelines for nutrition, physical activity, weight control, and other lifestyle choices that affect wellness, a glossary of related terms, and a directory of resources for further help and information / Angela Williams, managing editor.

Description: Sixth edition. | Detroit, MI: Omnigraphics, Inc., [2019]

Identifiers: LCCN 2019021359 (print) | LCCN 2019021833 (ebook) | ISBN 9780780817180 (ebook) | ISBN 9780780817173 (hard cover: alk. paper)

Subjects: LCSH: Men--Health and hygiene--Popular works.

Classification: LCC RA776.5 (ebook) | LCC RA776.5.M457 2019 (print) | DDC 613/.04234--dc23

LC record available at https://lccn.loc.gov/2019021359

Table of Contents

Preface xiii

Part I: Men's Health Basics

Chapter 1 — Sex-Specific Health Differences 3

    Section 1.1 — Differences in Men's and Women's Health: An Overview 4

    Section 1.2 — Why Women Live Longer than Men 10

    Section 1.3 — Alcohol Use and Risks to Men's Health 14

    Section 1.4 — Sex Differences in Substance Abuse 17

    Section 1.5 — PTSD Study: Men versus Women 20

Chapter 2 — Self-Examinations Recommended for Men 23

    Section 2.1 — Breast Self-Examination 24

    Section 2.2 — Oral Cancer Self-Examination 26

    Section 2.3 — Skin Cancer Self-Examination 28

    Section 2.4 — Testicular Self-Examination 30

Chapter 3 — Recommended Screening Tests for
Men 33

    Section 3.1 — Screening Tests for Men:
                What You Need and When 34

    Section 3.2 — Abdominal Aortic
                Aneurysm Screening 36

    Section 3.3 — Blood Pressure Screening 39

    Section 3.4 — Cholesterol Screening 42

    Section 3.5 — Colorectal Cancer Screening 46

    Section 3.6 — Osteoporosis Screening 51

    Section 3.7 — Prostate Cancer Screening 56

Chapter 4 — Vaccinations for Men 61

    Section 4.1 — Recommended
                Vaccinations for Adults 62

    Section 4.2 — Human Papillomavirus
                Vaccination Now
                Recommended for Young
                Men 65

    Section 4.3 — Seasonal Influenza
                Vaccination 67

Chapter 5 — Managing Common Disease Risk
Factors 71

    Section 5.1 — Preventing High Blood
                Pressure 72

    Section 5.2 — Preventing High
                Cholesterol 75

    Section 5.3 — Ensuring Adequate Sleep 77

    Section 5.4 — Managing Stress 81

Chapter 6 — Aim for a Healthy Weight 85

    Section 6.1 — Assessing Your Weight
                and Health Risk 86

    Section 6.2 — Understanding Body
                Mass Index 88

    Section 6.3 — Understanding
                Overweight and Obesity 92

Section 6.4 — Tips for Healthy
Weight Loss............................ 103

Section 6.5 — Guide to Selecting a
Weight-Loss Program 112

Chapter 7 — Nutrition Tips for Men 121

Section 7.1 — Healthy Eating for Men.......... 122

Section 7.2 — Nutrition Tips for Building
Strength and Increasing
Muscle Mass............................ 127

Chapter 8 — Physical Activity: Key to a Healthy Life 131

Section 8.1 — How Much Physical
Activity Do Adults Need? 132

Section 8.2 — The Benefits of Physical
Activity 139

Part II: Leading Causes of Death in Men

Chapter 9 — Causes of Death: A Statistical Overview............. 145

Section 9.1 — Leading Causes of Death
in the United States................. 146

Section 9.2 — Cancer among Men: Some
Statistics.................................. 151

Chapter 10 — Alzheimer Disease 153

Chapter 11 — Chronic Liver Disease 157

Section 11.1 — Viral Hepatitis 158

Section 11.2 — Cirrhosis.................................. 159

Chapter 12 — Chronic Obstructive Pulmonary
Disease 169

Chapter 13 — Colorectal Cancer... 173

Chapter 14 — Diabetes.. 181

Chapter 15 — Heart Disease... 199

Section 15.1 — Men and Heart Disease........... 200

Section 15.2 — Heart Failure 202

Section 15.3 — Coronary Artery Disease........ 215

Section 15.4 — Heart Attack 217

vii

Chapter 16—HIV and AIDS.. 225

Chapter 17—Influenza and Pneumonia 229

    Section 17.1 — Influenza 230

    Section 17.2 — Pneumonia 235

Chapter 18—Kidney Disease 249

Chapter 19—Liver Cancer... 273

Chapter 20—Lung Cancer.. 277

Chapter 21—Motor Vehicle Accidents.................................. 285

    Section 21.1 — Aggressive Driving 286

    Section 21.2 — Distracted Driving................. 288

    Section 21.3 — Drowsy Driving...................... 291

    Section 21.4 — Impaired Driving.................. 296

    Section 21.5 — Older Drivers 301

Chapter 22—Other Accidents and Injuries............................ 305

    Section 22.1 — Falls...................................... 306

    Section 22.2 — Fire-Related Injuries.............. 309

    Section 22.3 — Occupational Injuries............. 319

    Section 22.4 — Poisoning............................... 322

    Section 22.5 — Water-Related Accidents........ 325

Chapter 23—Penile Cancer 331

Chapter 24—Prostate Cancer 341

Chapter 25—Testicular Cancer.. 349

Chapter 26—Stroke 361

Chapter 27—Suicide 369

Part III: Sexual and Reproductive Concerns

Chapter 28—Kidney and Urological Disorders......................... 375

    Section 28.1 — Kidney Stones 376

    Section 28.2 — Urinary Incontinence
                in Men 388

Chapter 29—Penile Concerns 393

    Section 29.1 — Circumcision 394

    Section 29.2 — Balanitis................................ 395

    Section 29.3 — Penile Intraepithelial
                   Neoplasia.............................. 398

    Section 29.4 — Penile Trauma 400

    Section 29.5 — Peyronie Disease.................... 402

    Section 29.6 — Phimosis and
                   Paraphimosis 409

Chapter 30—Disorders of the Scrotum and Testicles.............. 413

    Section 30.1 — Epididymitis.......................... 414

    Section 30.2 — Hydrocele 418

    Section 30.3 — Inguinal Hernia 421

    Section 30.4 — Spermatocele.......................... 428

    Section 30.5 — Perineal Injury....................... 430

Chapter 31—Noncancerous Prostate Disorders........................ 439

    Section 31.1 — Benign Prostatic
                   Hyperplasia............................ 440

    Section 31.2 — Prostatitis.............................. 459

Chapter 32—Sexual Dysfunction... 467

Chapter 33—Male Infertility... 477

Chapter 34—Vasectomy and Vasectomy Reversal 481

Chapter 35—Nonsurgical Contraception 487

    Section 35.1 — Condoms................................. 488

    Section 35.2 — Withdrawal 490

Chapter 36—Safer Sex Guidelines 493

Chapter 37—Sexually Transmitted Diseases 497

    Section 37.1 — What Are Sexually
                   Transmitted Diseases? 498

    Section 37.2 — Chlamydia.............................. 507

    Section 37.3 — Genital Herpes....................... 509

    Section 37.4 — Gonorrhea 512

Section 37.5 — Hepatitis B 516

Section 37.6 — Human Papillomavirus 520

Section 37.7 — Pubic Lice 524

Section 37.8 — Scabies 526

Section 37.9 — Syphilis 533

Section 37.10 — Trichomoniasis 537

Part IV: Other Medical Issues of Concern to Men

Chapter 38 — Male-Linked Genetic Disorders 543

Section 38.1 — Color Vision Deficiency 544

Section 38.2 — Fragile X Syndrome 549

Section 38.3 — Hemophilia 554

Section 38.4 — Klinefelter Syndrome 566

Section 38.5 — Muscular Dystrophy 578

Chapter 39 — Breast Concerns in Men 585

Section 39.1 — Breast Cancer in Men 586

Section 39.2 — Gynecomastia 605

Chapter 40 — Osteoporosis in Men 609

Chapter 41 — Sleep Apnea 615

Chapter 42 — Male-Pattern Baldness 625

Chapter 43 — Mental-Health Concerns in Men 627

Section 43.1 — Men and Mental Health 628

Section 43.2 — Depression 629

Section 43.3 — Posttraumatic Stress
Disorder 637

Section 43.4 — Schizophrenia 640

Chapter 44 — Alcohol, Tobacco, and Drug Use in Men 645

Section 44.1 — Alcohol, Tobacco, and
Other Drugs 646

Section 44.2 — Excessive Alcohol Use
and Risks to Men's Health 647

Section 44.3 — Men's Health and
    Smoking.................................. 648

Section 44.4 — Anabolic Steroid Use 650

Chapter 45 — Violence against Men 653

Section 45.1 — Myths and Realities of
    Domestic Abuse against
    Men... 654

Section 45.2 — Sexual Assault of Men............ 657

Chapter 46 — Body Image and Eating Disorders in
Men... 661

Section 46.1 — Eating Disorders in Men 662

Section 46.2 — Muscle Dysmorphic
    Disorder.................................. 667

Chapter 47 — Male Menopause 671

Part V: Additional Help and Information

Chapter 48 — Glossary of Men's Health Terms.......................... 677

Chapter 49 — Directory of Resources That Provide
Information about Men's Health.......................... 685

Index... **693**

Preface

About This Book

The life expectancy gap between men and women has narrowed in recent years, but men still face many health disadvantages. Men are more likely than women to smoke and drink, engage in risky behaviors, and put off checkups and regular preventative care. Men also face a number of disorders unique to their gender, including prostate cancer, penile and testicular disorders, low testosterone, and sex-linked genetic disorders.

Men's Health Concerns Sourcebook, Sixth Edition discusses health issues that disproportionately affect men. It explains how men can help protect themselves and preserve their health with self-examinations, vaccinations, screening tests, and lifestyle choices. It provides facts about the specific diseases and injuries that comprise the list of leading causes of death in men and explains how men can avoid them or lessen their impact. Detailed information about sexual and reproductive concerns, prostate disorders, substance use, mental-health concerns, and other disorders affecting men is included. Lifestyle choices, nutrition, and physical activity for men are also covered. A glossary of related terms and a list of resources provide further help and information.

How to Use This Book

This book is divided into parts and chapters. Parts focus on broad areas of interest. Chapters are devoted to single topics within a part.

Part I: Men's Health Basics provides fundamental information about differences in men's and women's health, screening tests, self-examinations, and vaccinations that are recommended for men. It offers suggestions for managing common disease risk factors, including tips on weight management, nutrition, and physical activity.

Part II: Leading Causes of Death in Men describes the factors that contribute most significantly to men's mortality, including heart disease, cancer, diabetes, Alzheimer disease, liver and kidney disease, chronic obstructive pulmonary disease, and other respiratory illnesses. It discusses common injuries and accidents frequently associated with fatalities in men, including motor vehicle accidents, falls, occupational injuries, and suicide.

Part III: Sexual and Reproductive Concerns provides information about conditions that affect male reproductive organs, including urological disorders, prostate disorders, disorders of the scrotum and testicles, circumcision, and penile concerns. It offers suggestions for dealing with sexual dysfunction and male infertility. It includes facts about birth control methods, sexually transmitted diseases, and safer sex practices.

Part IV: Other Medical Issues of Concern to Men discusses male-linked genetic disorders, including color vision deficiency, hemophilia, and muscular dystrophy. It examines physical and mental-health concerns with gender differences in their expression or incidence rates. In addition, men's issues related to disorders traditionally associated with women, such as body image, breast cancer, and osteoporosis, are also addressed.

Part V: Additional Help and Information includes a glossary of terms related to men's health and a directory of resources offering additional help and support.

Bibliographic Note

This volume contains documents and excerpts from publications issued by the following U.S. government agencies: Centers for Disease Control and Prevention (CDC); *Eunice Kennedy Shriver* National Institute of Child Health and Human Development (NICHD); Genetics Home Reference (GHR); National Cancer Institute (NCI); National Eye Institute (NEI); National Heart, Lung, and Blood Institute (NHLBI); National Institute of Arthritis and Musculoskeletal and Skin Diseases (NIAMS); National Institute of Dental and Craniofacial Research

(NIDCR); National Institute of Diabetes and Digestive and Kidney Diseases (NIDDK); National Institute of Neurological Disorders and Stroke (NINDS); National Institute on Aging (NIA); National Institute on Drug Abuse (NIDA); National Institutes of Health (NIH); *NIH News in Health*; NIH Osteoporosis and Related Bone Diseases—National Resource Center (NIH ORBD—NRC), Office of Disease Prevention and Health Promotion (ODPHP); Substance Abuse and Mental Health Services Administration (SAMHSA); U.S. Bureau of Labor Statistics (BLS); U.S. Department of Agriculture (USDA); U.S. Department of Health and Human Services (HHS); U.S. Department of Veterans Affairs (VA); U.S. Fire Administration (FA); U.S. Food and Drug Administration (FDA); and U.S. Office of Personnel Management (OPM).

It may also contain original material produced by Omnigraphics and reviewed by medical consultants.

About the Health Reference Series

The *Health Reference Series* is designed to provide basic medical information for patients, families, caregivers, and the general public. Each volume takes a particular topic and provides comprehensive coverage. This is especially important for people who may be dealing with a newly diagnosed disease or a chronic disorder in themselves or in a family member. People looking for preventive guidance, information about disease warning signs, medical statistics, and risk factors for health problems will also find answers to their questions in the *Health Reference Series*. The *Series*, however, is not intended to serve as a tool for diagnosing illness, in prescribing treatments, or as a substitute for the physician/patient relationship. All people concerned about medical symptoms or the possibility of disease are encouraged to seek professional care from an appropriate healthcare provider.

A Note about Spelling and Style

Health Reference Series editors use *Stedman's Medical Dictionary* as an authority for questions related to the spelling of medical terms and the *Chicago Manual of Style* for questions related to grammatical structures, punctuation, and other editorial concerns. Consistent adherence is not always possible, however, because the individual volumes within the *Series* include many documents from a wide variety of different producers, and the editor's primary goal is to present material from each source as accurately as is possible. This sometimes means that information in different chapters or sections may follow other guidelines and alternate spelling authorities. For example, occasionally a copyright holder may require that eponymous terms be shown in possessive forms (Crohn's disease vs. Crohn disease) or that British spelling norms be retained (leukaemia vs. leukemia).

Medical Review

Omnigraphics contracts with a team of qualified, senior medical professionals who serve as medical consultants for the *Health Reference Series*. As necessary, medical consultants review reprinted and originally written material for currency and accuracy. Citations including the phrase "Reviewed (month, year)" indicate material reviewed by this team. Medical consultation services are provided to the *Health Reference Series* editors by:

Dr. Vijayalakshmi, MBBS, DGO, MD
Dr. Senthil Selvan, MBBS, DCH, MD
Dr. K. Sivanandham, MBBS, DCH, MS (Research), PhD

Our Advisory Board

We would like to thank the following board members for providing initial guidance on the development of this series:

- Dr. Lynda Baker, Associate Professor of Library and Information Science, Wayne State University, Detroit, MI

- Nancy Bulgarelli, William Beaumont Hospital Library, Royal Oak, MI

- Karen Imarisio, Bloomfield Township Public Library, Bloomfield Township, MI

- Karen Morgan, Mardigian Library, University of Michigan-Dearborn, Dearborn, MI

- Rosemary Orlando, St. Clair Shores Public Library, St. Clair Shores, MI

Health Reference Series *Update Policy*

The inaugural book in the *Health Reference Series* was the first edition of *Cancer Sourcebook* published in 1989. Since then, the *Series* has been enthusiastically received by librarians and in the medical community. In order to maintain the standard of providing high-quality health information for the layperson the editorial staff at Omnigraphics felt it was necessary to implement a policy of updating volumes when warranted.

Medical researchers have been making tremendous strides, and it is the purpose of the *Health Reference Series* to stay current with the most recent advances. Each decision to update a volume is made on an individual basis. Some of the considerations include how much new information is available and the feedback we receive from people who use the books. If there is a topic you would like to see added to the update list, or an area of medical concern you feel has not been adequately addressed, please write to:

Managing Editor
Health Reference Series
Omnigraphics
615 Griswold, Ste. 520
Detroit, MI 48226

Part One

Men's Health Basics

Chapter 1

Sex-Specific Health Differences

Chapter Contents

Section 1.1—Differences in Men's and Women's
        Health: An Overview 4

Section 1.2—Why Women Live Longer than Men 10

Section 1.3—Alcohol Use and Risks to Men's Health 14

Section 1.4—Sex Differences in Substance Abuse 17

Section 1.5—PTSD Study: Men versus Women 20

Section 1.1

Differences in Men's and Women's Health: An Overview

This section contains text excerpted from the following sources: Text under the heading "Sex and Gender" is excerpted from "Sex and Gender," *NIH News in Health*, National Institutes of Health (NIH), May 2016; Text under the heading "How Gender and Sex Influence Health and Disease" is excerpted from "How Sex/ Gender Influence Health and Disease (A–Z)," Office of Research on Women's Health (ORWH), National Institutes of Health (NIH), February 12, 2015. Reviewed June 2019.

Sex and Gender

Are you male or female? The answer to this seemingly simple question can have a major impact on your health. While both sexes are similar in many ways, researchers have found that sex and social factors can make a difference when it comes to your risk for disease, how well you respond to medications, and how often you seek medical care. That is why scientists are taking a closer look at the links between sex, gender, and health.

Many people use the words "sex" and "gender" interchangeably, but they are distinct concepts to scientists.

Defining differences: Sex is biological. It is based on your genetic makeup. Males have one X and one Y chromosome in every cell of the body. Females have two X chromosomes in every cell. These cells make up all your tissues and organs, including your skin, heart, stomach, muscles, and brain.

Gender is a social or cultural concept. It refers to the roles, behaviors, and identities that society assigns to girls and boys, women and men, and gender-diverse people. Gender is determined by how we see ourselves and each other, and how we act and interact with others.

There is a lot of diversity in how individuals and groups understand, experience, and express gender. Because gender influences our behaviors and relationships, it can also affect health.

Influences on health: "Sex and gender play a role in how health and disease affect individuals. There was a time when we studied men and applied those findings to women, but we've learned that there are distinct biological differences between women and men," explains Dr. Janine Austin Clayton, who heads research on women's health at the

National Institutes of Health (NIH). "Women and men have different hormones, different organs, and different cultural influences—all of which can lead to differences in health."

As scientists learn more about the biology of males and females, they are uncovering the influences of both sex and gender in many areas of health.

For instance, women and men can have different symptoms during a heart attack. For both men and women, the most common heart attack symptom is chest pain or discomfort. But, women are more likely than men to have shortness of breath, nausea and vomiting, fatigue, and pain in the back, shoulders, and jaw. Knowing about such differences can lead to better diagnoses and outcomes.

Men and women also tend to have different responses to pain. The National Institutes of Health-funded researchers recently learned that different cells in male and female mice drive pain processing. "Without studying both sexes, we wouldn't know if we're taking steps in the right direction toward appropriate clinical treatment for men and women," Clayton says. "Our differences also affect how we respond to medications, as well as which diseases and conditions we may be prone to and how those diseases progress in our bodies." For example, women metabolize nicotine faster than men, so nicotine-replacement therapies can be less effective in women.

Attention to addiction: Scientists are finding that addiction to nicotine and other drugs is influenced by sex as well. "When it comes to addiction, differences in sex and gender can be found across the board," says Dr. Sherry McKee, lead researcher at an NIH-funded center at Yale University that studies treatments for tobacco dependence. "There are different reasons men and women pick up a drug and keep using a drug, and in how they respond to treatment and experience relapse. Sex also influences disease risk in addiction. For example, women who smoke are more susceptible to lung and heart disease than men who smoke."

One NIH-funded research team has detected some of these differences in the brain. In a recent study, 16 people who smoke—eight men and eight women—underwent brain scans while smoking to create "movies" of how smoking affects dopamine, the chemical messenger that triggers feelings of pleasure in the brain.

These brain movies showed that smoking alters dopamine in the brain at different rates and in different locations in males and females.

Dopamine release in nicotine-dependent men occurred quickly in a brain area that reinforces the effect of nicotine and other drugs.

5

Women also had a rapid response but in a different brain region—the part associated with habit formation. "We were able to pinpoint a different brain response between male and female smokers, a finding that could be useful in developing sex-specific treatments to help smokers quit," says lead study researcher Dr. Kelly Cosgrove, a brain-imaging expert at Yale University.

Finding better ways to help men and women quit smoking is important for everyone's health. More than 16 million Americans have diseases caused by smoking. It is the leading cause of preventable death in the United States.

Autoimmune disorders: Scientists have found sex influences in autoimmune disorders as well. About 80 percent of those affected are women. But, autoimmune conditions in men are often more severe. For instance, more women than men get multiple sclerosis (MS), a disease in which the body's immune system attacks the brain and spinal cord. But, men seem more likely to get a progressive form of MS that gradually worsens and is more challenging to treat.

"Not only are women more susceptible to MS, but women also have many more considerations in the management of the disease, especially since it often begins during childbearing years," says Dr. Ellen Mowry, a specialist who studies MS at Johns Hopkins University.

"There are a lot of unanswered questions when it comes to the study of sex differences in MS and other autoimmune disorders," Mowry explains. "Researchers can learn a lot by studying women and men separately and together, considering possible risk or predictive factors that may differ based on sex or gender, and working collaboratively with other scientists to improve the likelihood of detecting these factors."

How Gender and Sex Influence Health and Disease

Research on sex and gender differences—research that spans basic studies on cells to large, clinical trials involving thousands of patients—aims to understand health differences between males and females at all levels. The knowledge will improve health for both women and men.

Arrhythmias

As an electrically controlled organ, the heart beats when a wave of electricity courses through heart muscle in a defined regular path. Any disruption of this path of conduction, called an "arrhythmia," causes the heart to beat irregularly. An arrhythmia can be very mild, even undetectable, or serious and fatal. Sex and gender differences are known to affect heart rhythms. Here are some examples.

- Certain medications, including the allergy drug Seldane and the gastrointestinal drug Propulsid (both of which have been taken off the market in the United States) trigger a potentially fatal heart arrhythmia more often in women than in men.

- A 2009 study showed that women are more likely than men to have complications from implantable cardiac defibrillators, devices that monitor heart rhythms and deliver shocks when needed to restore a normal heartbeat.

- Although men are more likely than women to experience a usually mild condition known as "atrial flutter" (heart palpitations), surgical treatment (ablation) of this arrhythmia affects women and men differently, according to a 2013 study.

Cardiovascular Risk

For the most part, an individual has direct control over whether she or he will develop heart disease, by managing behaviors that raise or reduce the chances that heart disease will take root in their body. National Institutes of Health-funded medical research that goes back decades has defined a core set of cardiovascular risk factors that individuals can manage with the help of a doctor. The risk factors include smoking, high cholesterol and triglycerides, high blood pressure, diabetes, and being overweight or obese.

Yet, even though everyone should pay attention to these risk factors that affect heart health, the risks differ between women and men in various ways that appear subtle, but can be very significant.

- In women, aspirin reduces risk of ischemic stroke, whereas in men, low-dose aspirin therapy reduces risk of heart attack.

- Cholesterol plaque in women may not build up into major artery blockages, but instead spreads evenly throughout the artery wall. This means that artery blockages can be more difficult to diagnose in women, who may not have outright symptoms but are still at high risk for heart attack.

Influenza

Influenza, more commonly called the "flu," is a viral infection of the nose, throat, and lungs. Flu symptoms may include muscle aches,

7

chills, cough, fever, headache, and sore throat. Research is underway to find out why the flu virus and vaccine affect men and women differently. For example, women are more likely than men to have severe flu symptoms. Men with high levels of testosterone produce fewer antibodies in response to the flu vaccine compared with men with low testosterone.

Lupus

Lupus is an autoimmune condition that causes inflammation and damage to various organs. Common symptoms include extreme fatigue, painful or swollen joints (arthritis), unexplained fever, skin rashes, hair loss, and kidney problems. Lupus develops slowly, with symptoms that come and go. The most common type, systemic lupus erythematosus, usually appears in the mid-teens, 30s or 40s. Women are more likely to get lupus than men, and African American, Hispanic, Asian, and American Indian women have a higher lupus risk than white women. Here are examples of how lupus can differ in women and men:

- Although more women than men get lupus and a related disorder, systemic sclerosis, men are more likely to have more severe disease.

- In contrast, women are more likely than men to develop lupus-related urinary tract infections (UTIs), hypothyroidism, depression, esophageal reflux, asthma, and fibromyalgia (FM).

- Among children and adults with lupus, males are at greater risk than females for kidney injury, kidney failure, and kidney-related death.

- Researchers have found a lupus-related gene (called *"IRAK1"*) on the X chromosome, which may help explain why women get the disease more often than men.

Osteoarthritis

Osteoarthritis (OA) is a condition that accompanies aging, as the body's bones and joints suffer wear and tear with time and lots of use. It is painful, and there is no cure. OA remains the leading cause of chronic disability in the United States, and it disproportionately affects postmenopausal women (PMW). Current treatment generally involves a mix of exercise, lifestyle modification (such as weight loss), and pain relievers. Researchers are hard at work looking for new clues about how to prevent and treat osteoarthritis. It is more common among women than men in every age group, but there are subtle differences worth knowing about.

- The severity of OA is usually significantly worse in women than it is in men.

- Black women and black men with OA are much less likely to undergo total knee replacement when compared to white men.

Stroke

A stroke is sort of like a heart attack in the brain. Strokes occur when blood flow to a part of the brain suddenly stops, starving brain cells of the oxygen they need to live. Clogged arteries can cause a so-called "ischemic stroke," in which fat and cholesterol form plaques in artery walls, allowing less blood to flow through freely.

While some of the risk factors for stroke are the same in men and women, such as family history of stroke, high blood pressure or cholesterol, smoking, and being overweight, certain aspects of stroke are unique to women. Researchers have identified several sex/gender differences, such as these:

- While men have a higher risk of stroke than women in general, women are usually older when they have strokes, and they are more likely to die of strokes than men.

- Women have a poorer quality of life (QOL) after a stroke than men.

- Women with a history of preeclampsia during pregnancy are 60 percent more likely to have a nonpregnancy-related stroke later in life.

- Women who suffer from migraines with visual components like flashing lights have a higher risk of having an ischemic stroke.

Vision Disorders

Vision disorders affect women disproportionately both in the United States and throughout the world. But in addition to affecting vision, eye changes can signal the presence of other conditions, especially autoimmune diseases such as lupus and rheumatoid arthritis (RA). Ocular manifestations of thyroid disease may be the first characteristic symptom that brings a woman to a physician's office to seek treatment. Here are some examples of how vision disorders affect women and men:

- Dry eye affects twice as many women than men over 50 years of age. Dry eye disease affects QOL, interfering with routine activities such as reading, working on a computer, and driving a car.

- Cataracts that cloud the eye's lens are more likely to occur in women than in men. In developing countries, women are less likely than men to receive cataract surgery.

- Brain-imaging studies of people with migraines, intense headaches that are twice as common in women than men and that often affect vision, have reported sex-specific patterns.

- Adult women experience about 25 percent more uncorrected visual impairment due to refractive error, which impedes the ability to focus, compared to adult men.

Section 1.2

Why Women Live Longer than Men

"Why Women Live Longer than Men,"
© 2017 Omnigraphics. Reviewed June 2019.

According to statistics compiled by the United Nations, women typically live 4.5 years longer than men worldwide. In 2013, the global average life expectancy for women was 71 years compared to 66.5 for men. This pattern has been observed in every country in the world, and it has held true the entire time that reliable birth and death records have existed.

Although social and lifestyle factors are believed to play a role in adult mortality rates, evidence suggests that biological and genetic factors are also involved. Significantly, studies have found sex-related differences in life expectancy among other primates—female gorillas, chimpanzees, and orangutans consistently outlive males of their species as well. By studying the various factors that may account for increased female longevity, scientists hope that they will identify ways to help both men and women live longer, healthier lives.

Biological Factors

Biologists have put forth a number of theories to explain why women live longer than men. Some of the major genetic and biological factors they believe may contribute to increased female longevity include the following.

- **Women carry two X chromosomes, while men have one X and one Y chromosome.**

  This biological difference means that men are more vulnerable to genetic mutations that can cause life-threatening health conditions. Whereas women may avoid the expression of genetic diseases by relying on a normal gene on the other X chromosome, men lack a second copy of the defective gene.

- **Women's bodies tend to be smaller in size than men's bodies.**

  Since larger people have more cells in their bodies, they may have a greater tendency to develop harmful cellular mutations. In addition, larger bodies use more energy, which creates wear and tear on organs and tissues and may increase the rate of long-term damage.

- **Women's immune system function declines at a slower rate than men's.**

  All people's immune function gradually declines with age. But, blood samples of healthy people have shown that the normal loss of white blood cells—which help protect the body from infection— occurs faster in men than in women. As a result, women may enjoy protection from illness to a more advanced age.

- **The male hormone testosterone may increase disease risk later in life.**

  Testosterone, which is secreted by the testicles, is the hormone primarily responsible for the development of male sex traits, such as deep voices and hairy chests. Although testosterone contributes to male strength and virility, it may also increase men's risk of developing cardiovascular disease and cancer later in life.

11

A modern analysis of records from nineteenth-century Korea revealed that eunuchs (men whose testicles are removed before puberty, and thus have significantly lower lifetime exposure to testosterone) lived an average of 20 years longer than typical Korean men and were far more likely to reach their hundredth birthday.

- **The female hormone estrogen may decrease disease risk later in life.**

  Estrogen, which is produced in the ovaries, is the hormone primarily responsible for female sex traits, such as breast development and menstruation. In contrast to testosterone, estrogen appears to protect against disease. Estrogen has antioxidant properties, meaning that it helps eliminate harmful chemicals that may cause cell damage. Studies have shown that when the ovaries are removed from female animals, the animals experience an increase in disease risk and a decrease in longevity.

- **Women develop heart disease a decade later than men.**

  Heart disease is the leading cause of death for both men and women in the United States. But, partly due to the protective effects of estrogen, which helps control cholesterol and prevent plaque formation in the arteries, women tend to develop heart disease 10 years later than men. In fact, women's risk of heart disease only begins to increase after menopause, when the production of estrogen declines. In addition, more than 4 times as many men as women smoke worldwide, and smoking is a major contributor to heart disease. Another theory to explain the delayed onset of cardiovascular illness in women is that women's heart rate tends to increase during the second half of the menstrual cycle. Some researchers claim that this increase offers the same health benefits as moderate exercise.

Lifestyle Factors

In addition to biological differences between men and women, studies have also suggested that sociological and lifestyle factors may contribute to women's longer lifespan. Some of the main factors that are believed to influence mortality rates include the following.

- **Men are more prone to risk-taking behavior.**

  According to the U.S. Centers for Disease Control and Prevention (CDC), unintentional injuries are the third-leading cause of death for American men. For women, on the other hand, unintentional injuries rank sixth. Scientists point out that the frontal lobe of the brain develops more slowly in males than in females. Since this part of the brain is involved in calculating risks and behaving responsibly, men are more likely to exhibit dangerous or risky behavior than women of the same age. As a result, studies show that men are less likely to wear seatbelts and more likely to drive aggressively and be involved in motor vehicle accidents.

- **Women have stronger social networks.**

Men are often socialized to hide their emotions and keep their concerns bottled up inside. For women, however, it is more culturally acceptable to express emotions and confide in friends or family members about sources of worry or stress. Studies have shown that strong social connections can decrease a person's risk of dying by 50 percent. Men can experience the protective nature of social ties by getting married—studies have also shown that married men tend to be healthier and live longer than single men.

- **Women take better care of their health.**

Another contributing factor to women's longevity is that they tend to take better care of their health. Men often ignore or deny symptoms of illness and avoid seeking medical attention. In fact, studies have shown that men are 24 percent less likely than women to have visited a doctor within the past year.

References

1. Bergland, Christopher. "Why Do Women Live Longer than Men?" *Psychology Today*, July 8, 2015.

2. Innes, Emma. "Women Live Longer than Men Because Their Immune Systems Age More Slowly," MailOnline, May 15, 2013.

3. Levine, Hallie. "5 Reasons Women Live Longer than Men," Health.com, October 13, 2014.

4. Zeilinger, Julie. "The Real Reason Women Live Longer than Men?" Huffington Post, August 3, 2013.

Section 1.3

Alcohol Use and Risks to Men's Health

This section includes text excerpted from "Fact
Sheets—Alcohol Use and Your Health," Centers for
Disease Control and Prevention (CDC), January 3, 2018.

Alcohol Use and Your Health

Drinking too much can harm your health. Excessive alcohol use led
to approximately 88,000 deaths and 2.5 million years of potential life
lost (YPLL) each year in the United States from 2006–2010, shortening
the lives of those who died by an average of 30 years. Further, excessive drinking was responsible for 1 in 10 deaths among working-age
adults between the ages of 20 and 64. The economic costs of excessive
alcohol consumption in 2010 were estimated at $249 billion, or $2.05
a drink.

What Is a "Drink"?

In the United States, a standard drink contains 0.6 ounces (14.0
grams or 1.2 tablespoons) of pure alcohol. Generally, this amount of
pure alcohol is found in:

- 12 ounces of beer (5 percent alcohol content)

- 8 ounces of malt liquor (7 percent alcohol content)

- 5 ounces of wine (12 percent alcohol content)

- 1.5 ounces of 80-proof (40 percent alcohol content) distilled
  spirits or liquor (e.g., gin, rum, vodka, whiskey)

What Is Excessive Drinking?

Excessive drinking includes binge drinking, heavy drinking, and
any drinking by pregnant women or people younger than the age of
21.

Binge drinking, the most common form of excessive drinking, is
defined as consuming:

- For women, four or more drinks during a single occasion

- For men, five or more drinks during a single occasion

Heavy drinking is defined as consuming:

- For women, 8 or more drinks per week

- For men, 15 or more drinks per week

Most people who drink excessively are not alcoholics or alcohol dependent.

What Is Moderate Drinking?

The Dietary Guidelines for Americans defines "moderate drinking" as "up to one drink per day for women and up to two drinks per day for men."

In addition, the Dietary Guidelines do not recommend that individuals who do not drink alcohol start drinking for any reason.

However, there are some people who should not drink any alcohol, including those who are:

- Younger than 21 years of age

- Driving, planning to drive, or participating in other activities requiring skill, coordination, and alertness

- Taking certain prescription or over-the-counter (OTC) medications that can interact with alcohol

- Suffering from certain medical conditions

- Recovering from alcoholism or are unable to control the amount they drink

By adhering to the Dietary Guidelines, you can reduce the risk of harm to yourself or others.

Short-Term Health Risks

Excessive alcohol use has immediate effects that increase the risk of many harmful health conditions. These are most often the result of binge drinking and include the following:

- Injuries, such as motor vehicle crashes, falls, drownings, and burns

- Violence, including homicide, suicide, sexual assault, and intimate partner violence

15

- Alcohol poisoning, a medical emergency that results from high blood alcohol levels

- Risky sexual behaviors, including unprotected sex or sex with multiple partners. These behaviors can result in unintended pregnancy or sexually transmitted diseases, including human immunodeficiency virus (HIV).

Long-Term Health Risks

Over time, excessive alcohol use can lead to the development of chronic diseases and other serious problems including:

- High blood pressure, heart disease, stroke, liver disease, and digestive problems

- Cancer of the breast, mouth, throat, esophagus, liver, and colon

- Learning and memory problems, including dementia and poor school performance

- Mental-health problems, including depression and anxiety

- Social problems, including lost productivity, family problems, and unemployment

- Alcohol dependence, or alcoholism

By not drinking too much, you can reduce the risk of these short- and long-term health risks.

Section 1.4

Sex Differences in Substance Abuse

This section includes text excerpted from "Gender Differences in
Primary Substance of Abuse across Age Groups," Substance
Abuse and Mental Health Services Administration (SAMHSA),
April 3, 2014. Reviewed June 2019.

National data consistently show that sex is an important factor to
consider when examining patterns of substance abuse, such as overall
prevalence rates and substances of choice. For example, males are
more likely than females to report marijuana and alcohol use, whereas
females are more likely than males to report nonmedical use of prescription drugs. Also, differences in substance abuse patterns among
men and women vary by age. Data from the 2011 National Survey
on Drug Use and Health show that men 18 years of age or older have
almost twice the rate of substance dependence as adult women, but
among youths between the ages of 12 and 17, the rate of substance
dependence for both sexes is the same (6.9%). Knowledge of how sex
can interact with age and patterns of substance abuse may be useful
to those responsible for the design of outreach, prevention, and treatment programs.

The Treatment Episode Data Set (TEDS) collects data on admissions to substance abuse treatment facilities across the United States
and can be used to examine differences in primary substance of abuse
among males and females by age. TEDS collects information on up to
three substances of abuse that led to the treatment episode. The main
substance abused by the client is known as the "primary substance of
abuse." For each admission, data on primary substance of abuse are
reported at the time of treatment entry. The analyses in this report
are based on TEDS data for 2011.

The Treatment Episode Data Set is a census of all admissions
to treatment facilities reported to the Substance Abuse and Mental
Health Services Administration (SAMHSA) by state substance abuse
agencies. Because TEDS involves actual counts rather than estimates,
statistical significance and confidence intervals are not applicable.

Overview and Demographic Characteristics

In 2011, about 609,000 of the 1.84 million admissions to substance
abuse treatment were female (33.1 percent), and 1.23 million were

17

male (66.9 percent). No meaningful sex differences were found by race/ethnicity. Specifically, the majority of female and male admissions (66.4 and 58.2 percent, respectively) were non-Hispanic White.

The percentages of female and male admissions that were non-Hispanic Black and Hispanic were similar.

Sex Profiles

No appreciable sex differences were found by primary substances of abuse overall. Alcohol was the most commonly reported primary substance of abuse by female (33.3%) and male (42.3%) admissions. Among females, alcohol was followed by heroin (15.3%), marijuana (14.6%), and prescription pain relievers (13.8%); among males, the next most frequently reported substances were marijuana (19.9%), heroin (15.0%), and prescription pain relievers (7.8%).

Differences in Primary Substance of Abuse

Analyses by sex and age were conducted for the six most commonly reported primary substances of abuse: alcohol, marijuana, heroin, prescription pain relievers, cocaine, and methamphetamine/amphetamines.

Alcohol and Marijuana

Compared with their male counterparts, a larger proportion of female admissions between the ages of 12 and 17 reported alcohol as their primary substance of abuse (21.7 vs. 10.5 percent). This pattern changed among adult admissions. Among admissions between the ages of 25 and 34, a smaller proportion of female admissions than male admissions reported alcohol as their primary substance of abuse (25.9 vs. 36.5 percent). Marijuana was reported as the primary substance of abuse less frequently by females than males among admissions between the ages of 12 and 17 (60.8 vs. 80.7 percent) and between the ages of 18 and 24 (22.1 vs. 33.4 percent). There was no variation by sex in primary marijuana abuse among admissions 25 years of age or older.

Methamphetamine/Amphetamines

The proportions of female and male admissions reporting methamphetamine/amphetamines as their primary substance of abuse were similar across all age groups with the exception of those between the ages of 18 and 24. Specifically, among admissions between the ages of 18 and 24, 8.9 percent of female admissions reported primary methamphetamine/amphetamine abuse compared with 3.7 percent of male admissions.

Prescription Pain Relievers

The highest proportions of primary abuse of prescription pain relievers (e.g., oxycodone) were found among admissions between the ages of 18 to 24 and 25 to 34. In the 25 to 34 age group, 19 percent of female admissions and 12.2 percent of male admissions reported prescription pain relievers as their primary substance of abuse. In terms of the effect size, however, the differences between male and female admissions in these age groups were negligible. The only meaningful difference by effect size between males and females was observed among admissions 65 years of age or older. Within the 65 years of age or older age group, the proportion of female admissions reporting primary abuse of prescription pain relievers was nearly 3 times that of their male counterparts (7.2 vs. 2.8 percent).

Discussion

This report highlights important differences in primary substance of abuse between males and females admitted to substance abuse treatment. These differences were found at various stages of life, from adolescence through older adulthood, particularly for abuse of alcohol, marijuana, methamphetamine/amphetamines, and prescription pain relievers. Although this report does not explain the potential reasons for these differences, it brings awareness to the fact that they exist. This may help inform the design of prevention, outreach, and treatment services for specific sex and age groups across multiple settings, including primary care. For example, other research shows that compared with men, women have been found to initiate use of methamphetamine at younger ages and have a greater vulnerability to methamphetamine dependence due to physiological factors. This research, coupled with the findings in this report, might suggest that age-appropriate methamphetamine prevention and outreach efforts directed towards adolescents and young women in particular may be important in areas with moderate to high rates of methamphetamine use.

Additionally, the findings related to differences in the abuse of prescription pain relievers between older adult males and females may warrant further investigation particularly in the context of older adults receiving medications in general medical settings. Further research is needed to understand who would benefit from programs that target particular sex and age groups compared with sex-specific programs and standard treatment.

Section 1.5

PTSD Study: Men versus Women

This section includes text excerpted from "PTSD Study: Men versus Women," U.S. Department of Veterans Affairs (VA), April 18, 2013. Reviewed June 2019.

"In the general population, women are twice as likely as men to develop posttraumatic stress disorder [PTSD]," noted Dr. Sonja Batten, the U.S. Department of Veterans Affairs' (VA) Deputy Chief Consultant for Specialty Mental Health. "But among recent returnees seeking care at VA, PTSD rates among men and women are the same. Statistics such as these suggest the need to better understand the role of gender [sex] in PTSD, particularly as it may impact our Veterans seeking care."

Researchers at the Department of Veterans Affairs are now taking some initial steps toward understanding this complex subject. To that end, Dr. Sabra Inslicht, a staff psychologist at the San Francisco VA Medical Center and an assistant professor of psychiatry at the University of California, San Francisco recently led a VA study that took a closer look at how men and women learn to fear. Her work was published in the October 2012 issue of the *Journal of Psychiatric Research*.

Men Are from Mars; Women Are from Venus

"If we can learn more about potential gender [sex] differences in the process of fear learning," Inslicht said, "it may help us develop more targeted treatments that are geared more precisely to the unique needs of men and women."

For their study, Inslicht and her team recruited 18 men and 13 women who had been diagnosed with PTSD. These participants were all shown various images on a computer screen. Electrodes were attached to their palms, so researchers could measure participants' physiological response to each image.

After certain images appeared, the test subject received a small electrical shock. Gradually, the test subject came to associate these particular images with something unpleasant. "They learned to anticipate the impending shock," Inslicht said. "They learned the danger cues. We call this 'fear conditioning.'"

Researchers carefully monitored test subjects' skin conductive responses—that is, how sweaty their palms got—to measure the body's stress reaction to the image on the screen.

"We discovered that women responded more strongly to the visual cues than men when they saw a particular image that they knew was going to be followed by an electric shock," Inslicht explained. "This suggests that women conditioned more robustly than men. In our future work, we'd like to get a better understanding as to why these differences may occur."

Fight or Flight

"To some extent, learning to fear is important for survival," the researcher said. "When we are threatened by something dangerous, we tend to react with a stress response or 'fight-or-flight' response. It helps keep us safe by mobilizing our bodies to either fight or flee a threat, thus enabling us to protect ourselves from harm in dangerous situations."

Inslicht said this "fight or flight" response, however, can sometimes persist even in nonthreatening situations. "For example," she said, "if you witnessed a suicide bombing while on patrol in a crowded marketplace in Afghanistan, you might develop a fear of crowded places. While you're on patrol and in potential danger, a heightened level of vigilance can be protective. However, if that response persists even after returning home and to a safe place, it can become problematic.

"When you're unable to turn it off in safe situations, the stress becomes prolonged," she continued. "This can cause wear and tear on both the mind and the body. When this heightened reactivity starts to negatively impact your daily life, we begin to worry about posttraumatic stress." But, if fear conditioning does in fact occur differently in men and women, then might not the process known as "fear extinction" also be affected by sex differences?

21

"Fear extinction happens," Inslicht said, "when you are gradually exposed to the previously learned danger cues, such as crowds, and you gradually come to realize that the cue will not be followed by a stressful or potentially traumatic event. This results in the diminishing of the fear response. Since extinction learning is believed to be important for recovery from PTSD, a deeper understanding of this process could alter our strategy for how we treat PTSD in men and women."

Much More to Learn

Inslicht said her small study leaves a number of questions unanswered, and that more in-depth research is needed.

"For example, all our study participants had PTSD," she said, "so we couldn't arrive at any conclusions regarding whether women, as a general rule, condition more strongly than men do, or whether this difference is found only among women who have already developed PTSD."

"Finally, we did not examine what may drive the gender [sex] differences that we found," the researcher noted. "For example, there may be biological differences such as particular hormones and neuropeptides that may mediate these effects."

Inslicht said the research community is only just beginning to understand fear learning and extinction mechanisms and their relationship to PTSD.

"Ultimately, however, this line of research may result in advances for treatment," she concluded. "There may be ways that we can enhance extinction learning—perhaps through medications or with other modifications to existing behavioral treatments."

Chapter 2

Self-Examinations Recommended for Men

Chapter Contents

Section 2.1—Breast Self-Examination 24

Section 2.2—Oral Cancer Self-Examination 26

Section 2.3—Skin Cancer Self-Examination 28

Section 2.4—Testicular Self-Examination................................... 30

Section 2.1

Breast Self-Examination

"Breast Self-Examination,"
© 2016 Omnigraphics. Reviewed June 2019.

Many people are not aware that men can develop breast cancer. Males do have breast tissue, however, and malignant (cancerous) cells can develop there—just as they can in any other part of the body. Although less than one percent of all cases of breast cancer occur in males, several factors may increase the risk of male breast cancer, including:

- Inherited gene mutations, such as *BRCA1* or *BRCA2*;

- Family history of breast cancer;

- Exposure to radiation;

- High levels of estrogen;

- Advanced age (most cases are detected in men between the ages of 60 and 70).

Since early detection of male breast cancer can lead to improved treatment options and prognosis, many healthcare practitioners and cancer-prevention organizations recommend that men with an increased risk of breast cancer perform monthly breast self-examinations.

Breast self-examination is a technique people can use to visually and manually check their own breast tissue for lumps or other changes. People who conduct regular self-exams become familiar with the normal appearance and feel of their breast tissue, which enables them to recognize changes and discover lumps that may require medical attention. Some of the changes that should be checked by a doctor include:

- Hard lumps or new areas of thickness, which may or may not be painful;

- Discharge of fluid from the nipples;

- Dimpling, puckering, rashes, or other changes to the skin;

- Changes to the size or shape of the breast.

How to Perform a Breast Self-Examination

Doctors recommend that men at risk of breast cancer perform a regular breast self-examination once per month. It should cover the entire surface area of each breast, from the collarbone down to the abdomen and from the armpit across to the center of the chest. Perhaps the easiest way for men to examine their breast area is in the shower. Using soap and water to create a slippery surface allows the fingers to slide easily over the breast tissue.

The main steps in performing a male breast self-examination are as follows:

1. Raise your right arm, and place it behind or on top of your head.

2. Use the pads of the three middle fingers on your left hand to examine your right breast.

3. Move your fingers in small circles, about the size of a quarter.

4. Begin under the armpit, and work from top to bottom along the outer part of your breast.

5. After completing one vertical strip, move over one finger width and begin a new strip, working from bottom to top. Do not lift the fingers between rows.

6. Check the entire breast area in an up-and-down pattern, as if mowing a lawn.

7. Repeat the process by using the left hand to examine the right breast.

8. Gently squeeze each nipple between your fingers to check for any fluid discharge, puckering, or retraction.

9. After stepping out of the shower and drying off, visually examine your breasts in front of a mirror. They should appear symmetrical in size and shape, and the skin should not show signs of dimpling, puckering, or rashes.

Men who find a lump or notice other changes in their breast tissue during a self-examination should not become alarmed. Around 80 percent of all breast lumps are not cancerous. In addition, most lumps or inflammation detected in male breasts are due to a benign condition called "gynecomastia." This condition is commonly associated with the hormonal changes of puberty, but it may also occur as a side effect of certain medications. Still, any hard lumps or other areas of concern should be checked by a medical practitioner.

References

1. "Check Yourself for Male Breast Cancer," MaleCare, 2016.

2. Stephan, Pam. "Male Breast Self-Examination," VeryWell, December 16, 2014.

Section 2.2

Oral Cancer Self-Examination

This section contains text excerpted from the following sources: Text in this section begins with excerpts from "Oral Cancer," MedlinePlus, National Institutes of Health (NIH), August 18, 2016; Text under the heading "How Oral Cancer Self-Examination Is Done?" is excerpted from "The Oral Cancer Exam," National Institute of Dental and Craniofacial Research (NIDCR), September 2018.

Oral cancer can form in any part of the mouth. Most oral cancers begin in the flat cells that cover the surfaces of your mouth, tongue, and lips. Anyone can get oral cancer, but the risk is higher if you are male, use tobacco, drink lots of alcohol, have human papillomavirus (HPV), or have a history of head or neck cancer. Frequent sun exposure is also a risk factor for lip cancer.

Symptoms of oral cancer include:

- White or red patches in your mouth

- A mouth sore that will not heal

- Bleeding in your mouth

- Loose teeth

- Problems or pain with swallowing

- A lump in your neck

- An earache

Tests to diagnose oral cancer include a physical exam, endoscopy, biopsy, and imaging tests. Oral cancer treatments may include surgery, radiation therapy, and chemotherapy. Some patients have a combination of treatments.

How Oral Cancer Self-Examination Is Done?

An oral cancer exam is painless and quick—it takes only a few minutes. Your regular dental checkup is an excellent opportunity to have the exam.

Here is what to expect:

1. Preparing for the exam: If you have dentures (plates) or partials, you will be asked to remove them.

2. Your healthcare provider will inspect your face, neck, lips, and mouth to look for any signs of cancer.

3. With both hands, she or he will feel the area under your jaw and the side of your neck, checking for lumps that may suggest cancer.

4. She or he will then look at and feel the insides of your lips and cheeks to check for possible signs of cancer, such as red and/or white patches.

5. Next, your provider will have you stick out your tongue so it can be checked for swelling or abnormal color or texture.

6. Using gauze, she or he will then gently pull your tongue to one side, then the other, to check the base of your tongue. The underside of your tongue will also be checked.

7. In addition, she or he will look at the roof and floor of your mouth, as well as the back of your throat.

8. Finally, your provider will put one finger on the floor of your mouth and, with the other hand under your chin, gently press down to check for lumps or sensitivity.

Section 2.3

Skin Cancer Self-Examination

"Skin Cancer Self-Examination,"
© 2016 Omnigraphics. Reviewed June 2019.

When potential skin cancers are found and treated early, they can usually be cured. Thus, early detection is thus a major priority. Doctors and cancer-fighting organizations recommend conducting a thorough, head-to-toe skin cancer self-examination every month as a way to help people notice changes in their skin and identify suspicious moles, growths, or lesions that should be checked by a physician.

Medical professionals have developed two main strategies to help people recognize malignant melanoma—the deadliest form of skin cancer—as well as nomelanoma skin cancers, such as basal cell carcinoma and squamous cell carcinoma. These early recognition strategies, the ABCDEs, and the Ugly Duckling sign can be applied by individuals examining their own skin, as well as by healthcare professionals.

How to Conduct a Skin Cancer Self-Examination

Medical practitioners and skin cancer awareness organizations recommend that people conduct a head-to-toe self-examination once per month to check for unusual moles or lesions on their skin. A complete examination should include the following areas:

1. **Face**—use a mirror to examine the nose, mouth, and ears.

2. **Scalp**—use a blow dryer to expose various sections of the scalp for inspection or ask a friend or family member to help.

3. **Hands**—check the palms as well as the backs of the hands, and look between the fingers and under the fingernails.

4. **Arms**—begin by inspecting the wrists and forearms, then use a mirror to check the elbows, upper arms, and underarms.

5. **Chest**—examine the neck, collarbone, chest, and torso.

6. **Back**—using a full-length mirror and a hand mirror, check the back of the neck, shoulders, upper back, and lower back.

7. **Genitals**—use a hand mirror to examine the buttocks and genital area.

8. **Legs**—inspect the front and back of each leg, including thigh, shin, calf, and ankle.

9. **Feet**—check the top and bottom of each foot, as well as between the toes and under toenails.

What to Look for in a Skin Cancer Self-Examination

Most people have ordinary, harmless moles or spots on their skin. Also known as "nevi," moles are common skin growths in which pigment cells form a cluster. A typical nevus may appear black, brown, tan, pink, or red. It may be flat or slightly raised, and it may be round or oval in shape. The goal of a skin cancer self-examination is to identify atypical moles (dysplastic nevi) that may be precancerous or cancerous. The two main strategies to help people distinguish between harmless and suspicious moles are the ABCDEs, and the Ugly Duckling sign.

The ABCDEs

The acronym ABCDE is a valuable tool for helping people evaluate moles, spots, and other skin growths. Each letter represents a specific warning sign that a mole may potentially be cancerous and should be checked by a doctor:

A. **Asymmetry**—benign (noncancerous) moles tend to be symmetrical, meaning that the two halves match; asymmetry is a warning sign for melanoma.

B. **Border irregularity**—typical moles tend to have smooth, regular borders, while melanomas usually have rough, uneven, notched, or scalloped edges.

C. **Color variation**—benign moles tend to be all one color, while melanomas often have a number of different shades of brown, tan, black, red, or white.

D. **Diameter**—benign moles are typically smaller than 6 millimeters in diameter (about the size of the eraser on a pencil), while melanomas tend to be larger in diameter.

E. **Evolution**—the appearance of common moles tends to remain the same over time, so any changes or evolution in a mole's size, shape, color, or other characteristics (such as itching, crusting, bleeding, or failing to heal) should be considered a warning sign.

The Ugly Duckling Sign

Although the ABCDEs are helpful in identifying potential skin cancers, even experts may find it challenging to distinguish melanomas from harmless moles that display some of the warning signs. Given the importance of early detection, skin cancer specialists developed a second tool—the Ugly Duckling sign—to aid in screening and diagnosis.

The Ugly Duckling sign is based on the fact that all of the moles on the skin of a specific person tend to resemble one another. Whether a person has a dozen moles or a hundred moles, most will be of a similar shape, color, and size. As a result, part of the skin cancer self-examination should involve comparing each mole to surrounding moles and looking for outliers—or "ugly ducklings"—that do not fit into the usual pattern. For instance, a mole that stands out because it is larger or a different color than the others should be considered suspicious and checked by a doctor.

References

1. "Do You Know Your ABCDEs?" Skin Cancer Foundation, 2016.

2. Scope, Alon, and Ashfaq A. Marghoob. "The Ugly Duckling Sign: An Early Melanoma Recognition Tool for Clinicians and the Public," Skin Cancer Foundation, August 29, 2011.

3. "Step-by-Step Self-Examination," Skin Cancer Foundation, 2016.

Section 2.4

Testicular Self-Examination

"Testicular Self-Examination," © 2016
Omnigraphics. Reviewed June 2019.

Although testicular cancer has a relatively low rate of occurrence, accounting for just 1 percent of malignancies in all men, it is the most common neoplasm, or abnormal growth, in adolescent males and young men under 35 years of age. Testicular cancer is easily diagnosable and can be successfully treated, with a high survival rate of more than 10 years in nearly 90 percent of patients. As with most types of cancer, the prognosis is particularly good with early detection. While significant advances have been made in developing treatments for testicular cancer in the last few decades, the benefits of early detection through self-examination have not received much attention, often resulting in delays before medical attention is sought.

Importance of Testicular Self-Examination

In the absence of a standard or routine screening for testicular cancer, the condition is most often detected either by a doctor during a routine physical examination or by an individual during the course of a self-exam. The outlook for testicular cancer depends on whether or not the disease has metastasized to lymph nodes, tissues, and organs, and this underscores the importance of early detection by testicular self-examination (TSE).

Early detection involves the diagnosis of testicular cancer through stages 1 and 2. Stage 1 refers to a "localized" tumor restricted to the primary site, the testes. Stage 2 is the term for a "regional" tumor, one that has spread to other areas. An early diagnosis resulting from a self-exam can greatly enhance treatment outcomes and also reduce the side effects commonly associated with chemotherapy, radiation, and surgery.

How to Perform a Testicular Self-Examination

It is important to perform a self-examination every month. This allows you to familiarize yourself with the size, shape, and consistency of your testes and to sensitize you to any abnormality in the future. This also helps you to distinguish the epididymis—a highly coiled duct behind the testis for the temporary storage of sperm—from an abnormal lump or growth. Further, it is quite normal for most men to have testicular asymmetry. Differently sized testes with one hanging lower than the other is a normal anatomical feature and should not be construed as a sign of abnormality.

The ideal time to perform a self-exam is right after a warm shower when the scrotum is relaxed and can be easily drawn back to examine the testicles.

Testicular self-examination is a simple procedure that takes no more than a couple of minutes:

- Hold the penis away from the scrotum to enable close examination of the testes.

- Hold the testicles between your thumb and fingers and roll gently.

- Feel each testicle for any painless lump, usually grain or pea-sized, in the front or sides, taking care not to confuse a lump with supporting tissues and blood vessels.

- If you detect any thickening, discomfort, or pain in the testicles or groin, contact your healthcare professional immediately.

Studies show that men often delay seeking medical attention because early symptoms are typically mild, and many men tend to believe that a lump is benign or harmless and may go away on its own. Concerns about loss of sexuality, or sterility, may also get in the way of seeking professional help when an abnormality is detected.

While the majority of scrotal and testicular irregularities may not be associated with malignancy, it is important for all men—especially those who carry a high risk for testicular tumors—to perform regular self-exams. A family history of testicular cancer and previous history of malignant tumors in one or both of the testes are regarded as high-risk factors, as are conditions such as cryptorchidism, a common birth defect associated with undescended testes.

References

1. "How to Perform a Testicular Self-Examination," The Nemours Foundation/KidsHealth®, 2012.

2. "Testicular Examination and Testicular Self-Examination (TSE)," Healthwise, Incorporated, June 4, 2014.

3. "SEER Stat Fact Sheets: Testis Cancer," National Institutes of Health (NIH), April 2016.

Chapter 3

Recommended
Screening Tests for Men

Chapter Contents

Section 3.1—Screening Tests for Men: What You
    Need and When 34

Section 3.2—Abdominal Aortic Aneurysm Screening................. 36

Section 3.3—Blood Pressure Screening 39

Section 3.4—Cholesterol Screening 42

Section 3.5—Colorectal Cancer Screening................................... 46

Section 3.6—Osteoporosis Screening 51

Section 3.7—Prostate Cancer Screening 56

Section 3.1

Screening Tests for Men: What You Need and When

This section includes text excerpted from "Men: Stay Healthy at Any Age," U.S. Office of Personnel Management (OPM), August 15, 2010. Reviewed June 2019.

Get the Screenings You Need

Screenings are tests that look for diseases before you have symptoms. Blood pressure checks and tests for high cholesterol are examples of screenings. You can get some screenings, such as blood pressure readings, in your doctor's office. Others—such as a colonoscopy, a test for colorectal cancer—need special equipment, so you may need to go to a different office. After a screening test, ask when you will see the results and who you should talk to about them.

Abdominal aortic aneurysm. If you are between the ages of 65 and 75 and have ever been a smoker, talk to your doctor or nurse about being screened for abdominal aortic aneurysm (AAA). AAA is a bulging in your abdominal aorta, the largest artery in your body. An AAA may burst, which can cause dangerous bleeding and death.

Colorectal cancer. Have a screening test for colorectal cancer starting at the age of 50. If you have a family history of colorectal cancer, you may need to be screened earlier. Several different tests can detect this cancer. Your doctor can help you decide which is best for you.

Depression. Your emotional health is as important as your physical health. Talk to your doctor or nurse about being screened for depression especially if during the last two weeks:

- You have felt down, sad, or hopeless.

- You have felt little interest or pleasure in doing things.

Diabetes. Get screened for diabetes if your blood pressure is higher than 135/80 or if you take medication for high blood pressure. Diabetes (high blood sugar) can cause problems with your heart, brain, eyes, feet, kidneys, nerves, and other body parts.

High blood pressure. Starting at the age of 18, have your blood pressure checked at least every 2 years. High blood pressure is 140/90

34

or higher. High blood pressure can cause strokes, heart attacks, kidney and eye problems, and heart failure.

High cholesterol. If you are 35 years of age or older, have your cholesterol checked. Have your cholesterol checked starting at 20 years of age if:

- You use tobacco.
- You are obese.
- You have diabetes or high blood pressure.
- You have a personal history of heart disease or blocked arteries.
- A man in your family had a heart attack before the age of 50 or a woman had a heart attack before the age of 60.

Human immunodeficiency virus (HIV). Talk with your health-care team about HIV screening if any of these apply to you:

- You have had unprotected sex with multiple partners.
- You have sex with men.
- You use or have used injection drugs.
- You exchange sex for money or drugs, or you have sex partners who do.
- You have or had a sex partner who is HIV-infected or injects drugs.
- You are being treated for a sexually transmitted disease (STD).
- You had a blood transfusion between 1978 and 1985.
- You have any other concerns.

Syphilis. Ask your doctor or nurse whether you should be screened for syphilis.

Overweight and obesity. The best way to learn if you are over-weight or obese is to find your body mass index (BMI). You can find your BMI by entering your height and weight into an online BMI calculator. A BMI between 18.5 and 25 indicates a normal weight. Persons with a BMI of 30 or higher may be obese. If you are obese, talk to your doctor or nurse about seeking intensive counseling and getting help with changing your behaviors to lose weight. Being overweight or obese can lead to diabetes and cardiovascular disease.

It Is Your Body

You know your body better than anyone else. Always tell your doctor or nurse about any changes in your health, including your vision and hearing. Ask them about being checked for any condition you are concerned about, not just the ones here. If you are wondering about diseases such as prostate cancer or skin cancer, for example, ask about them.

Section 3.2

Abdominal Aortic Aneurysm Screening

This section includes text excerpted from "Talk to Your Doctor about Abdominal Aortic Aneurysm," Office of Disease Prevention and Health Promotion (ODPHP), U.S. Department of Health and Human Services (HHS), May 29, 2019.

The Basics

If you are a man between the ages of 65 and 75 and have ever smoked, ask your doctor about getting screened (tested) for an abdominal aortic aneurysm (AAA).

Am I at Risk for an Abdominal Aortic Aneurysm?

Men over the age of 65 who have smoked at any point in their lives have the highest risk of an AAA. Both men and women can have an AAA, but it is more common in men.

Risk factors for an AAA include:

- Family history—for example, if a parent or sibling had an AAA

- Smoking

- Older age

- High blood pressure

- High cholesterol

- Heart disease or vascular disease (problems with blood vessels)

36

What Is an Abdominal Aortic Aneurysm?

The aorta is your body's main artery. An artery is a blood vessel (or tube) that carries blood from your heart. The aorta carries blood from your heart to your abdomen, pelvis, and legs.

If the wall of your aorta is weak, it can swell like a balloon. This balloon-like swelling is called an "aneurysm." An AAA is an aneurysm that occurs in the part of the aorta running through the abdomen.

Why Do I Need to Talk to the Doctor?

Aneurysms usually grow slowly and without any symptoms. When aneurysms grow large enough to rupture (burst), they can cause dangerous bleeding inside the body that can lead to death.

If an abdominal aortic aneurysm is found early, it can be treated before it bursts. That is why it is so important to talk to your doctor about your risk.

How Do I Know If I Have an Abdominal Aortic Aneurysm?

To screen (test) for an AAA, your doctor may order an ultrasound. An ultrasound uses sound waves to look inside the body. It can help your doctor see if there is any swelling of the aorta. Most types of ultrasounds are painless.

What Are the Symptoms of an Abdominal Aortic Aneurysm?

There are usually no symptoms of AAA until it is a medical emergency. Blood vessels such as the aorta can swell up slowly over time, so it is important to talk with your doctor about AAA to see if you need to get tested.

A ruptured aneurysm can cause dangerous bleeding that can lead to death. If this happens, you may suddenly have:

- Pain in your lower back, abdomen, or legs
- Nausea (feeling like you are going to throw up)
- Vomiting (throwing up)
- Clammy (sweaty) skin

If you have a ruptured aneurysm, you will need to have surgery right away.

Take Action

Take these steps to lower your risk for AAA.

Talk with Your Doctor about Your Risk for an Abdominal Aortic Aneurysm

Here are some questions you might want to ask your doctor or nurse:

- Do I need to get screened for an AAA?
- How can I get help to quit smoking?
- What are my blood pressure and cholesterol numbers?
- What other steps can I take to keep my heart and blood vessels healthy?

What about the Cost of Screening

Under the Affordable Care Act, the healthcare reform law passed in 2010, insurance plans must cover AAA screening for men between the ages of 65 and 75 who have smoked. This means that you may be able to get screened at no cost to you.

- If you have Medicare, find out about Medicare coverage for AAA screening.
- If you have private insurance, talk to your insurance provider about what is included in your plan. Ask about the Affordable Care Act.

Make Changes to Lower Your Risk for an Abdominal Aortic Aneurysm

It is never too late to take steps to lower your risk for an AAA.

Quit Smoking

Quitting smoking is the most important thing you can do to lower your risk for an AAA.

If you smoke, now is the time to quit. Call 800-QUIT-NOW (800-784-8669) for free support and help setting up a plan to quit.

Check Your Blood Pressure

Get your blood pressure checked. If your blood pressure is high, you can help lower it by getting active, watching your weight, and eating less sodium (salt).

Get Your Cholesterol Checked

Find out what your cholesterol levels are. If your cholesterol is high, start a heart-healthy eating plan. This means eating foods low in saturated fat, *trans* fat, and cholesterol.

Aim for 2 hours and 30 minutes of physical activity every week.

Section 3.3

Blood Pressure Screening

This section includes text excerpted from "Get Your Blood Pressure Checked," Office of Disease Prevention and Health Promotion (ODPHP), U.S. Department of Health and Human Services (HHS), April 19, 2019.

The Basics

One in three American adults have high blood pressure. High blood pressure increases your risk for serious health problems, including stroke and heart attack.

Get your blood pressure checked regularly starting at 18 years of age, and do your best to keep track of your blood pressure numbers.

How Often Do I Need to Get My Blood Pressure Checked?

- If you are 40 years of age or older, or if you are at a higher risk for high blood pressure, get your blood pressure checked once a year.

- If you are between the ages of 18 and 40 and you are not at an increased risk for high blood pressure, get your blood pressure checked every 3 to 5 years.

What Puts Me at Higher Risk for High Blood Pressure?

Your risk for high blood pressure goes up as you get older. You are also at an increased risk for high blood pressure if you:

- Are African American

- Are overweight or obese

- Do not get enough physical activity

- Drink too much alcohol

- Do not eat a healthy diet

- Have kidney failure, diabetes, or some types of heart disease

What Is Blood Pressure?

Blood pressure is how hard your blood pushes against the walls of your arteries when your heart pumps blood. Arteries are the tubes that carry blood away from your heart. Every time your heart beats, it pumps blood through your arteries to the rest of your body.

What Is Hypertension?

"Hypertension" is the medical term for high blood pressure. High blood pressure usually has no symptoms, so it is sometimes called a "silent killer." The only way to know if you have high blood pressure is to get tested.

What Do Blood Pressure Numbers Mean?

A blood pressure test measures how hard your heart is working to pump blood through your body.

Blood pressure is measured with two numbers. The first number is the pressure in your arteries when your heart beats. The second number is the pressure in your arteries between beats, when your heart relaxes.

Compare your blood pressure to these numbers:

- Normal blood pressure is lower than 120/80 (said "120 over 80").

- High blood pressure is 140/90 or higher.

- Blood pressure that is between normal and high (for example, 130/85) is called "elevated blood pressure" or "prehypertension."

How Can I Get My Blood Pressure Checked?

To test your blood pressure, a nurse or doctor will put a cuff around your upper arm. The nurse or doctor will pump the cuff with air until it feels tight, then slowly let it out. This will not take more than a few minutes.

You can find out what your blood pressure numbers are right after the test is over. If the test shows that your blood pressure is high, ask the doctor what to do next.

Blood pressure can go up and down, so you may need to get it checked it more than once.

Can I Check My Blood Pressure by Myself

Yes. Many shopping malls, pharmacies, and grocery stores have blood pressure machines you can use in the store. You can also buy a home blood pressure monitor at a drugstore. If the test shows that your blood pressure is high, talk to your doctor.

What If I Have High Blood Pressure?

If you have high blood pressure, you may need medicine to control it. Take these steps to lower your blood pressure:

- Eat healthy, including foods that are low in saturated fat and sodium.

- Get active. Aim for 2 hours and 30 minutes a week of moderate aerobic activity.

- Watch your weight by eating healthy and getting active.

- Remember to take medicines as prescribed (ordered) by your doctor.

Small changes can add up. For example, losing just 10 pounds can help lower your blood pressure.

Take Action

To prevent or lower high blood pressure, start by getting your blood pressure checked as soon as possible.

Check Your Blood Pressure Regularly

Make sure a doctor or nurse checks your blood pressure at your next visit. Write down your blood pressure numbers so you will remember them.

You can also find blood pressure machines at many shopping malls, pharmacies, and grocery stores. Most of these machines are free to use.

If you want to check your blood pressure at home, you can buy a home blood pressure monitor at a drugstore.

What about the Cost of Testing

Under the Affordable Care Act, the healthcare reform law passed in 2010, insurance plans must cover blood pressure testing. Depending on your insurance, you may be able to get your blood pressure checked by a doctor or nurse at no cost to you.

Section 3.4

Cholesterol Screening

This section includes text excerpted from "Get Your Cholesterol Checked," Office of Disease Prevention and Health Promotion (ODPHP), U.S. Department of Health and Human Services (HHS), September 26, 2018.

The Basics

It is important to get your cholesterol checked regularly. Too much cholesterol in your blood can cause a heart attack or a stroke.

The good news is that it is easy to get your cholesterol checked. If your cholesterol is high, you can take steps to lower it, such as eating healthy, getting more physical activity, and taking medicine if your doctor recommends it.

How Often Do I Need to Get My Cholesterol Checked?

The general recommendation is to get your cholesterol checked every four to six years. Some people may need to get their cholesterol checked more or less, often depending on their risk for developing heart disease.

For example, high cholesterol can run in families. If someone in your family has high cholesterol or takes medicine to control their cholesterol, you might need to get tested more often. Talk to your doctor about what is best for you.

What Is Cholesterol?

Cholesterol is a waxy substance (material) that is found naturally in your blood. Your body makes cholesterol and uses it to do important things, such as making hormones and digesting fatty foods.

You also raise your cholesterol by eating foods, such as egg yolks, fatty meats, and cheese.

If you have too much cholesterol in your body, it can build up inside your blood vessels and make it hard for blood to flow through them. Over time, this can lead to heart disease and heart attack or stroke.

How Can I Tell If I Have High Cholesterol?

Most people who have high cholesterol do not have any signs or symptoms. That is why it is so important to get your cholesterol checked.

How Can I Get My Cholesterol Checked?

Your doctor will check your cholesterol levels with a blood test called a "lipid profile." For this test, a nurse will take a small sample of blood from your finger or arm.

Be sure to ask your doctor how to get ready for the test. For example, you may need to fast (not eat or drink anything except water) for 9 to 12 hours before the test.

There are other blood tests that can check cholesterol, but a lipid profile gives the most information.

What Do the Test Results Mean?

If you get a lipid profile test, the results will show 4 numbers. A lipid profile measures:

- Total cholesterol
- Low-density lipoprotein (LDL) cholesterol

- High-density lipoprotein (HDL) cholesterol

- Triglycerides

Total cholesterol is a measure of all the cholesterol in your blood. It is based on the LDL, HDL, and triglycerides numbers.

Low-density lipoprotein cholesterol is the "bad" type of cholesterol that can block your arteries. Therefore, a lower level is better for you.

High-density lipoprotein cholesterol is the "good" type of cholesterol. It helps clear LDL cholesterol out of your arteries. Therefore, a higher level is better for you. Having a low HDL cholesterol level can increase your risk for heart disease.

Triglycerides are a type of fat in your blood that can increase your risk for heart attack and stroke.

What Can Cause Unhealthy Cholesterol Levels?

Low-density lipoprotein cholesterol levels tend to increase as people get older. Other causes of high LDL cholesterol levels include:

- Family history of high LDL cholesterol

- High blood pressure or type 2 diabetes

- Smoking

- Being overweight

- Not getting enough physical activity

- Eating too much saturated fat, *trans* fat, and cholesterol, and not enough fruits and vegetables

- Taking certain medicines, such as medicines to lower blood pressure

Causes of low HDL (good) cholesterol levels include:

- Smoking

- Being overweight

- Not getting enough physical activity

- Eating too much sugar and starch (called "carbohydrates")

- Not eating enough fruits, vegetables, and unsaturated fat (such as olive oil)

What If My Cholesterol Levels Are Not Healthy?

As your low-density lipoprotein cholesterol gets higher, so does your risk of heart disease. Take these steps to lower your cholesterol and reduce your risk of heart disease:

- Eat heart-healthy foods.

- Get active.

- Stay at a healthy weight.

- If you smoke, quit.

- If you have type 2 diabetes or high blood pressure, take steps to manage it.

- Ask your doctor about taking medicine to lower your risk of heart attack and stroke.

Take Action

Find out what your cholesterol levels are. If your cholesterol is high or you are at risk for heart disease, take steps to control your cholesterol levels.

Make an Appointment to Get Your Cholesterol Checked

Call your doctor's office or health center to schedule the test. Be sure to ask for a complete lipid profile and find out what instructions you will need to follow before the test. For example, you may need to fast for 9 to 12 hours before the test.

What about Cost

Cholesterol testing is covered under the Affordable Care Act, the healthcare reform law passed in 2010. Depending on your insurance plan, you may be able to get your cholesterol checked at no cost to you.

Even if you do not have insurance, you can still get your cholesterol checked.

Keep Track of Your Cholesterol Levels

Remember to ask the doctor or nurse for your cholesterol levels each time you get your cholesterol checked. Write the levels down to keep track of your progress.

Section 3.5

Colorectal Cancer Screening

This section includes text excerpted from "Get Tested for
Colorectal Cancer," Office of Disease Prevention and Health
Promotion (ODPHP), U.S. Department of Health and
Human Services (HHS), April 29, 2019.

The Basics

If you are between the ages of 50 and 75, get tested regularly for
colorectal cancer. A special test (called a "screening test") can help
prevent colorectal cancer or find it early, when it may be easier to treat.

You may need to get tested before the age of 50 if colorectal cancer
runs in your family. Talk with your doctor and ask about your risk
for colorectal cancer.

How Often Should I Get Screened?

How often you need to get screened will depend on:

• Your risk for colorectal cancer

• Which screening test you choose

How Do I Decide Which Test to Take?

There are different ways to test for colorectal cancer. Your doctor
can help you decide which test you would prefer.

Before you talk with your doctor about which test to get, it can be
helpful to think about your values and preferences.

Together, you and your doctor can make a screening plan that is
right for you.

What Are the Different Kinds of Tests?

Several different kinds of tests can be used to screen for colorectal
cancer. The main types are:

• Stool-based tests

• Tests that look directly inside the colon and rectum

Stool tests are done at home. You collect a stool sample and send
it to a lab for testing. Then the lab sends the results to your doctor.

Tests that look directly at your colon and rectum, such as a colonoscopy, are done in a doctor's office or hospital. For these tests, you need to take a laxative to clean out your bowels before the appointment. You will get anesthesia before the test, and you will need someone to drive you home after the test.

Your doctor will tell you how to get ready for your test, including if you need to avoid certain foods beforehand.

Does It Hurt to Get a Colonoscopy?

Preparing for a colonoscopy can be unpleasant, but most people agree that the benefits to their health outweigh any discomfort. And getting anesthesia means that you will not have any pain or feel uncomfortable during the test.

What Is Colorectal Cancer?

Colorectal cancer is a cancer that develops in the colon or the rectum. The colon is the longest part of the large intestine. The rectum is the bottom part of the large intestine.

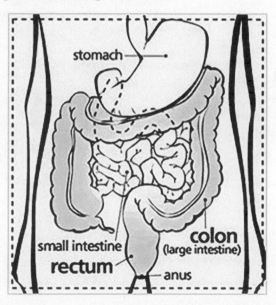

Figure 3.1. *Human Colorectal Tract*

As with other types of cancer, colorectal cancer can spread to other parts of your body.

Am I at Risk for Colorectal Cancer?

The risk of developing colorectal cancer increases as you get older. That is why screening is recommended for everyone between the ages of 50 and 75.

Other risk factors are:

- Having certain types of polyps (growths) inside the colon

- Having a personal or family history of colorectal cancer

- Smoking cigarettes

- Being overweight or obese

- Not getting enough physical activity

- Drinking too much alcohol

- Having certain health conditions, such as Crohn's disease, that cause chronic inflammation (ongoing irritation) of the small intestine and colon

Take Control—Act Early

If you start getting screened at 50 years of age, you have a good chance of preventing colorectal cancer or finding it when it can be treated more easily.

If your doctor finds polyps inside your colon during the test, she or he can remove them before they become cancer.

If your doctor finds cancer during the test, you can take steps to get treatment right away.

Take Action

The best way to prevent colorectal cancer or to find it early is to get tested, starting at 50 years of age.

Talk with Your Doctor about Getting Screened

You can ask your doctor the following questions about colorectal cancer screening.

- What is my risk for colorectal cancer?

- When do you recommend that I start getting tested?

- What are the different types of screening tests for colorectal cancer?

- Which screening test do you recommend for me? Why?

- How often do I need to get tested?

- What does happen during the test? How do I prepare?

- Does the test have any risks or side effects?

- How long will it take to get the results?

- What can I do to reduce my risk of colorectal cancer?

What about Cost

Under the Affordable Care Act, the healthcare reform law passed in 2010, most health insurance plans must cover screening for colorectal cancer. Depending on your plan, you may be able to get screened at no cost to you.

- If you have private insurance, talk to your insurance company to find out what is included in your plan.

- If you have Medicare, find out about Medicare coverage for different colorectal cancer screening tests

- If you do not have insurance, you can still get important screening tests.

Get Support

If you are nervous about getting a colorectal cancer test, get support.

- Ask a family member or friend to go with you when you talk to the doctor.

- Talk with people you know who have been screened to learn what to expect.

Give Support

Do you know someone 50 years of age or older who has not been tested for colorectal cancer yet?

Quit Smoking

People who smoke are more likely to get colorectal cancer. If you smoke, make a plan to quit today.

Watch Your Weight

Being overweight increases your chance of developing colon cancer. Find out how to control your weight.

Get Active

Regular exercise may help reduce your risk of colorectal cancer. Take steps to get moving today.

Drink Alcohol Only in Moderation

Drinking too much alcohol may increase your risk of colorectal cancer. If you choose to drink, have only a moderate (limited) amount. This means:

- No more than one drink a day for women
- No more than two drinks a day for men

Talk with Your Doctor about Taking Aspirin Every Day

Taking aspirin every day can lower your risk of colorectal cancer, heart attack, and stroke. But, it is not right for everyone. If you are between the ages of 50 and 59 and have risk factors for heart disease, ask your doctor if daily aspirin is right for you.

Section 3.6

Osteoporosis Screening

This section includes text excerpted from "Get
a Bone Density Test," Office of Disease Prevention and
Health Promotion (ODPHP), U.S. Department of
Health and Human Services (HHS), May 28, 2019.

The Basics

A bone density test measures how strong bones are. The test will tell you if you have osteoporosis, or weak bones.

Women are at higher risk for osteoporosis than men, and this risk increases with age.

- If you are a woman age 65 or older, schedule a bone density test.

- If you are a woman age 64 or younger and you have gone through menopause, ask your doctor if you need a bone density test.

If you are at risk for osteoporosis, your doctor or nurse may recommend you get a bone density test every two years.

Even though women are at a higher risk for osteoporosis, men can get osteoporosis too. If you are a man over 65 years of age and you are concerned about your bone strength, talk with your doctor or nurse.

What Is Osteoporosis?

Osteoporosis is a bone disease. It means that your bones are weak and more likely to break. People with osteoporosis most often break bones in the hip, spine, and wrist.

There are no signs or symptoms of osteoporosis. You might not know you have the disease until you break a bone. That is why it is so important to get a bone density test to measure your bone strength.

What Happens during a Bone Density Test

A bone density test is similar to an X-ray or scan of your body. A bone density test does not hurt, and you do not need to do anything to prepare for it. It only takes about 15 minutes.

Am I at Risk for Osteoporosis?

Anyone can get osteoporosis, but it is most common in older women. The older you are, the greater your risk for osteoporosis.

These things can also increase your risk for osteoporosis:

- Hormone changes (especially for women who have gone through menopause)

- Not getting enough calcium and Vitamin D

- Taking certain medicines

- Smoking cigarettes or drinking too much alcohol

- Not getting enough physical activity

What If I Have Osteoporosis?

If you have osteoporosis, you can still slow down bone loss. Finding and treating this disease early can keep you healthier and more active, lowering your chances of breaking a bone.

Depending on the results of your bone density test, you may need to:

- Add more calcium and vitamin D to your diet.

- Exercise more to strengthen your bones.

- Take medicine to stop bone loss.

Your doctor can tell you what steps are right for you. It does not matter how old you are; it is not too late to build stronger bones.

Take Action

Take these steps to protect your bone health.

Schedule a Bone Density Test If Your Doctor Recommends It

Ask your doctor if you are at risk for osteoporosis and find out when to start getting bone density tests.

What about Cost?

Screening for osteoporosis is covered under the Affordable Care Act, the healthcare reform law passed in 2010. Depending on your insurance plan, you may be able to get screened at no cost to you.

- Check with your insurance company to find out what is included in your plan.

- If you have Medicare, find out about Medicare coverage for bone density tests.

- If you do not have health insurance, you can still get a bone density test.

Get Enough Calcium

Calcium helps keep your bones strong. Good sources of calcium include:

- Low-fat or fat-free milk, cheese, and yogurt
- Almonds
- Broccoli and greens
- Tofu with added calcium
- Orange juice with added calcium
- Calcium pills

Dairy Products

Look for fat-free or low-fat dairy products.

- Fat-free or low-fat (1%) milk
- Fat-free or low-fat yogurt (choose options with no added sugars)
- Low-fat cheese (3 grams of fat or less per serving)
- Soymilk with added calcium, vitamin A, and vitamin D

Vegetables

You can also get calcium from vegetables, such as:

- Soybeans (edamame)
- Kale
- Turnip greens
- Chinese cabbage (bok choy)
- Collard greens
- Broccoli

If you buy canned vegetables, watch out for sodium. Read the nutrition facts label, and choose the option with the least sodium.

If you buy frozen vegetables, check the nutrition facts label and choose ones without butter or cream sauces.

Foods with Added Calcium

Check the nutrition facts label to look for foods that have 10 percent or more of the daily value of calcium added, such as:

- Breakfast cereal

- Tofu

- 100 percent orange juice

- Soymilk, almond milk, or rice milk

Foods with Vitamin D

Also be sure to look for foods with vitamin D. Vitamin D helps your body absorb (take in) calcium.

- Vitamin D is added to some foods, such as milk, breakfast cereals, and juice. Check the nutrition facts label.

- You can also get some vitamin D from many types of fish, such as salmon, tuna, and trout.

Get Enough Vitamin D

Vitamin D helps your body absorb (take in) calcium.

Your body makes vitamin D when you are out in the sun. You can also get vitamin D from:

- Salmon or tuna

- Fat-free or low-fat milk and yogurt with added vitamin D

- Breakfast cereals and juices with added vitamin D

- Vitamin D pills

Get Active

Physical activity can help slow down bone loss. Weight-bearing activities (such as running or doing jumping jacks) help keep your bones strong.

- Aim for 2 hours and 30 minutes a week of moderate aerobic activity. If you are new to exercise, start with 10 minutes of activity at a time.

- Do strengthening activities at least 2 days a week. These include lifting weights or using resistance bands (long rubber strips that stretch).

- Find an exercise buddy, or go walking with friends. You will be more likely to stick with it if you exercise with other people.

Find Activities That Work for You

You do not need special equipment or a gym membership to stay active. Check with your local community center or senior center to find fun, low-cost, or free exercise options. If you have a health condition or a disability, be as active as you can be. Your doctor can help you choose activities that are right for you.

Stay Away from Cigarettes and Alcohol

Smoking cigarettes and drinking too much alcohol can weaken your bones.

If you drink alcohol, drink only in moderation. This means no more than one drink a day for women and no more than two drinks a day for men.

Take Steps to Prevent Falls

Falls can be especially serious for people with weak bones. You can make small changes to lower your risk of falling, such as doing exercises that improve your balance. For example, try walking backward or standing up from a sitting position without using your hands.

Section 3.7

Prostate Cancer Screening

This section includes text excerpted from "Prostate Cancer
Screening (PDQ®)—Patient Version," National
Cancer Institute (NCI), April 10, 2019.

What Is Screening?

Screening is looking for cancer before a person has any symptoms. This can help find cancer at an early stage. When abnormal tissue or cancer is found early, it may be easier to treat. By the time symptoms appear, cancer may have begun to spread.

Scientists are trying to better understand which people are more likely to get certain types of cancer. They also study the things we do and the things around us to see if they cause cancer. This information helps doctors recommend who should be screened for cancer, which screening tests should be used, and how often the tests should be done.

It is important to remember that your doctor does not necessarily think that you have cancer if she or he suggests a screening test. Screening tests are given when you have no cancer symptoms. Screening tests may be repeated on a regular basis.

If a screening test result is abnormal, you may need to have more tests done to find out if you have cancer. These are called "diagnostic tests."

General Information about Prostate Cancer
Prostate Cancer Is a Disease in Which Malignant Cells Form in the Tissues of the Prostate

The prostate is a gland in the male reproductive system located just below the bladder (the organ that collects and empties urine) and in front of the rectum (the lower part of the intestine). It is about the size of a walnut and surrounds part of the urethra (the tube that empties urine from the bladder). The prostate gland produces fluid that makes up part of semen.

As men age, the prostate may get bigger. A bigger prostate may block the flow of urine from the bladder and cause problems with sexual function. This condition is called "benign prostatic hyperplasia" (BPH), and although it is not cancer, surgery may be needed to correct it. The symptoms of benign prostatic hyperplasia or of other problems in the prostate may be similar to symptoms of prostate cancer.

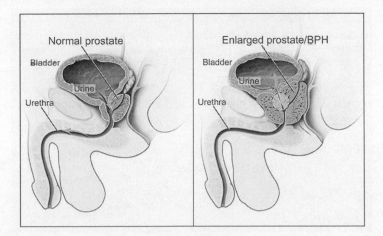

Figure 3.2. *Normal Prostate and Benign Prostatic Hyperplasia*

A normal prostate does not block the flow of urine from the bladder. An enlarged prostate presses on the bladder and urethra and blocks the flow of urine.

Prostate Cancer Is the Most Common Nonskin Cancer among Men in the United States

Prostate cancer is found mainly in older men. Although the number of men with prostate cancer is large, most men diagnosed with this disease do not die from it. Prostate cancer causes more deaths in men than any other cancer except lung cancer. Prostate cancer occurs more often in African American men than in White men. African American men with prostate cancer are more likely to die from the disease than White men with prostate cancer.

Different Factors Increase or Decrease the Risk of Developing Prostate Cancer

Anything that increases a person's chance of developing a disease is called a "risk factor." Anything that decreases your chance of getting a disease is called a "protective factor."

Prostate Cancer Screening
Tests Are Used to Screen for Different Types of Cancer When a Person Does Not Have Symptoms

Scientists study screening tests to find those with the fewest harms and most benefits. Cancer screening trials also are meant to show whether early detection helps a person live longer or decreases a person's chance of dying from the disease. For some types of cancer, the chance of recovery is better if the disease is found and treated at an early stage.

There Is No Standard or Routine Screening Test for Prostate Cancer

Although there are no standard or routine screening tests for prostate cancer, the following tests are being used or studied to screen for it:

Digital Rectal Exam

A digital rectal exam (DRE) is an exam of the rectum. The doctor or nurse inserts a lubricated, gloved finger into the lower part of the rectum to feel the prostate for lumps or anything else that seems unusual.

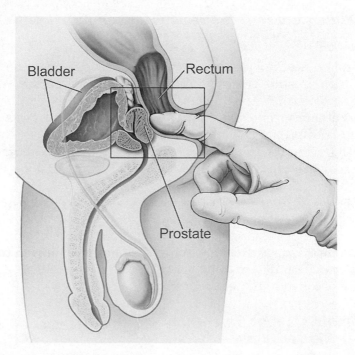

Figure 3.3. *Digital Rectal Exam*

The doctor inserts a gloved, lubricated finger into the rectum and feels the rectum, anus, and prostate (in males) to check for anything abnormal.

Prostate-Specific Antigen Test

A prostate-specific antigen (PSA) test is a test that measures the level of PSA in the blood. PSA is a substance made mostly by the prostate that may be found in an increased amount in the blood of men who have prostate cancer. The level of PSA may also be high in men who have an infection or inflammation of the prostate or benign prostatic hyperplasia (BPH; an enlarged, but noncancerous, prostate).

A prostate-specific antigen test or a digital rectal exam may be able to detect prostate cancer at an early stage, but it is not clear whether early detection and treatment decrease the risk of dying from prostate cancer.

Studies are being done to find ways to make PSA testing more accurate for early cancer detection.

A Prostate Cancer Gene 3 RNA Test May Be Used for Certain Patients

If a man had a high PSA level and a biopsy of the prostate did not show cancer and the PSA level remains high after the biopsy, a prostate cancer gene 3 (PCA3) RNA test may be done. This test measures the amount of PCA3 RNA in the urine after a DRE. If the PCA3 RNA level is higher than normal, another biopsy may help diagnose prostate cancer.

Risks of Prostate Cancer Screening
Screening Tests Have Risks

Decisions about screening tests can be difficult. Not all screening tests are helpful, and most have risks. Before having any screening test, you may want to discuss the test with your doctor. It is important to know the risks of the test and whether it has been proven to reduce the risk of dying from cancer.

The Risks of Prostate Screening
Finding Prostate Cancer May Not Improve Health or Help a Man Live Longer

Screening may not improve your health or help you live longer if you have cancer that has already spread to the area outside of the prostate or to other places in your body.

Some cancers never cause symptoms or become life-threatening, but if found by a screening test, the cancer may be treated. Finding these cancers is called "overdiagnosis." It is not known if treatment of these cancers would help you live longer than if no treatment were given.

Treatments for prostate cancer, such as radical prostatectomy and radiation therapy, may have long-term side effects in many men. The most common side effects are erectile dysfunction (ED) and urinary incontinence.

Some studies of patients with newly diagnosed prostate cancer showed that these patients had a higher risk of death from cardiovascular (heart and blood vessel) disease or suicide. The risk was greatest in the first weeks or months after diagnosis.

Follow-Up Tests

If a prostate-specific antigen test is higher than normal, a biopsy of the prostate may be done. Complications from a biopsy of the prostate may include fever, pain, blood in the urine or semen, and urinary tract infection (UTI). Even if a biopsy shows that a patient does not have prostate cancer, he may worry more about developing prostate cancer in the future.

False-Negative Test Results Can Occur

Screening test results may appear to be normal even though prostate cancer is present. A man who receives a false-negative test result (one that shows that there is no cancer when there really is) may delay seeking medical care even if he has symptoms.

False-Positive Test Results Can Occur

Screening test results may appear to be abnormal even though no cancer is present. A false-positive test result (one that shows there is cancer when there really is not) can cause anxiety and is usually followed by more tests, (such as a biopsy) which also have risks.

Your doctor can advise you about your risk for prostate cancer and your need for screening tests.

Chapter 4

Vaccinations for Men

Chapter Contents

Section 4.1—Recommended Vaccinations for Adults.................. 62

Section 4.2—Human Papillomavirus Vaccination
               Now Recommended for Young Men 65

Section 4.3—Seasonal Influenza Vaccination 67

Section 4.1

Recommended Vaccinations for Adults

This section includes text excerpted from "Vaccines for Adults,"
Vaccines.gov, U.S. Department of Health and
Human Services (HHS), December 2017.

Every year, thousands of adults in the United States get sick and
are hospitalized from vaccine-preventable diseases. Getting vaccinated
will help you stay healthy, so you will miss less work and also have
more time for your family and friends.

And did you know that when you get vaccinated, you also help protect your family and your community? Because of community immunity, vaccines help keep diseases from spreading to people who may
not be able to get certain vaccines, such as newborn babies.

Adults Between the Ages of 19 and 26

Young adults need vaccines too. Vaccines protect young adults
from getting serious and even deadly diseases. They may be especially important if you are living in close quarters with others—such
as in college dorms—and sharing bedrooms, bathrooms, and food.
This can make you more likely to come into contact with dangerous
germs.

By getting vaccinated, you can help keep yourself, your family, and
your community healthy.

Which Vaccines Are Recommended for Adults Between the Ages of 19 and 26?

It is important for young adults to get vaccines that protect
against diseases such as the flu and whooping cough. You also need
to be up to date on meningococcal and human papillomavirus (HPV)
vaccines.

You may also need other vaccines—for example, if you are planning
to travel outside the United States.

Make Sure Your Childhood Vaccines Are up to Date

In addition to getting the vaccinations you need now as a young
adult, it is important to make sure you have had all of your childhood
vaccinations.

It is also a good idea to ask your doctor about any childhood shots that you may have missed or new vaccines that are now available.

Adults Between the Ages of 27 and 64

Did you know that it is just as important for you to stay on top of your vaccinations now as it was when you were a child?

You need a flu shot every year, and you may need additional doses of some vaccines to help you stay protected from diseases. As you age, or your lifestyle or health conditions change, you may need protection from different diseases.

Getting vaccinated can help keep you, your family, and your community healthy.

Adults 65 Years of Age and Older

Vaccines are especially important for older adults. As you get older, your immune system weakens, and it can be more difficult to fight off infections. You are more likely to get diseases such as the flu, pneumonia, and shingles, and you are more likely to have complications that can lead to long-term illness, hospitalization, and even death.

If you have an ongoing health condition, such as diabetes or heart disease, getting vaccinated is especially important. Vaccines can protect you from serious diseases (and related complications), so you can stay healthy as you age.

Getting vaccinated can help keep you, your family, and your community healthy.

Does Medicare Cover Vaccines for Older Adults?

Medicare Part B covers vaccines that protect against the flu and pneumococcal disease—and the hepatitis B vaccine if you are at increased risk for hepatitis B. It also covers vaccines that you might need after an injury (such as the tetanus vaccine) or coming into contact with a disease (such as the rabies vaccine).

Medicare Part D plans generally cover more vaccines than Part B. But depending on your Medicare Part D plan, you may have out-of-pocket costs for these vaccines. Contact Medicare to find out what is covered.

I Have Gotten All My Childhood Vaccines. Why Do I Need More?

Adults need vaccines for several reasons. For example:

- Some vaccines are recommended only for adults, who are more at risk for certain diseases, such as shingles.

- Protection from childhood vaccines wears off over time, so you need additional doses of certain vaccines to stay protected.

- You may not have gotten some of the newer vaccines that are now available.

- Some viruses, such as the virus that causes the flu, can change over time.

- You may be at an increased risk for diseases based on travel plans, your job, or health conditions.

How Do I Know Which Vaccinations I Have Had and Which Ones I Need?

To find out which vaccinations you have had, you will need to find your vaccination record. Your vaccination record is the history of all the vaccines you have had as a child and as an adult. To find your vaccination record:

- Ask your parents or caregivers if they have your vaccination record.

- Contact current or previous doctors, and ask for your record.

- Contact your state health department. Some states have registries (immunization information systems (IISs)) that can provide information about your vaccination records.

- If you cannot find your record, ask your doctor if you should get some vaccinations again.

Section 4.2

Human Papillomavirus Vaccination Now Recommended for Young Men

This section includes text excerpted from "HPV (Human Papillomavirus)," Vaccines.gov, U.S. Department of Health and Human Services (HHS), January 2018.

Why Is the Human Papillomavirus Vaccine Important?

Human papillomavirus (HPV) infections are so common that nearly all men and women get at least 1 type of HPV at some point in their lives, and the complications can be serious. About 17,500 women and 9,300 men get cancer caused by HPV infections in the United States every year. Many of these cancers do not cause symptoms until they have gotten serious and hard to treat.

Getting vaccinated against HPV can protect your child from HPV infections that cause cancer.

What Is Human Papillomavirus?

Human papillomavirus is a group of more than 150 viruses. Many people who get HPV have no symptoms. Some people who get HPV develop warts in their genital area.

Some human papillomavirus infections do not go away and can cause cancer, including:

- Cervical cancer

- Cancer of the penis (penile cancer)

- Cancer of the anus (anal cancer) or rectum (rectal cancer)

- Cancer of the throat (oropharyngeal cancer), including the base of the tongue and tonsils

Human papillomavirus spreads through intimate skin-to-skin contact. Most of the time, it spreads when a person who has an HPV infection has vaginal, oral, or anal sex. And since HPV may not cause symptoms, people can have it and spread it to others without knowing.

Who Needs to Get the Human Papillomavirus Vaccine

Everyone needs to get the HPV vaccine—preteens, teens, and young adults can get it from the age of 9 through 26 years of age.

Preteens and Teens Ages 9 through 14

Preteens and teens need 2 doses of the HPV vaccine as part of their routine vaccine schedule. They get the second dose about 6 to 12 months after the first dose. Preteens usually get the HPV vaccine at the age of 11 or 12, though vaccination can start as early as at 9 years of age.

Teens and Young Adults Ages 15 through 26

If you did not get the HPV vaccine as a preteen, you can still get it. Teens and young adults need three doses of the HPV vaccine. They need to get the second dose one to two months after the first dose—and the third dose six months after the first dose.

Some people may need to get the HPV vaccine at other ages. Talk with your doctor about how to protect your family from HPV.

Who Should Not Get the Human Papillomavirus Vaccine?

You should not get the HPV vaccine if you have had a life-threatening allergic reaction to the HPV vaccine or any ingredient in the vaccine.

Be sure to tell your doctor before getting vaccinated if you:

- Have any serious allergies, including an allergy to yeast

- Are pregnant

What Are the Side Effects of Human Papillomavirus Vaccine?

Side effects are usually mild and go away in a few days. They may include:

- Pain, redness, and swelling where the shot was given

- Fever

- Headache

It is very unlikely that the HPV vaccine could cause a serious reaction. Keep in mind that getting the HPV vaccine is much safer than getting cancer caused by an HPV infection.

Section 4.3

Seasonal Influenza Vaccination

This section includes text excerpted from "Flu (Influenza),"
Vaccines.gov, U.S. Department of Health and
Human Services (HHS), January 18, 2018.

Every year, millions of people get the flu. The good news is that the seasonal flu vaccine can lower the risk of getting the flu by about half. Getting the yearly flu vaccine is the best way to protect yourself from the flu.

What Is the Flu?

The flu is caused by a virus. Common symptoms of the flu include:

- Fever and chills
- Cough
- Sore throat
- Runny or stuffy nose
- Muscle or body aches
- Headache
- Feeling very tired

Some people with the flu may throw up or have diarrhea (watery poop)—this is more common in children than adults. It is also important to know that not everyone with the flu will have a fever.

The flu is worse than the common cold. It is a common cause of problems like sinus or ear infections. It can also cause serious complications like:

- Pneumonia (lung infection)

- Worsening of long-term health problems, like asthma or heart failure

- Inflammation of the brain or heart

- Sepsis, a life-threatening inflammatory condition

The flu is contagious, meaning it can spread from person to person. The flu can spread when:

- Someone with the flu coughs, sneezes, or talks—and droplets from their mouth or nose get into the mouths or noses of people nearby

- Someone touches a surface that has flu virus on it and then touches their mouth, nose, or eyes

People can spread the flu before they know they are sick—and while they have the flu.

Why Is the Flu Vaccine Important?

Most people who get the flu have a mild illness. But for some, it can be serious—and even deadly. Serious complications from the flu are more likely in babies and young children, pregnant women, older adults, and people with certain long-term health conditions—like diabetes or asthma.

Getting vaccinated every year is the best way to lower your chances of getting the flu. Flu vaccines can't cause the flu. Keep in mind that getting the flu vaccine also protects the people around you. So when you and your family get vaccinated, you help keep yourselves and your community healthy.

This is especially important if you spend time with people who are at risk for serious illness from the flu-like young children or older adults.

Who Needs to Get the Flu Vaccine
Everyone Age 6 Months and Older

Everyone needs to get the flu vaccine every year. It's part of the routine vaccine schedules for children, teens, and adults.

It's important to get the flu vaccine every year. That's important for two reasons: first, immunity (protection) decreases with time.

Additionally, the flu viruses are constantly changing—so the vaccine is often updated to give the best protection.

People at Increased Risk for Complications from the Flu

It's especially important for people who are at high risk of developing complications from the flu to get the vaccine every year. People at high risk for complications from the flu include:

- Pregnant women

- Adults age 65 years and older

- Children younger than 5 years—and especially children younger than 2 years

- People with long-term health conditions like asthma, diabetes, or cancer

Healthcare Professionals and Caregivers

It's also very important for people who spend a lot of time with people at high risk for complications from the flu to get the vaccine—for example, healthcare professionals and caregivers.

Talk with your doctor about how to protect your family from the flu.

Who Should Not Get the Flu Vaccine?

Children younger than 6 months should not get the flu vaccine. Be sure to tell your doctor before getting vaccinated if you:

- Have had a life-threatening allergic reaction to a dose of the flu vaccine or any ingredient in the vaccine (like eggs or gelatin)

- Have had Guillain-Barré Syndrome (an immune system disorder)

If you are sick, you may need to wait until you are feeling better to get the flu vaccine.

What Are the Side Effects of Flu Vaccines?

Side effects are usually mild and go away in a few days. These side effects are not the flu—the flu vaccine cannot cause the flu.

Side effects from the flu vaccine may include:

- Pain, swelling, or redness where the shot was given
- Headache
- Muscle aches
- Fever
- Upset stomach

Serious side effects from the flu vaccine are very rare.

Like any medicine, there's a very small chance that the flu vaccine could cause a serious reaction. Keep in mind that getting the flu vaccine is much safer than getting the flu.

Chapter 5

Managing Common Disease Risk Factors

Chapter Contents

Section 5.1—Preventing High Blood Pressure 72

Section 5.2—Preventing High Cholesterol 75

Section 5.3—Ensuring Adequate Sleep 77

Section 5.4—Managing Stress 81

Section 5.1

Preventing High Blood Pressure

This section includes text excerpted from "How to
Prevent High Blood Pressure," MedlinePlus, National
Institutes of Health (NIH), February 28, 2017.

What Is Blood Pressure?

Blood pressure is the force of your blood pushing against the walls of
your arteries. Each time your heart beats, it pumps blood into the arteries.
Your blood pressure is highest when your heart beats, pumping the blood.
This is called "systolic pressure." When your heart is at rest, between
beats, your blood pressure falls. This is called "diastolic pressure."

Your blood pressure reading uses these two numbers. Usually, the
systolic number comes before or above the diastolic number.

How Do I Know If My Blood Pressure Is High?

High blood pressure usually has no symptoms. So, the only way to
find out if you have high blood pressure is to get regular blood pressure
checks from your healthcare provider. Your provider will use a gauge,
a stethoscope or electronic sensor, and a blood pressure cuff. For most
adults, blood pressure readings will be in one of four categories:

Normal blood pressure means:

- Your systolic pressure is less than 120.

- Your diastolic pressure is less than 80.

Prehypertension means:

- Your systolic pressure is between 120 to 139.

- Your diastolic pressure is between 80 to 89.

Stage 1 high blood pressure means:

- Your systolic pressure is between 140 to 159.

- Your diastolic pressure is between 90 to 99.

Stage 2 high blood pressure means:

- Your systolic pressure is 160 or higher.

- Your diastolic pressure is 100 or higher.

For children and teens, the healthcare provider compares the blood pressure reading to what is normal for other kids who are the same age, height, and sex.

People with diabetes or chronic kidney disease should keep their blood pressure below 130/80.

Why Do I Need to Worry about Prehypertension and High Blood Pressure?

Prehypertension means that you are likely to end up with high blood pressure unless you take steps to prevent it.

When your blood pressure stays high over time, it causes the heart to pump harder and work overtime, possibly leading to serious health problems, such as a heart attack, stroke, heart failure, and kidney failure.

What Are the Different Types of High Blood Pressure?

There are two main types of high blood pressure: primary and secondary high blood pressure.

- **Primary,** or essential, high blood pressure is the most common type of high blood pressure. For most people who get this kind of blood pressure, it develops over time as you get older.

- **Secondary** high blood pressure is caused by another medical condition or use of certain medicines. It usually gets better after you treat the cause or stop taking the medicines that are causing it.

Who Is at Risk for High Blood Pressure?

Anyone can develop high blood pressure, but there are certain factors that can increase your risk:

- **Age.** Blood pressure tends to rise with age.

- **Race/ethnicity.** High blood pressure is more common in African American adults.

- **Weight.** People who are overweight or obese are more likely to develop prehypertension or high blood pressure.

73

- **Sex.** Before the age of 55, men are more likely than women to develop high blood pressure. After the age of 55, women are more likely than men to develop it.

- **Lifestyle.** Certain lifestyle habits can raise your risk for high blood pressure, such as eating too much sodium or not enough potassium, lack of exercise, drinking too much alcohol, and smoking.

- **Family history.** A family history of high blood pressure raises the risk of developing prehypertension or high blood pressure.

How Can I Prevent High Blood Pressure?

You can help prevent high blood pressure by having a healthy lifestyle. This means:

- **Eating a healthy diet.** To help manage your blood pressure, you should limit the amount of sodium that you eat and increase the amount of potassium in your diet. It is also important to eat foods that are lower in fat, as well as plenty of fruits, vegetables, and whole grains. The Dietary Approaches to Stop Hypertension (DASH) diet is an example of an eating plan that can help you to lower your blood pressure.

- **Getting regular exercise.** Exercise can help you maintain a healthy weight and lower your blood pressure. You should try to get moderate-intensity aerobic exercise at least 2 and a half hours per week, or vigorous-intensity aerobic exercise for 1 hour and 15 minutes per week. Aerobic exercise, such as brisk walking, is an exercise in which your heart beats harder and you use more oxygen than usual.

- **Being at a healthy weight.** Being overweight or obese increases your risk for high blood pressure. Maintaining a healthy weight can help you control high blood pressure and reduce your risk for other health problems.

- **Limiting alcohol.** Drinking too much alcohol can raise your blood pressure. It also adds extra calories, which may cause weight gain. Men should have no more than two drinks per day, and women only one.

- **Not smoking.** Cigarette smoking raises your blood pressure and puts you at a higher risk for heart attack and stroke. If you do not smoke, do not start. If you do smoke, talk to your healthcare provider for help in finding the best way for you to quit.

- **Managing stress.** Learning how to relax and manage stress can improve your emotional and physical health and lower high blood pressure. Stress management techniques include exercising, listening to music, focusing on something calm or peaceful, and meditating.

If you already have high blood pressure, it is important to prevent it from getting worse or causing complications. You should get regular medical care and follow your prescribed treatment plan. Your plan will include healthy lifestyle habit recommendations and possibly medicines.

Section 5.2

Preventing High Cholesterol

This section includes text excerpted from "Control Your Cholesterol," *NIH News in Health*, National Institutes of Health (NIH), February 15, 2019.

Have you had your cholesterol checked? Most adults should have a cholesterol test every 4 to 6 years. That is because nearly 78 million American adults have high levels of the type of cholesterol that is linked to heart disease and stroke.

Cholesterol is a waxy, fat-like substance that your body needs to function properly. It travels through your bloodstream to reach the cells that need it. Your cells use cholesterol for many important functions, such as making hormones and digesting fatty foods.

But, too much cholesterol in your blood can cause waxy buildup called "plaques" in blood vessels. "These plaques can eventually become inflamed and rupture, leading to a clot," explains cholesterol expert Dr. Ronald Krauss at the University of California, San Francisco Benioff Children's Hospital in Oakland.

If a clot blocks blood flow through an artery in the heart, it can cause a heart attack. "Or, if this happens in the artery of the brain, it can cause a stroke," he says.

Cholesterol travels through the bloodstream in particles called "lipoproteins." There are different types of lipoproteins that have different effects.

Low-density lipoproteins, or LDLs, contribute to plaques. LDL cholesterol is sometimes called "bad cholesterol."

"Many people in this country have too many of these LDL particles in the blood," Krauss says. Studies have found that lowering LDL cholesterol levels reduces heart disease and stroke.

The most common cause of high LDL cholesterol is an unhealthy lifestyle. Excess body weight and eating a lot of animal fats are linked to high levels of LDL cholesterol. The genes that you inherit from your parents, other medical conditions, and certain medicines can also cause high cholesterol. You may also have heard about "good cholesterol": high-density lipoproteins, or HDL. HDL particles absorb cholesterol and carry it to the liver. The liver then flushes it from the body. That is why scientists previously thought that raising levels of HDL cholesterol might lower your risk for heart disease and stroke.

But, recent research suggests that HDL cholesterol works better in some people than others. And clinical trials have not found that medicines aimed at raising HDL cholesterol reduce the risk of heart attack. There is still a lot to learn about HDL.

Lab tests can measure the different types of cholesterol in your blood. How often you should get tested depends on your age and other risk factors, including a family history of high cholesterol or heart disease.

If tests show that you have a high level of LDL cholesterol, your doctor may order additional tests. You can try to lower it by eating a heart-healthy diet, being physically active, and losing excess weight.

For some people, lifestyle changes are not enough to lower LDL cholesterol. Your biological makeup can be a strong influence on cholesterol buildup, too. In these cases, a type of drug known as a "statin" is the usual treatment. Doctors may combine statins with other drugs.

If your LDL cholesterol is very high, Krauss says that it is important that your family members get tested too. If your genes put you at risk for high cholesterol, your close relatives might have a similar risk.

Talk to your doctor about getting tested. And remember that heart-healthy lifestyle changes can not only lower cholesterol levels but also bring many long-term health benefits.

Section 5.3

Ensuring Adequate Sleep

This section includes text excerpted from "Get
Enough Sleep," Office of Disease Prevention and Health
Promotion (ODPHP), U.S. Department of Health and
Human Services (HHS), July 18, 2018.

The Basics

It is important to get enough sleep. Sleep helps keep your mind
and body healthy.

How Much Sleep Do I Need?

Most adults need seven to eight hours of good quality sleep on a
regular schedule each night. Make changes to your routine if you
cannot find enough time to sleep.

Getting enough sleep is not only about total hours of sleep. It is also
important to get good, quality sleep on a regular schedule so that you
feel rested when you wake up.

If you often have trouble sleeping—or if you often still feel tired
after sleeping—talk with your doctor.

Why Is Getting Enough Sleep Important?

Getting enough sleep has many benefits. It can help you:

- Get sick less often

- Stay at a healthy weight

- Lower your risk for serious health problems, such as diabetes
  and heart disease

- Reduce stress and improve your mood

- Think more clearly and do better in school and at work

- Get along better with people

- Make good decisions and avoid injuries. For example, sleepy
  drivers cause thousands of car accidents every year.

Does It Matter When I Sleep?

Yes. Your body sets your "biological clock" according to the pattern of daylight where you live. This helps you naturally get sleepy at night and stay alert during the day.

If you have to work at night and sleep during the day, you may have trouble getting enough sleep. It can also be hard to sleep when you travel to a different time zone.

Why Can I Not Fall Asleep?

Many things can make it harder for you to sleep, including:

- Stress or anxiety

- Pain

- Certain health conditions, such as heartburn or asthma

- Some medicines

- Caffeine (usually from coffee, tea, and soda)

- Alcohol and other drugs

- Untreated sleep disorders, such as sleep apnea or insomnia

If you are having trouble sleeping, try making changes to your routine to get the sleep you need. You may want to:

- Change what you do during the day. For example, get your physical activity in the morning instead of at night.

- Create a comfortable sleep environment, and make sure that your bedroom is dark and quiet.

- Set a bedtime routine, and go to bed at the same time every night.

How Can I Tell If I Have a Sleep Disorder?

Sleep disorders can cause many different problems. Keep in mind that it is normal to have trouble sleeping every now and then. People with sleep disorders generally experience these problems on a regular basis.

Common signs of sleep disorders include:

- Trouble falling or staying asleep

- Still feeling tired after a good night's sleep
- Sleepiness during the day that makes it difficult to do everyday activities, such as driving a car or concentrating at work
- Frequent loud snoring
- Pauses in breathing or gasping while sleeping
- Itchy feelings in your legs or arms at night that feel better when you move or massage the area
- Trouble moving your arms and legs when you wake up

If you have any of these signs, talk to a doctor or nurse. You may need to be tested or treated for a sleep disorder.

Take Action

Making small changes to your daily routine can help you get the sleep you need.

Change What You Do during the Day

- Try to spend some time outdoors every day.
- Plan your physical activity for earlier in the day, not right before you go to bed.
- Stay away from caffeine (including coffee, tea, and soda) late in the day.
- If you have trouble sleeping at night, limit daytime naps to 20 minutes or less.
- If you drink alcohol, drink only in moderation. This means no more than one drink a day for women and no more than two drinks a day for men. Alcohol can keep you from sleeping well.
- Do not eat a big meal close to bedtime.
- Quit smoking. The nicotine in cigarettes can make it harder for you to sleep.

Create a Good Sleep Environment

- Make sure that your bedroom is dark. If there are streetlights near your window, try putting up light-blocking curtains.

- Keep your bedroom quiet.
- Consider keeping electronic devices—such as televisions, computers, and smartphones—out of the bedroom.

Set a Bedtime Routine

- Go to bed at the same time every night.
- Get the same amount of sleep each night.
- Avoid eating, talking on the phone, or reading in bed.
- Avoid using computers or smartphones, watching television, or playing video games at bedtime.

If you are still awake after staying in bed for more than 20 minutes, get up. Do something relaxing, such as reading or meditating, until you feel sleepy.

If You Are Concerned about Your Sleep, See a Doctor

Talk with a doctor or nurse if you have any of the following signs of a sleep disorder:

- Frequent, loud snoring
- Pauses in breathing during sleep
- Trouble waking up in the morning
- Pain or itchy feelings in your legs or arms at night that feel better when you move or massage the area
- Trouble staying awake during the day

Even if you are not aware of problems like these, talk with a doctor if you feel like you often have trouble sleeping.

Section 5.4

Managing Stress

This section includes text excerpted from "Manage
Stress," Office of Disease Prevention and Health
Promotion (ODPHP), U.S. Department of Health and
Human Services (HHS), September 26, 2018.

The Basics

Not all stress is bad. But chronic (ongoing) stress can lead to health problems.

Preventing and managing chronic stress can lower your risk for serious conditions, such as heart disease, obesity, high blood pressure, and depression.

You can prevent or reduce stress by:

* Planning ahead

* Deciding which tasks need to be done first

* Preparing for stressful events

Some stress is hard to avoid. You can find ways to manage stress by:

* Noticing when you feel stressed

* Taking time to relax

* Getting active and eating healthy

* Talking to friends and family

What Are the Signs of Stress?

When people are under stress, they may feel:

* Worried

* Angry

* Irritable

* Depressed

* Unable to focus

81

Stress also affects your body. Physical signs of stress include:

- Headaches
- Back pain
- Problems sleeping
- Upset stomach
- Weight gain or loss
- Tense muscles
- Frequent or more serious colds

What Causes Stress

Change is often a cause of stress. Even positive changes, such as having a baby or getting a job promotion, can be stressful.
Stress can be short term or long term.
Common causes of short-term stress:

- Needing to do a lot in a short amount of time
- Experiencing many small problems in the same day, like a traffic jam or running late
- Getting lost
- Having an argument

Common causes of long-term stress:

- Problems at work or at home
- Money problems
- Caring for someone with a serious illness
- Chronic illness
- Death of a loved one

What Are the Benefits of Managing Stress?

Over time, chronic stress can lead to health problems. Managing stress can help you:

- Sleep better
- Control your weight
- Get sick less often

- Feel better faster when you do get sick

- Have less neck and back pain

- Be in a better mood

- Get along better with family and friends

Take Action

You cannot always avoid stress, but you can take steps to deal with your stress in a positive way. Follow these nine tips for preventing and managing stress.

Being prepared and feeling in control of your situation might help lower your stress.

1. **Plan your time.**

   Think ahead about how you are going to use your time. Write a to-do list and figure out what is most important, then do that thing first. Be realistic about how long each task will take.

2. **Prepare yourself.**

   Prepare ahead of time for stressful events, such as a job interview or a hard conversation with a loved one.

   - Stay positive.

   - Picture what the room will look like and what you will say.

   - Have a back-up plan.

3. **Relax with deep breathing or meditation.**

   Deep breathing and meditation are two ways to relax your muscles and clear your mind.

4. **Relax your muscles.**

   Stress causes tension in your muscles. Try stretching or taking a hot shower to help you relax.

5. **Get active.**

   Regular physical activity can help prevent and manage stress. It can also help relax your muscles and improve your mood.

   Aim for 2 hours and 30 minutes a week of physical activity. Try going for a bike ride or taking a walk.

- Be sure to exercise for at least 10 minutes at a time.

- Do strengthening activities, such as crunches or lifting weights, at least two days a week.

6. **Eat healthy.**

Give your body plenty of energy by eating healthy, including vegetables, fruits, and lean sources of protein.

7. **Drink alcohol only in moderation.**

Avoid using alcohol or other drugs to manage stress. If you choose to drink, drink only in moderation. This means no more than one drink a day for women and no more than two drinks a day for men.

8. **Talk to friends and family.**

Tell your friends and family if you are feeling stressed. They may be able to help.

9. **Get help if you need it.**

Stress is a normal part of life. But if your stress does not go away or keeps getting worse, you may need help. Over time, stress can lead to serious problems, such as depression or anxiety.

- If you are feeling down or hopeless, talk to a doctor about depression.

- If you are feeling anxious, find out how to get help for anxiety.

- If you have lived through an unsafe event, find out about treatment for posttraumatic stress disorder (PTSD).

A mental-health professional (such as a psychologist or social worker) can help treat these conditions with talk therapy (called "psychotherapy") or medicine.

Lots of people need help dealing with stress—it is nothing to be ashamed of.

Chapter 6

Aim for a Healthy Weight

Chapter Contents

Section 6.1—Assessing Your Weight and Health Risk 86

Section 6.2—Understanding Body Mass Index 88

Section 6.3—Understanding Overweight and Obesity 92

Section 6.4—Tips for Healthy Weight Loss 103

Section 6.5—Guide to Selecting a Weight-Loss
Program 112

Section 6.1

Assessing Your Weight and Health Risk

This section includes text excerpted from "Healthy Weight," Centers
for Disease Control and Prevention (CDC), October 2, 2018.

When it comes to weight loss, there is no lack of fad diets promising fast results. But, such diets limit your nutritional intake, can be unhealthy, and tend to fail in the long run.

The key to achieving and maintaining a healthy weight is not about short-term dietary changes. It is about a lifestyle that includes healthy eating, regular physical activity, and balancing the number of calories you consume with the number of calories your body uses.

Staying in control of your weight contributes to good health now and as you age.

Assessing Your Weight

A high amount of body fat can lead to weight-related diseases and other health issues, and being underweight can also put one at risk for health issues. Body mass index (BMI) and waist circumference are two measures that can be used as screening tools to estimate weight status in relation to potential disease risk. However, BMI and waist circumference are not diagnostic tools for disease risks. A trained healthcare provider should perform other health assessments in order to evaluate disease risk and diagnose disease status.

How to Measure and Interpret Weight Status
Adult Body Mass Index

Body mass index is a person's weight in kilograms divided by the square of height in meters. A high BMI can be an indicator of high body fatness and having a low BMI can be an indicator of having too low body fatness. BMI can be used as a screening tool but is not diagnostic of the body fatness or health of an individual.

- If your BMI is less than 18.5, it falls within the underweight range.

- If your BMI is 18.5 to 24.9, it falls within the normal or healthy weight range.

- If your BMI is 25.0 to 29.9, it falls within the overweight range.

- If your BMI is 30.0 or higher, it falls within the obese range.

Weight that is higher than what is considered as a healthy weight for a given height is described as "overweight" or "obese." Weight that is lower than what is considered as healthy for a given height is described as "underweight."

How to Measure Height and Weight for Body Mass Index

Height and weight must be measured in order to calculate BMI. It is most accurate to measure height in meters and weight in kilograms. However, the BMI formula has been adapted for height measured in inches and weight measured in pounds. These measurements can be taken in a healthcare provider's office or at home using a tape measure and scale.

Waist Circumference

Another way to estimate your potential disease risk is to measure your waist circumference. Excessive abdominal fat may be serious because it places you at a greater risk for developing obesity-related conditions, such as type 2 diabetes, high blood pressure, and coronary artery disease. Your waistline may be telling you that you have a higher risk of developing obesity-related conditions if you are:

- A man whose waist circumference is more than 40 inches

Waist circumference can be used as a screening tool but is not diagnostic of the body fatness or health of an individual. A trained healthcare provider should perform appropriate health assessments in order to evaluate an individual's health status and risks.

Section 6.2

Understanding Body Mass Index

This section includes text excerpted from "What Is BMI?" Centers for Disease Control and Prevention (CDC), August 29, 2017.

What Is Body Mass Index?

Body mass index (BMI) is a person's weight in kilograms divided by the square of height in meters. BMI does not measure body fat directly, but research has shown that BMI is moderately correlated with more direct measures of body fat obtained from skinfold thickness measurements, bioelectrical impedance, densitometry (underwater weighing), dual-energy X-ray absorptiometry (DXA), and other methods. Furthermore, BMI appears to be as strongly correlated with various metabolic and disease outcome as are these more direct measures of body fatness. In general, BMI is an inexpensive and easy-to-perform method of screening for a weight category, such as being underweight, of normal or healthy weight, overweight, and obese.

How Is Body Mass Index Used?

A high BMI can be an indicator of high body fatness. BMI can be used as a screening tool but is not diagnostic of the body fatness or health of an individual.

To determine if a high BMI is a health risk, a healthcare provider would need to perform further assessments. These assessments might include skinfold thickness measurements, evaluations of diet, physical activity, family history, and other appropriate health screenings.

What Are the Body Mass Index Trends for Adults in the United States?

The prevalence of an adult BMI greater than or equal to 30 kg/m2 (obese status) has greatly increased since the 1970s. Recently, however, this trend has leveled off, except for older women. Obesity has continued to increase in adult women who are 60 years of age and older.

Why Is Body Mass Index Used to Measure Overweight and Obesity?

Body Mass Index can be used for population assessment of individuals that are overweight and obese. Because the BMI calculation requires only height and weight, it is inexpensive and easy to use for clinicians and for the general public. BMI can be used as a screening tool for body fatness but is not diagnostic.

What Are Some of the Other Ways to Assess Excess Body Fatness Besides Body Mass Index?

Other methods to measure body fatness include skinfold thickness measurements (with calipers), underwater weighing, bioelectrical impedance, dual-energy X-ray absorptiometry (DXA), and isotope dilution. However, these methods are not always readily available, and they are either expensive or need to be conducted by highly trained personnel. Furthermore, many of these methods can be difficult to standardize across observers or machines, complicating comparisons across studies and time periods.

How Is Body Mass Index Calculated?

Body mass index is calculated the same way for both adults and children. The calculation is based on the following formulas:

Table 6.1. BMI Calculation

Measurement Units	Formula and Calculation
Kilograms and meters (or centimeters)	Formula: weight (kg) / [height (m)]^2 With the metric system, the formula for BMI is weight in kilograms divided by height in meters squared. Because height is commonly measured in centimeters, divide height in centimeters by 100 to obtain height in meters. Example: Weight = 68 kg, Height = 165 cm (1.65 m) Calculation: $68 \div (1.65)^2 = 24.98$
Pounds and inches	Formula: weight (lb) / [height (in)]^2 x 703 Calculate BMI by dividing weight in pounds (lbs) by height in inches (in) squared and multiplying by a conversion factor of 703. Example: Weight = 150 lbs, Height = 5'5" (65") Calculation: $[150 \div (65)^2]$ x 703 = 24.96

How Is Body Mass Index Interpreted for Adults?

For adults 20 years of age and older, BMI is interpreted using standard weight status categories. These categories are the same for men and women of all body types and ages.

The standard weight status categories associated with BMI ranges for adults are shown in the following table.

Table 6.2. BMI Interpretation

BMI	Weight Status
Below 18.5	Underweight
18.5 – 24.9	Normal or Healthy Weight
25.0 – 29.9	Overweight
30.0 and Above	Obese

For example, here are the weight ranges, the corresponding BMI ranges, and the weight status categories for a person who is 5′ 9″.

Table 6.3. Weight and the Corresponding BMI Range

Height	Weight Range	BMI	Weight Status
	124 lbs or less	Below 18.5	Underweight
	125 lbs to 168 lbs	18.5 to 24.9	Normal or Healthy Weight
	169 lbs to 202 lbs	25.0 to 29.9	Overweight
5′ 9″	203 lbs or more	30 or higher	Obese

Is Body Mass Index Interpreted the Same Way for Children and Teens as It Is for Adults?

Body mass index is interpreted differently for children and teens, even though it is calculated using the same formula as adult BMI. Children and teen's BMI need to be age and sex-specific because the amount of body fat changes with age, and the amount of body fat differs between girls and boys. The Centers for Disease Control and Prevention (CDC) BMI-for-age growth charts take into account these differences and visually show BMI as a percentile ranking. These percentiles were determined using representative data of the U.S. population of youth between 2 and 19 years of age that was collected in various surveys from 1963–65 to 1988–94.

Obesity among youth between the ages of 2 and 19 years of age is defined as a BMI at or above the 95th percentile of children of the same age and sex in this 1963 to 1994 reference population. For example, a 10-year-old boy of average height (56 inches) who weighs 102 pounds would have a BMI of 22.9 kg/m². This would place the boy in the 95th percentile for BMI—meaning that his BMI is greater than that of 95 percent of similarly aged boys in this reference population—and he would be considered to be obese.

How Good Is Body Mass Index as an Indicator of Body Fatness?

The correlation between the BMI and body fatness is fairly strong, but even if two people have the same BMI, their level of body fatness may differ.

In general:

- At the same BMI, women tend to have more body fat than men.

- At the same BMI, Blacks have less body fat than Whites, and Asians have more body fat than Whites.

- At the same BMI, older people, on average, tend to have more body fat than younger adults.

- At the same BMI, athletes have less body fat than do nonathletes.

- The accuracy of BMI as an indicator of body fatness also appears to be higher in persons with higher levels of BMI and body fatness. While a person with a very high BMI (e.g., 35 kg/m²) is very likely to have high body fat, a relatively high BMI can be the results of either high body fat or high lean body mass (muscle and bone). A trained healthcare provider should perform appropriate health assessments in order to evaluate an individual's health status and risks.

If an Athlete or Other Person with a Lot of Muscle Has a Body Mass Index Over 25, Is That Person Still Considered to Be Overweight?

According to the BMI weight status categories, anyone with a BMI between 25 and 29.9 would be classified as overweight, and anyone with a BMI over 30 would be classified as obese.

However, athletes may have a high BMI because of increased muscularity rather than increased body fatness. In general, a person who has a high BMI is likely to have body fatness and would be considered to be overweight or obese, but this may not apply to athletes. A trained healthcare provider should perform appropriate health assessments in order to evaluate an individual's health status and risks.

Section 6.3

Understanding Overweight and Obesity

This section includes text excerpted from "Overweight and Obesity," National Heart, Lung, and Blood Institute (NHLBI), February 23, 2017.

Overweight and obesity are increasingly common conditions in the United States. They are caused by the increase in the size and the amount of fat cells in the body. Doctors measure body mass index (BMI) and waist circumference to screen and diagnose overweight and obesity. Obesity is a serious medical condition that can cause complications, such as metabolic syndrome, high blood pressure, atherosclerosis, heart disease, diabetes, high blood cholesterol, cancers, and sleep disorders. Treatment depends on the cause and severity of your condition and whether you have complications. Treatments include lifestyle changes, such as heart-healthy eating and increased physical activity, and the U.S. Food and Drug Administration (FDA)-approved weight-loss medicines. For some people, surgery may be a treatment option.

*What Are the Health Consequences of Obesity for Adults?**

People who are obese are at an increased risk for many diseases and health conditions, including the following:

- All causes of death (mortality)
- High blood pressure (hypertension)
- High low-density lipoprotein (LDL) cholesterol, low high-density lipoprotein (HDL) cholesterol, or high levels of triglycerides (dyslipidemia)

- Type 2 diabetes

- Coronary heart disease

- Stroke

- Gallbladder disease

- Osteoarthritis (a breakdown of cartilage and bone within a joint)

- Sleep apnea and breathing problems

- Chronic inflammation and increased oxidative stress

- Some cancers (endometrial, breast, colon, kidney, gallbladder, and liver)

- Low quality of life

- Mental illness, such as clinical depression, anxiety, and other mental disorders

- Body pain and difficulty with physical functioning

* Excerpted from "What Is BMI?" Centers for Disease Control and Prevention (CDC), August 29, 2017.

Causes of Overweight and Obesity

Energy imbalances, some genetic or endocrine medical conditions, and certain medicines are known to cause overweight or obesity.

Energy Imbalances Cause the Body to Store Fat

Energy imbalances can cause overweight and obesity. An energy imbalance means that your energy intake does not equal your energy outtake. This energy is measured in calories. Energy in is the amount of calories you get from food and drinks. Energy out is the amount of calories that your body uses for things, such as breathing, digesting, being physically active, and regulating body temperature.

Overweight and obesity develop over time when you take in more calories than you use, or when energy in is more than your energy out. This type of energy imbalance causes your body to store fat.

Your body uses certain nutrients, such as carbohydrates or sugars, proteins, and fats, from the foods you eat to:

- Make energy for immediate use to power routine daily body functions and physical activity.

- Store energy for future use by your body. Sugars are stored as glycogen in the liver and muscles. Fats are stored mainly as triglyceride in fat tissue.

The amount of energy that your body gets from the food you eat depends on the type of foods you eat, how the food is prepared, and how long it has been since you last ate.

The body has three types of fat tissue—white, brown, and beige—that it uses to fuel itself, regulate its temperature in response to cold, and store energy for future use.

- White fat tissue can be found around the kidneys and under the skin in the buttocks, thighs, and abdomen. This fat type stores energy, makes hormones, that control the way the body regulates urges to eat or stop eating, and makes inflammatory substances that can lead to complications.

- Brown fat tissue is located in the upper back area of human infants. This fat type releases stored energy as heat energy when a baby is cold. It also can make inflammatory substances. Brown fat can be seen in children and adults.

- Beige fat tissue is seen in the neck, shoulders, back, chest and abdomen of adults and resembles brown fat tissue. This fat type, which uses carbohydrates and fats to produce heat, increases when children and adults are exposed to cold.

Medical Conditions

Some genetic syndromes and endocrine disorders can cause overweight or obesity.

Genetic Syndromes

Several genetic syndromes are associated with overweight and obesity, including the following.

- Prader-Willi syndrome

- Bardet-Biedl syndrome

- Alström syndrome

- Cohen syndrome

The study of these genetic syndromes has helped researchers understand obesity.

Endocrine Disorders

Because the endocrine system produces hormones that help maintain energy balances in the body, the following endocrine disorders or tumor affecting the endocrine system can cause overweight and obesity.

- **Hypothyroidism.** People with this condition have low levels of thyroid hormones. These low levels are associated with decreased metabolism and weight gain, even when food intake is reduced. People with hypothyroidism also produce less body heat, have a lower body temperature, and do not efficiently use stored fat for energy.

- **Cushing syndrome.** People with this condition have high levels of glucocorticoids, such as cortisol, in the blood. High cortisol levels make the body feel like it is under chronic stress. As a result, people have an increase in appetite and the body will store more fat. Cushing syndrome may develop after taking certain medicines or because the body naturally makes too much cortisol.

- **Tumors.** Some tumors, such as craniopharyngioma, can cause severe obesity because the tumors develop near parts of the brain that control hunger.

Medicines for Overweight and Obesity

Medicines, such as antipsychotics, antidepressants, antiepileptics, and antihyperglycemics, can cause weight gain and lead to overweight and obesity.

Talk to your doctor if you notice weight gain while you are using one of these medicines. Ask if there are other forms of the same medicine or other medicines that can treat your medical condition but have less of an effect on your weight. Do not stop taking the medicine without talking to your doctor.

Several parts of your body, such as your stomach, intestines, pancreas, and fat tissue, use hormones to control how your brain decides if you are hungry or full. Some of these hormones are insulin, leptin, glucagon-like peptide (GLP-1), peptide YY, and ghrelin.

Risk Factors for Overweight and Obesity

There are many risk factors for overweight and obesity. Some risk factors can be changed, such as unhealthy lifestyle habits and environments. Other risk factors, such as age, family history and genetics, race and ethnicity, and sex, cannot be changed. Healthy lifestyle changes can decrease your risk for developing overweight and obesity.

Unhealthy Lifestyle Habits

Lack of physical activity, unhealthy eating patterns, not enough sleep, and high amounts of stress can increase your risk for overweight and obesity.

Lack of Physical Activity

Lack of physical activity due to high amounts of TV, computer, videogame or other screen usage has been associated with a high BMI. Healthy lifestyle changes, such as being physically active and reducing screen time, can help you aim for a healthy weight.

Unhealthy Eating Behaviors

Some unhealthy eating behaviors can increase your risk for overweight and obesity.

- Eating more calories than you use. The amount of calories you need will vary based on your sex, age, and physical activity level. Find out your daily calorie needs or goals with the Body Weight Planner.

- Eating too much saturated and *trans* fats

- Eating foods high in added sugars

Not Enough Sleep

Many studies have seen a high BMI in people who do not get enough sleep. Some studies have seen a relationship between sleep and the way our bodies use nutrients for energy and how lack of sleep can affect hormones that control hunger urges.

High Amounts of Stress

Acute stress and chronic stress affect the brain and trigger the production of hormones, such as cortisol, that control our energy balances and hunger urges. Acute stress can trigger hormone changes that make you not want to eat. If the stress becomes chronic, hormone changes can make you eat more and store more fat.

Age

Childhood obesity remains a serious problem in the United States, and some populations are more at risk for childhood obesity than others. The risk of unhealthy weight gain increases as you age. Adults who have a healthy BMI often start to gain weight in young adulthood and continue to gain weight until 60 to 65 years of age, when they tend to start losing weight.

Unhealthy Environments

Many environmental factors can increase your risk for overweight and obesity:

- Social factors, such as having a low socioeconomic status or an unhealthy social or unsafe environment in the neighborhood

- Built environment factors, such as easy access to unhealthy fast foods, limited access to recreational facilities or parks, and few safe or easy ways to walk in your neighborhood

- Exposure to chemicals known as "obesogens" that can change hormones and increase fatty tissue in our bodies

Family History and Genetics

Genetic studies have found that overweight and obesity can run in families, so it is possible that our genes or deoxyribonucleic acid (DNA) can cause these conditions. Research studies have found that certain DNA elements are associated with obesity.

Did you know obesity can change your DNA and the DNA you pass on to your children?

Eating too much or eating too little during a pregnancy can change a baby's DNA and can affect how a child stores and uses fat later in life. Also, studies have shown that obese fathers have DNA changes in their sperm that can be passed on to their children.

Race or Ethnicity

Overweight and obesity is highly prevalent in some racial and ethnic minority groups. Rates of obesity in American adults are highest in Blacks, followed by Hispanics, then Whites. This is true for men or women. While Asian men and women have the lowest rates of unhealthy BMIs, they may have high amounts of unhealthy fat in the abdomen. Samoans may be at risk for overweight and obesity because they may carry a DNA variant that is associated with increased BMI but not with common obesity-related complications.

Sex

In the United States, obesity is more common in Black or Hispanic women than in Black or Hispanic men. A person's sex may also affect the way the body stores fat. For example, women tend to store less unhealthy fat in the abdomen than men do.

Overweight and obesity is also common in women with polycystic ovary syndrome (PCOS). This is an endocrine condition that causes large ovaries and prevents proper ovulation, which can reduce fertility.

Screening and Prevention of Overweight and Obesity

Children and adults should be screened at least annually to see if they have a high or increasing body mass index (BMI), which allows doctors to recommend healthy lifestyle changes to prevent overweight and obesity.

Screening for a High or Increasing Body Mass Index

To screen for overweight and obesity, doctors measure BMI using calculations that depend on whether you are a child or an adult. After reading the information below, talk to your doctor or your child's doctor to determine if you or your child has a high or increasing BMI.

- **Children:** A healthy weight is usually when your child's BMI is at the 5th percentile up to the 85th percentile, based on growth charts for children who are the same age and sex.

- **Adults:** A healthy weight for adults is usually when your BMI is 18.5 to less than 25. To figure out your BMI, use the National Heart, Lung, and Blood Institute's online BMI calculator and compare it with the table below. You can also download the BMI calculator app for iPhone and Android.

Weight Category	Body Mass Index	
	Children	Adults
Underweight	Below 5th percentile*	Below 18.5
Healthy weight	5th percentile to less than 85th percentile	18.5 to 24.9
Overweight	85th percentile to less than 95th percentile	25 to 29.9
Obese	95th percentile or above	30 or above

Figure 6.1. *Body Mass Index Calculator*

*Body mass index (BMI) is used to determine if you or your child are underweight, healthy, or overweight or obese. Children are underweight if their BMI is below the 5th percentile, healthy weight if their BMI is between the 5th to less than the 85th percentile, overweight if their BMI is the 85th percentile to less than the 95th percentile, and obese if their BMI is the 95th percentile or above. Adults are underweight if their BMI is below 18.5, healthy weight if their BMI is 18.5 to 24.9, overweight if their BMI is 25 to 29.9, and obese if their BMI is 30 or above. *A child's BMI percentile is calculated by comparing your child's BMI to growth charts for children who are the same age and sex as your child.*

Healthy Lifestyle Changes to Prevent Overweight and Obesity

If your BMI indicates that you are getting close to being overweight, or if you have certain risk factors, your doctor may recommend you adopt healthy lifestyle changes to prevent you from becoming overweight and obese. Changes include healthy eating, being physically active, aiming for a healthy weight, and getting healthy amounts of sleep.

Signs and Symptoms of Overweight and Obesity

There are no specific symptoms of overweight and obesity. The signs of overweight and obesity include a high body mass index and an unhealthy body fat distribution that can be estimated by measuring your waist circumference.

Diagnosis of Overweight and Obesity

Your doctor may diagnose overweight and obesity based on your medical history, physical exams that confirm you have a high body mass index and possibly a high waist circumference, and tests to rule out other medical conditions.

Confirming a High Body Mass Index

To diagnose overweight and obesity, doctors measure your BMI using calculations that depend on whether you are a child or an adult.

- **Children:** A healthy weight is usually when your child's BMI is at the 5th percentile up to less than the 85th percentile based on growth charts for children who are the same age and sex.

- **Adults:** A healthy weight for adults is usually when your BMI is 18.5 to less than 25. You can also download the BMI calculator app for iPhone and Android. Even if your BMI is in the healthy range, it is possible to be diagnosed as obese if you have a large waist circumference that suggests increased amounts of fat in your abdomen that can lead to complications.

Medical History

Your doctor will ask about your eating and physical activity habits, family history, and will see if you have other risk factors Your doctor may ask if you have any other signs or symptoms. This information can help determine if you have other conditions that may be causing you to be overweight or obese or if you have complications from being overweight or obese.

Physical Exam

During your physical exam, your doctor will measure your weight and height to calculate your BMI. Your doctor may also measure your waist circumference to estimate the amount of unhealthy fat in your abdomen. In adults, a waist circumference over 35 inches for women who are not pregnant or 40 inches for men can help diagnose obesity and assess risk of future complications. If you are of South Asian or Central and South American descent, your doctor may use smaller waist circumference values to diagnose your obesity. People from these backgrounds often do not show signs of a large waist circumference even though they may have unhealthy amounts of fat deep in their abdomens and may be diagnosed with obesity.

Tests to Identify Other Medical Conditions

Your doctor may order some of the following tests to identify medical conditions that may be causing your overweight and obesity.

- **Blood tests.** Blood tests that check your thyroid hormone levels can help rule out hypothyroidism as a cause of your overweight or obesity. Cortisol and adrenocorticotropic hormone (ACTH) tests can rule out Cushing syndrome. Total testosterone and dehydroepiandrosterone sulfate (DHEAS) tests can help rule out polycystic ovary syndrome (PCOS).

Living with Overweight and Obesity

If you have been diagnosed with overweight and obesity, it is important that you continue your treatment. Read about tips to help you aim for a healthy weight; the benefit of finding and continuing a behavioral weight-loss program; and ways your doctor may monitor if your condition is stable, worsening, or improving and assess your risk for complications.

Tips to Aim for a Healthy Weight

Changing lifestyle habits takes time and patience. Follow these tips to help you maintain the healthy lifestyle changes your doctor recommended to aim for a healthy weight.

- **Set specific goals.** An example of a specific goal is to "walk 30 minutes, 5 days a week." Be realistic about your time and abilities.

- **Set doable goals that do not change too much at once.** Consecutive goals that can move you ahead in small steps, are the best way to reach a distant point. When starting a new lifestyle, try to avoid changing too much at once. Slow changes lead to success. Remember, quick weight loss methods do not provide lasting results.

- **Learn from your slips.** Everyone slips, especially when learning something new. Do not worry if work, the weather, or your family causes you to have an occasional slip. Remember that changing your lifestyle is a long-term process.

- **Celebrate your success.** Reward yourself along the way as you meet your goals. Instead of eating out to celebrate your success, try a night at the movies, go shopping for workout clothes, visit the library or bookstore, or go on a hike.

- **Identify temptations.** Learn what environments or social activities, such as watching TV or going out with friends, may be keeping you from meeting your goals. Once you have identified them, use creative strategies to help keep you on track.

- **Plan regular physical activity with a friend.** Find a fun activity that you both enjoy, such as Zumba, jogging, biking or swimming. You are more likely to stick with that activity if you and a friend have committed to it.

Find and Continue a Behavioral Weight-Loss Program

Some people find it is easier to aim and maintain a healthy weight when they have support from a weight-loss specialist or other individuals who also are trying to lose weight. Behavioral weight-loss programs can provide this support, and they can help you set goals that are specific to your needs. Your weight-loss specialist usually reviews or modifies your goals every six months based on your progress and overall health.

When you are choosing a behavioral weight-loss program, you may want to consider whether the program should:

- Offer the service of multiple professionals, such as registered dietitians, doctors, nurses, psychologists, and exercise physiologists

- Provide goals that have been customized for you that consider things, such as the types of food you like, your schedule, your physical fitness, and your overall health

- Provide individual or group counseling to help you change your eating patterns and personal unhealthy habits

- Teach long-term strategies to deal with problems that can lead to future weight gain, such as stress or slipping back into unhealthy habits

When selecting a program, you may want to ask about:

- The percentage of people who complete the program

- The average weight loss for people who finish the program

- Possible side effects

- Fees or costs for additional items, such as dietary supplements

Monitoring Your Condition and Its Health Risks

You should visit your healthcare provider periodically to monitor for possible complications, which if left untreated can be life-threatening. Your doctor may do any of the following to monitor your condition.

- Assess your weight loss since your last visit. A weight loss of approximately five percent in an overweight patient may improve the function of the fat tissue and help lower bad cholesterol and other substances that can predispose to complications.

- Measure your waist circumference if you are an adult. If your waist circumference is greater than 35 inches for women or greater than 40 inches for men, you may be at risk for heart disease, stroke, or type 2 diabetes. South Asians and South and Central Americans have a higher risk of complications, so waist circumference should be smaller than 35 for man and 31 for women. To correctly measure your waist, stand and place a tape measure around your middle, just above your hip bones. Measure your waist just after you breathe out.

- Order blood tests to screen for complications. A lipid panel test can check if you have high cholesterol or triglyceride levels in your blood. A liver function test can determine if your liver is working properly. A fasting glucose test can find out if you have prediabetes or diabetes.

Section 6.4

Tips for Healthy Weight Loss

This section includes text excerpted from "Losing Weight," Centers for Disease Control and Prevention (CDC), February 13, 2018.

What Is Healthy Weight Loss?

It is natural for anyone trying to lose weight to want to lose it very quickly. But, evidence shows that people who lose weight gradually and steadily (about one to two pounds per week) are more successful at keeping weight off. Healthy weight loss is not just about a diet or program. It is about an ongoing lifestyle that includes long-term changes in daily eating and exercise habits.

Once you have achieved a healthy weight, by relying on healthful eating and physical activity most days of the week (about 60 to 90 minutes, moderate intensity), you are more likely to be successful at keeping the weight off over the long term.

Losing weight is not easy, and it takes commitment. But if you are ready to get started, we have got a step-by-step guide to help get you on the road to weight loss and better health.

Even Modest Weight Loss Can Mean Big Benefits

The good news is that no matter what your weight loss goal is, even a modest weight loss, such as 5 to 10 percent of your total body weight, is likely to produce health benefits, such as improvements in blood pressure, blood cholesterol, and blood sugars.

For example, if you weigh 200 pounds, a 5 percent weight loss equals 10 pounds, bringing your weight down to 190 pounds. While this weight may still be in the "overweight" or "obese" range, this modest weight loss can decrease your risk factors for chronic diseases related to obesity.

So even if the overall goal seems large, see it as a journey rather than just a final destination. You will learn new eating and physical activity habits that will help you live a healthier lifestyle. These habits may help you maintain your weight loss over time.

In addition to improving your health, maintaining a weight loss is likely to improve your life in other ways. For example, a study of participants in the National Weight Control Registry (NWCR) found that those who had maintained a significant weight loss reported improvements in not only their physical health, but also their energy levels, physical mobility, general mood, and self-confidence.

Losing Weight: Getting Started

Losing weight takes more than desire. It takes commitment and a well-thought-out plan. Here is a step-by-step guide to getting started.

Step 1: Make a Commitment

Making the decision to lose weight, change your lifestyle, and become healthier is a big step to take. Start simply by making a commitment to yourself. Many people find it helpful to sign a written contract committing to the process. This contract may include things like the amount of weight you want to lose, the date you would like to lose the weight by, the dietary changes you will make to establish healthy eating habits, and a plan for getting regular physical activity.

Writing down the reasons why you want to lose weight can also help. It might be because you have a family history of heart disease, or because you want to see your kids get married, or simply because you want to feel better in your clothes. Post these reasons where they serve as a daily reminder of why you want to make this change.

Step 2: Take Stock of Where You Are

Consider talking to your healthcare provider. She or he can evaluate your height, weight, and explore other weight-related risk factors you may have. Ask for a follow-up appointment to monitor changes in your weight or any related health conditions.

Keep a food diary for a few days, in which you write down everything you eat. By doing this, you become more aware of what you are eating and when you are eating. This awareness can help you avoid mindless eating.

Next, examine your current lifestyle. Identify things that might pose challenges to your weight loss efforts. For example, does your work or travel schedule make it difficult to get enough physical activity? Do you find yourself eating sugary foods because that is what you buy for your kids? Do your coworkers frequently bring high-calorie items, such as doughnuts, to the workplace to share with everyone? Think through things you can do to help overcome these challenges.

Finally, think about aspects of your lifestyle that can help you lose weight. For example, is there an area near your workplace where you and some coworkers can take a walk at lunchtime? Is there a place in your community, such as a YMCA, with exercise facilities for you and child care for your kids?

Step 3: Set Realistic Goals

Set some short-term goals and reward your efforts along the way. If your long-term goal is to lose 40 pounds and to control your high blood pressure, some short-term eating and physical activity goals might be to start eating breakfast, taking a 15-minute walk in the evenings, or having a salad or vegetable with supper.

Focus on two or three goals at a time. Great, effective goals are:

- Specific

- Realistic

- Forgiving (less than perfect)

For example, "Exercise More" is not a specific goal. But if you say, "I will walk 15 minutes, 3 days a week for the first week," you are setting a specific and realistic goal for the first week.

Remember, small changes every day can lead to big results in the long run. Also, remember that realistic goals are achievable goals. By achieving your short-term goals day-by-day, you will feel good about your progress and be motivated to continue. Setting unrealistic goals, such as losing 20 pounds in 2 weeks, can leave you feeling defeated and frustrated.

Being realistic also means expecting occasional setbacks. Setbacks happen when you get away from your plan for whatever reason—maybe the holidays, longer work hours, or another life change. When setbacks happen, get back on track as quickly as possible. Also take some time to think about what you would do differently if a similar situation happens, to prevent setbacks.

Keep in mind everyone is different—what works for someone else might not be right for you. Just because your neighbor lost weight by taking up running does not mean running is the best option for you. Try a variety of activities—walking, swimming, tennis, or group exercise classes—to see what you enjoy most and can fit into your life. These activities will be easier to stick with over the long term.

Step 4: Identify Resources for Information and Support

Find family members or friends who will support your weight-loss efforts. Making lifestyle changes can feel easier when you have others you can talk to and rely on for support. You might have coworkers or neighbors with similar goals, and together you can share healthful recipes and plan group exercise.

Joining a weight loss group or visiting a healthcare professional, such as a registered dietitian, can help.

Step 5: Continually Check in with Yourself to Monitor Your Progress

Revisit the goals you set for yourself and evaluate your progress regularly. If you set a goal to walk each morning but are having trouble

106

fitting it in before work, see if you can shift your work hours or if you can get your walk in at lunchtime or after work. Evaluate which parts of your plan are working well and which ones need tweaking. Then rewrite your goals and plan accordingly.

If you are consistently achieving a particular goal, add a new goal to help you continue on your pathway to success.

Reward yourself for your successes. Recognize when you are meeting your goals, and be proud of your progress. Use nonfood rewards, such as a bouquet of freshly picked flowers, a sports outing with friends, or a relaxing bath. Rewards help keep you motivated on the path to better health.

Improving Your Eating Habits

When it comes to eating, we have strong habits. Some are good ("I always eat breakfast"), and some are not so good ("I always clean my plate"). Although many of our eating habits were established during childhood, it does not mean it is too late to change them.

Making sudden, radical changes to eating habits, such as eating nothing but cabbage soup, can lead to short-term weight loss. However, such radical changes are neither healthy nor a good idea, and they will not be successful in the long run. Permanently improving your eating habits requires a thoughtful approach in which you reflect, replace, and reinforce.

- Reflect on all of your specific eating habits, both bad and good, and your common triggers for unhealthy eating.

- Replace your unhealthy eating habits with healthier ones.

- Reinforce your new, healthier eating habits.

Reflect

1. Create a list of your eating habits. Keeping a food diary for a few days, in which you write down everything you eat and the time of day you ate it, will help you uncover your habits. For example, you might discover that you always seek a sweet snack to get you through the mid-afternoon energy slump. It is good to note how you were feeling when you decided to eat, especially if you were eating when you were not hungry. Were you tired? Stressed out?

107

2. Highlight the habits on your list that may be leading you to overeat. Common eating habits that can lead to weight gain are:

    -   Eating too fast

    -   Always cleaning your plate

    -   Eating when not hungry

    -   Eating while standing up (may lead to eating mindlessly or too quickly)

    -   Always eating dessert

    -   Skipping meals (or maybe just breakfast)

3. Look at the unhealthy eating habits you have highlighted. Be sure you have identified all the triggers that cause you to engage in those habits. Identify a few you would like to work on improving first. Do not forget to pat yourself on the back for the things you are doing right. Maybe you almost always eat fruit for dessert, or you drink low-fat or fat-free milk. These are good habits! Recognizing your successes will help encourage you to make more changes.

4. Create a list of "cues" by reviewing your food diary to become more aware of when and where you are "triggered" to eat for reasons other than hunger. Note how you are typically feeling at those times. Often an environmental "cue," or a particular emotional state, is what encourages eating for nonhunger reasons.

    Common triggers for eating when not hungry are:

    -   Opening up the cabinet and seeing your favorite snack food

    -   Sitting at home watching television

    -   Before or after a stressful meeting or situation at work

    -   Coming home after work and having no idea what is for dinner

    -   Having someone offer you a dish they made "just for you"

    -   Walking past a candy dish on the counter

    -   Sitting in the break room beside the vending machine

    -   Seeing a plate of doughnuts at the morning staff meeting

- Swinging through your favorite drive-through every morning

- Feeling bored or tired and thinking food might offer a pick-me-up

5. Circle the "cues" on your list that you face on a daily or weekly basis. Going home for the Thanksgiving holiday may be a trigger for you to overeat, and eventually, you want to have a plan for as many eating cues as you can. But for now, focus on the ones you face more often.

6. Ask yourself these questions for each "cue" you have circled:

- Is there anything I can do to avoid the cue or situation? This option works best for cues that do not involve others. For example, could you choose a different route to work to avoid stopping at a fast food restaurant on the way? Is there another place in the break room where you can sit so you are not next to the vending machine?

- For things I cannot avoid, can I do something differently that would be healthier? Obviously, you cannot avoid all situations that trigger your unhealthy eating habits, such as staff meetings at work. In these situations, evaluate your options. Could you suggest or bring healthier snacks or beverages? Could you offer to take notes to distract your attention? Could you sit farther away from the food so it will not be as easy to grab something? Could you plan ahead and eat a healthy snack before the meeting?

Replace

1. Replace unhealthy habits with new, healthy ones. For example, in reflecting upon your eating habits, you may realize that you eat too fast when you eat alone. So, make a commitment to share a lunch each week with a colleague, or have a neighbor over for dinner one night a week. Other strategies might include putting your fork down between bites or minimizing other distractions (i.e., watching the news during dinner) that might keep you from paying attention to how quickly—and how much—you are eating.

2. Eat more slowly. If you eat too quickly, you may "clean your plate" instead of paying attention to whether your hunger is satisfied.

3. Eat only when you are truly hungry instead of when you are tired, anxious, or feeling an emotion besides hunger. If you find yourself eating when you are experiencing an emotion besides hunger, such as boredom or anxiety, try to find a noneating activity to do instead. You may find that a quick walk or phone call with a friend helps you feel better.

4. Plan meals ahead of time to ensure that you eat a healthy well-balanced meal.

Reinforce

Reinforce your new healthy habits, and be patient with yourself. Habits take time to develop. It does not happen overnight. When you do find yourself engaging in an unhealthy habit, stop as quickly as possible and ask yourself: Why do I do this? When did I start doing this? What changes do I need to make? Be careful not to berate yourself or think that one mistake ruins a whole day's worth of healthy habits. You can do it! It just takes one day at a time.

Keeping It Off

If you have recently lost excess weight, congratulations! It is an accomplishment that will likely benefit your health now and in the future. Now that you have lost weight, let us talk about some ways to maintain that success.

The following tips are some of the common characteristics among people who have successfully lost weight and maintained that loss over time.

Watch Your Diet

• Follow a healthy and realistic eating pattern. You have embarked on a healthier lifestyle, now the challenge is maintaining the positive eating habits you have developed along the way. In studies of people who have lost weight and kept it off for at least a year, most continued to eat a diet lower in calories as compared to their preweight loss diet.

• Keep your eating patterns consistent. Follow a healthy eating pattern regardless of changes in your routine. Plan ahead for weekends, vacations, and special occasions. By making a plan, it is more likely you will have healthy foods on hand for when your routine changes.

- Eat breakfast every day. Eating breakfast is a common trait among people who have lost weight and kept it off. Eating a healthful breakfast may help you avoid getting "over-hungry" and then overeating later in the day.

Be Active

Get daily physical activity. People who have lost weight and kept it off typically engage in 60 to 90 minutes of moderate intensity physical activity most days of the week while not exceeding calorie needs. This does not necessarily mean 60 to 90 minutes at one time. It might mean 20 to 30 minutes of physical activity 3 times a day. For example, a brisk walk in the morning, at lunchtime, and in the evening. Some people may need to talk to their healthcare provider before participating in this level of physical activity.

Stay on Course

- Monitor your diet and activity. Keeping a food and physical activity journal can help you track your progress and spot trends. For example, you might notice that your weight creeps up during periods when you have a lot of business travel or when you have to work overtime. Recognizing this tendency can be a signal to try different behaviors, such as packing your own healthful food for the plane and making time to use your hotel's exercise facility when you are traveling. Or if working overtime, maybe you can use your breaks for quick walks around the building.

- Monitor your weight. Check your weight regularly. When managing your weight loss, it is a good idea to keep track of your weight so you can plan accordingly and adjust your diet and exercise plan as necessary. If you have gained a few pounds, get back on track quickly.

Get support from family, friends, and others. People who have successfully lost weight and kept it off often rely on support from others to help them stay on course and get over any "bumps." Sometimes, having a friend or partner who is also losing weight or maintaining a weight loss can help you stay motivated.

Section 6.5

Guide to Selecting a Weight-Loss Program

This section includes text excerpted from "Choosing a Safe and Successful Weight-Loss Program," National Institute of Diabetes and Digestive and Kidney Diseases (NIDDK), July 2017.

Do you think you need to lose weight? Have you been thinking about trying a weight-loss program?

You are not alone. More than 70 percent of U.S. adults are overweight or have obesity—and many of them try to lose the extra pounds through different kinds of weight-loss programs. A number of these programs are advertised in magazines and newspapers, as well as on the radio, TV, and Internet. But are they safe? And will they work for you?

Here you will find tips on how to choose a program that may help you lose weight safely and keep it off over time. You will also learn how to talk with a healthcare professional about your weight.

Your healthcare professional may be able to help you make lifestyle changes to reach and maintain a healthy weight. However, if you are having trouble making these lifestyle changes—or if these changes are not enough to help you reach and stay at a healthy weight—you may want to consider a weight-loss program or other types of treatment.

Where Do I Start?

Talking with a healthcare professional about your weight is an important first step. Sometimes, healthcare professionals may not address issues, such as healthy eating, physical activity, and weight during general office visits. You may need to raise these issues yourself. If you feel uneasy talking about your weight, bring your questions with you and practice talking about your concerns before your office visit. Aim to work with your healthcare professional to improve your health.

Prepare for Your Visit

Before your visit with a healthcare professional, think about the following questions:

- How can I change my eating habits so I can be healthier and reach a healthy weight?

- How much and what type of physical activity do I think I need to be healthier and reach a healthy weight?

- Could I benefit from seeing a nutrition professional or weight-loss specialist, or joining a weight-loss program?

You can be better prepared for a visit with a healthcare professional if you:

- Write down all of your questions ahead of time

- Record all of the medicines and dietary supplements you take, or bring them with you

- Write down the types of diets or programs you have tried in the past to lose weight

- Bring a pen and paper, smartphone, or other mobile device to read your questions and take notes

During your visit, a healthcare professional may:

- Review any medical problems you have and medicines you take to see whether they may be affecting your weight or your ability to lose weight

- Ask you about your eating, drinking, and physical activity habits

- Determine your body mass index to see whether you are overweight or have obesity

People who are overweight have a BMI between 25.0 and 29.9. People with obesity have a BMI of 30.0 or higher, and those with extreme obesity have a BMI of 40.0 or higher.

If a healthcare professional says you should lose weight, you may want to ask for a referral to a weight-loss program, dietitian, or weight-loss specialist. If you decide to choose a weight-loss program on your own, consider talking with the healthcare professional about the program before you sign up, especially if you have any health problems.

Questions to Ask a Healthcare Professional

You may want to ask a healthcare professional the following questions:

- What is a healthy weight or BMI for me?

- Will losing weight improve my general health, as well as specific health problems I have?

113

- Could any of my medical conditions or medications be causing weight gain or making it harder for me to lose weight?

- Are there any types or amounts of physical activity I should not do because of my health?

- What dietary approaches do you recommend I try or avoid?

What Should I Look for in a Weight-Loss Program?

To reach and stay at a healthy weight over the long term, you must focus on your overall health and lifestyle habits, not just on what you eat. Successful weight-loss programs should promote healthy behaviors that help you lose weight safely, that you can stick with every day, and that help you keep the weight off.

Safe and successful weight-loss programs should include:

- Behavioral treatment, also called "lifestyle counseling," that can teach you how to develop and stick with healthier eating and physical activity habits—for example, keeping food and activity records or journals

- Information about getting enough sleep, managing stress, and the benefits and drawbacks of weight-loss medicines

- Ongoing feedback, monitoring, and support throughout the program, either in person, by phone, online, or through a combination of these approaches

- Slow and steady weight-loss goals—usually one to two pounds per week (though weight loss may be faster at the start of a program)

- A plan for keeping the weight off, including goal setting, self-checks such as keeping a food journal, and counseling support

The most successful weight-loss programs provide 14 sessions or more of behavioral treatment over at least 6 months—and are led by trained staff.

Some commercial weight-loss programs have all of these components for a safe and successful weight-loss program. Check for these features in any program you are thinking about trying.

Although these diets may help some people lose a lot of weight quickly—for example, 15 pounds in a month and they may not help people keep the weight off long term. These diets also may have related health risks, the most common being gallstones.

For people who are overweight or have obesity, experts recommend a beginning weight-loss goal of 5 to 10 percent of your starting weight within 6 months. If you weigh 200 pounds, that would amount to a loss of 10 pounds, which is 5 percent of starting weight, to 20 pounds, which is 10 percent of starting weight, in 6 months.

Changing your lifestyle is not easy, but adopting healthy habits that you do not give up after a few weeks or months may help you maintain your weight loss.

What If the Program Is Offered Online

Many weight-loss programs are now being offered partly or completely online and through apps for mobile devices. Researchers are studying how well these programs work on their own or together with in-person programs, especially long term. However, experts suggest that these weight-loss programs should provide the following:

- Organized, weekly lessons, offered online or by podcast, and tailored to your personal goals

- Support from a qualified staff person to meet your goals

- A plan to track your progress on changing your lifestyle habits, such as healthy eating and physical activity, using tools, such as cellphones, activity counters, and online journals

- Regular feedback on your goals, progress, and results provided by a counselor through email, phone, or text messages

- The option of social support from a group through bulletin boards, chat rooms, or online meetings

Whether a program is online or in person, you should get as much background as you can before you decide to join.

Weight-Loss Programs to Avoid

Avoid weight-loss programs that make any of the following promises:
- Lose weight without diet or exercise!
- Lose weight while eating as much as you want of all your favorite foods!
- Lose 30 pounds in 30 days!
- Lose weight in specific problem areas of your body!

115

Other warning signs to look out for include:

- Very small print, asterisks, and footnotes, which may make it easy to miss important information
- Before-and-after photos that seem too good to be true
- Personal endorsements that may be made up

What Questions Should I Ask about a Weight-Loss Program?

Weight-loss program staff should be able to answer questions about the program's features, safety, costs, and results. Find out if the program you are interested in is based on current research about what works for reaching and maintaining a healthy weight.

A first and very important question to ask of commercial weight-loss programs is, "Has your company published any reports in peer-reviewed, scientific journals about the safety and effectiveness of your program?"

If the response is "yes," ask for a copy of the report or how you could get it. If the answer is "no," the program is harder to evaluate and may not be as favorable a choice as programs that have published such information. If you have questions about the findings, discuss the report with your healthcare professional.

Here are some other questions you may want to ask:

What Does the Program Include?
Eating

- Am I expected to follow a specific meal plan?
- Am I encouraged to write down what I eat each day?
- Do I have to buy special meals or supplements? If so, what are the daily or weekly costs?
- Does the program offer healthy meal-plan suggestions that I could stick with?
- If the program requires special foods, can I make changes based on my likes, dislikes, and any food allergies I may have?

Physical Activity

- Does the program include a physical activity plan?

- Does the program offer ways to help me be more physically active and stay motivated?

Counseling

- Does the program offer one-on-one or group counseling to help me develop and stick with my healthier habits?
- Does the program include a trained coach or counselor to help me overcome roadblocks and stay on track?

Weight Maintenance

- Does the program include a plan to help me keep off the weight I have lost?
- What does that program include? Will there be ongoing counseling support?

Other Features

- How long is the actual weight-loss program?
- How long is the weight-loss maintenance program?
- Does the program require that I take any kind of medicine?
- Can I speak with a doctor or certified health professional if I need to?
- Can I change the program to meet my lifestyle, work schedule, and cultural needs?
- Will the program help me cope with such issues as stress or social eating, getting enough sleep, changes in work schedules, lack of motivation, and injury or illness?
- Is the program in person? Is there an online part to the program?

What Kind of Education or Training Do Staff Members Have?

These questions are especially important if you are considering a medically supervised program that encourages quick weight loss (three or more pounds a week for several weeks):

- Does a doctor or other certified health professional run or oversee the program?

117

- Does the program include specialists in nutrition, physical activity, behavior change, and weight loss?

- What type of certifications, education, experience, and training do staff members have? How long, on average, have most of the staff been working with the program?

Does the Program or Product Carry Any Risks?

- Could the program cause health problems or be harmful to me in any way?

- Is there ongoing input and follow-up to ensure my safety while I am in the program?

- Will the program's doctor or staff work with my healthcare professional if needed—for example, to address how the program may affect an ongoing medical issue?

How Much Does the Program Cost?

- What is the total cost of the program, from beginning to end?

- Are there costs that are not included in that total, such as membership fees or fees for:

  - Weekly visits?

  - Food, meal replacements, supplements, or other products?

  - Medical tests?

  - Counseling sessions?

  - Follow-up to maintain the weight I have lost?

What Results Do People in the Program Typically Achieve?

- How much weight does the average person lose?

- How long does the average person keep the weight off?

- Do you have written information on these and other program results?

- Are the results of the program published in a peer-reviewed scientific journal?

What If I Need More Help Losing Weight?

If a weight-loss program is not enough to help you reach a healthy weight, ask your healthcare professional about other types of weight-loss treatments. Prescription medicines to treat overweight and obesity, combined with healthy lifestyle changes, may help some people reach a healthy weight. For some people who have extreme obesity, bariatric surgery may be an option.

Chapter 7

Nutrition Tips for Men

Chapter Contents

Section 7.1—Healthy Eating for Men 122

Section 7.2—Nutrition Tips for Building Strength
        and Increasing Muscle Mass 127

Section 7.1

Healthy Eating for Men

This section includes text excerpted from
"Eat Healthy," Office of Disease Prevention and Health
Promotion (ODPHP), U.S. Department of Health
and Human Services (HHS), February 21, 2019.

The Basics

Eating healthy means following a healthy eating pattern that includes a variety of nutritious foods and drinks. It also means getting the number of calories that is right for you (not eating too much or too little).

Use Your Calories to Eat a Variety of Healthy Foods

To eat healthy, be sure to choose:

- Vegetables
- Fruits
- Whole grains
- Fat-free or low-fat dairy products
- A variety of foods with protein, including seafood, lean meats and poultry, eggs, beans, peas, nuts, seeds, and soy products

Limit Certain Nutrients and Ingredients
Sodium

Sodium is found in table salt, but most of the sodium we eat comes from packaged food or food that is prepared in restaurants.

Added Sugars

Added sugars include syrups and sweeteners that manufacturers add to products, such as sodas, yogurt, and cereals—as well as things you add, such as sugar in your coffee.

Saturated Fats

Saturated fats come from animal products, such as cheese, fatty meats and poultry, whole milk, butter, and many sweets and snack foods. Some plant products, such as palm and coconut oils, also have saturated fats.

Refined Grains and Starches

Refined grains and starches are in foods such as cookies, white bread, and some snack foods.

A Healthy Eating Pattern Can Help Keep You Healthy

Eating healthy is good for your overall health, and there are many ways to do it.

Making smart food choices can also help you manage your weight and lower your risk for certain chronic (long-term) diseases.

When you eat healthy, you can reduce your risk for:

- Obesity
- Heart disease
- Type 2 diabetes
- High blood pressure
- Some types of cancer

Take Action

Making small changes to your eating habits can make a big difference for your health over time. Here are some tips and tools you can use to get started.

Keep a Food Diary

Knowing what you eat now will help you figure out what you want to change. Print a food diary and write down:

- When you eat
- What and how much you eat
- Where you are and who you are with when you eat
- How you are feeling when you eat

For example, you might write something such as: "Tuesday 3:30 p.m., two chocolate chip cookies, at work with Mary, feeling stressed."

Shop Smart at the Grocery Store

The next time you go food shopping:

- Make a shopping list ahead of time. Only buy what is on your list.

- Do not shop while you are hungry; eat something before you go to the store.

Use these tips to make healthy choices:

- Try a variety of vegetables and fruits in different colors.

- Choose fat-free or low-fat dairy products.

- Replace old favorites with options that are lower in calories, sodium, added sugars, and saturated fat.

- Choose foods with whole grains, such as 100 percent whole-wheat or whole-grain bread, cereal, and pasta.

- Buy lean cuts of meat and poultry. Eat a variety of foods with protein, such as fish, shellfish, beans, and nuts.

- Save money by getting fruits and vegetables in season or on sale.

Read the Nutrition Facts Label

Understanding the Nutrition Facts label on food packages can help you make healthy choices.

First, look at the serving size and the number of servings per package—there may be more than 1 serving.

Then, check out the calories. Calories tell you how much energy is in one serving of a food. In general:

- 100 calories per serving is moderate

- 400 calories per serving is high

To stay at a healthy weight, you need to balance the calories you eat and drink with the calories you burn.

Next, look at the percent daily value (% DV) column. The DV column shows you if a food is higher or lower in certain nutrients. Look for foods that are:

- Lower in added sugars, sodium, and saturated fat (5% DV or less)

- Higher in fiber, calcium, potassium, iron, and vitamin D (20% DV or more)

You can also use the DV column to compare food products. Just be sure to check and see if the serving size is the same.

The picture below shows an example of a nutrition facts label.

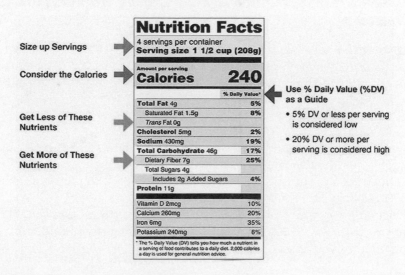

Figure 7.1. *Nutrition Facts Label*

Be a Healthy Family

Parents and caregivers are important role models for healthy eating. You can teach kids how to choose and prepare healthy snacks and meals.

- Turn cooking into a fun activity for the whole family.

- Make healthy snacks.

Eat Healthy Away from Home

You can make smart food choices wherever you are—at work, in your favorite restaurant, or out running errands. Try these tips for eating healthy even when you are away from home:

- At lunch, have a sandwich on whole-grain bread instead of white bread.

- Skip the soda, and drink water instead.

- In a restaurant, choose dishes that are steamed, baked, or grilled instead of fried.

- On a long drive or shopping trip, pack healthy snacks, such as fruit, unsalted nuts, or low-fat string cheese sticks.

If You Are Worried about Your Eating Habits, Talk to a Doctor

If you need help making healthier food choices, ask your doctor for help. Your doctor may refer you to a registered dietitian. A registered dietitian is a health professional who helps people with healthy eating.

What about Cost?

Under the Affordable Care Act, the healthcare reform law passed in 2010, most health plans must cover diet counseling for people at a higher risk for chronic diseases, such as type 2 diabetes and high blood pressure.

Depending on your insurance, you may be able to get diet counseling at no cost to you. Check with your insurance company to find out what is included in your plan.

Manage Your High Blood Pressure or Diabetes

If you or a loved one has high blood pressure, type 2 diabetes, or heart disease, talk with your doctor or a registered dietitian about how to stay healthy.

Section 7.2

Nutrition Tips for Building Strength and Increasing Muscle Mass

This section includes text excerpted from "Healthy Muscles Matter," National Institute of Arthritis and Musculoskeletal and Skin Diseases (NIAMS), September 3, 2017.

Basic Facts about Muscles

Did you know you have more than 600 muscles in your body? These muscles help you move, lift things, pump blood through your body, and even help you breathe.

When you think about your muscles, you probably think most about the ones you can control. These are your voluntary muscles, which means you can control their movements. They are also called "skeletal muscles" because they attach to your bones and work together with your bones to help you walk, run, pick up things, play an instrument, throw a baseball, kick a soccer ball, push a lawnmower, or ride a bicycle. The muscles of your mouth and throat even help you talk.

Keeping your muscles healthy will help you to be able to walk, run, jump, lift things, play sports, and do all the other things you love to do. Exercising, getting enough rest, and eating a balanced diet will help to keep your muscles healthy for life.

Why Healthy Muscles Matter to You

Healthy muscles let you move freely and keep your body strong. They help you to enjoy playing sports, dancing, walking the dog, swimming, and other fun activities. And they help you do those other (not so fun) things that you have to do, such as making the bed, vacuuming the carpet, or mowing the lawn.

Strong muscles also help to keep your joints in good shape. For example, if the muscles around your knee get weak, you may be more likely to injure that knee. Strong muscles also help you keep your balance, so you are less likely to slip or fall.

And remember, the activities that make your skeletal muscles strong will also help to keep your heart muscle strong.

Different Kinds of Muscles Have Different Jobs

Skeletal muscles are connected to your bones by tough cords of tissue called "tendons." As the muscle contracts, it pulls on the tendon, which moves the bone. Bones are connected to other bones by ligaments, which are similar to tendons and help hold your skeleton together.

Smooth muscles are also called "involuntary muscles" since you have no control over them. Smooth muscles work in your digestive system to move food along and push waste out of your body. They also help keep your eyes focused without your having to think about it.

Did you know that your heart is also a muscle? It is a specialized type of involuntary muscle. It pumps blood through your body, changing its speed to keep up with the demands you put on it. It pumps more slowly when you are sitting or lying down, and faster when you are running or playing sports and your skeletal muscles need more blood to help them do their work.

What Can Go Wrong?

Almost everyone has had sore muscles after exercising or working too much. Some soreness can be a normal part of healthy exercise. But, in other cases, muscles can become strained. Muscle strain can be mild (the muscle has just been stretched too much) to severe (the muscle actually tears). Maybe you lifted something that was too heavy, and the muscles in your arms were stretched too far. Lifting heavy things in the wrong way can also strain the muscles in your back. This can be very painful and can even cause an injury that will last a long time and make it hard to do everyday things.

The tendons that connect the muscles to the bones can also be strained if they are pulled or stretched too much. If ligaments are stretched or pulled too much, the injury is called a "sprain." Most people are familiar with the pain of a sprained ankle.

Contact sports, such as soccer, football, hockey, and wrestling, can often cause strains. Sports in which you grip something, such as gymnastics or tennis, can lead to strains in your hand or forearm.

How Can I Keep My Muscles More Healthy?
Physical Activity

When you make your muscles work by being physically active, they respond by growing stronger. They may even get bigger by adding more muscle tissue. This is how bodybuilders get such big muscles, but your muscles can be healthy without getting that big.

There are lots of activities you can do for your muscles. Walking, jogging, lifting weights, playing tennis, climbing stairs, jumping, and dancing are all good ways to exercise your muscles. Swimming and biking will also give your muscles a good workout. It is important to get different kinds of activities to work all your muscles. Any activity that makes you breathe harder and faster will help exercise the heart muscle as well.

Get 60 minutes of physical activity every day. It does not have to be all at once, but it does need to be in at least 10-minute increments to count toward your 60 minutes of physical activity per day.

Eat a Healthy Diet

You really do not need a special diet to keep your muscles in good health. Eating a balanced diet will help manage your weight and provide a variety of nutrients for your muscles and overall health. A balanced diet:

- Emphasizes fruits; vegetables; whole grains; and fat-free or low-fat dairy products, such as milk, cheese, and yogurt

- Includes protein from lean meats, poultry, seafood, beans, eggs, and nuts

- Is low in solid fats, saturated fats, cholesterol, salt, added sugars, and refined grains

- Is as low as possible in *trans* fats

- Balances calories taken in through food with calories burned in physical activity to help maintain a healthy weight

As you grow and become an adult, iron is an important nutrient. Not getting enough iron can cause anemia, which can make you feel weak and tired because your muscles do not get enough oxygen. This can also keep you from getting enough activity to keep your muscles healthy. You can get iron from foods such as lean beef, chicken, and turkey; beans and peas; spinach; and iron-enriched breads and cereals. You can also get iron from dietary supplements, but it is always good to check with a doctor first.

Some people think that supplements will make their muscles bigger and stronger. However, supplements, such as creatine, can cause serious side effects, and protein and amino acid supplements are no better than getting protein from your food. Using steroids to increase your muscles is illegal (unless a doctor has prescribed them for a medical problem) and can have dangerous side effects. No muscle-building supplement can take the place of good nutrition and proper training.

Prevent Injuries

To help prevent sprains, strains, and other muscle injuries:

- Warm up and cool down. Before exercising or playing sports, warm-up exercises, such as stretching and light jogging, may make it less likely that you will strain a muscle. They are called "warm-up exercises" because they make the muscles warmer and more flexible. Cool-down exercises loosen muscles that have tightened during exercise.

- Wear the proper protective gear for your sport, such as pads or helmets. This will help reduce your risk for injuring your muscles or joints.

- Remember to drink lots of water while you are playing or exercising, especially in warm weather. If your body's water level gets too low (dehydration), you could get dizzy or even pass out. Dehydration can cause many medical problems.

- Do not try to "play through the pain." If something starts to hurt, stop exercising or playing. You might need to see a doctor, or you might just need to rest the injured part for a while.

- If you have been inactive, "start low and go slow" by gradually increasing how often and how long activities are done. Increase physical activity gradually over time.

- Be careful when you lift heavy objects. Keep your back straight, and bend your knees to lift the object. This will protect the muscles in your back and put most of the weight on the strong muscles in your legs. Get someone to help you lift something heavy.

Start Now

Keeping your muscles healthy will help you have more fun and enjoy the things you do. Healthy muscles will help you look your best and feel full of energy. Start good habits now, while you are young, and you will have a better chance of keeping your muscles healthy for the rest of your life.

Chapter 8

Physical Activity: Key to a Healthy Life

Chapter Contents

Section 8.1—How Much Physical Activity Do
　　　　　Adults Need? 132

Section 8.2—The Benefits of Physical Activity 139

Section 8.1

How Much Physical Activity Do Adults Need?

This section includes text excerpted from "Physical Activity
Basics," ChooseMyPlate.gov, U.S. Department of
Agriculture (USDA), January 2, 2018.

Being physically active can improve your health today, tomorrow,
and in the future. However, most people do not do enough physical
activity. People of all types, shapes, sizes, and abilities can benefit
from being physically active. The more you do, the greater the health
benefits and the better you will feel. The information and tips below
can help you learn ways to add physical activity to your life.

What Is Physical Activity?

Physical activity simply means movement of the body that uses
energy. Walking, gardening, briskly pushing a baby stroller, climbing the stairs, playing soccer, or dancing the night away are all good
examples of being active. For health benefits, physical activity should
be moderate or vigorous intensity.

Moderate Physical Activities

- Walking briskly (about 3½ miles per hour)
- Bicycling (less than 10 miles per hour)
- General gardening (raking, trimming shrubs)
- Dancing
- Golf (walking and carrying clubs)
- Water aerobics
- Canoeing
- Tennis (doubles)

Vigorous Physical Activities

- Running/jogging (5 miles per hour)
- Walking very fast (4½ miles per hour)
- Bicycling (more than 10 miles per hour)

- Heavy yard work, such as chopping wood
- Swimming (freestyle laps)
- Aerobics
- Basketball (competitive)
- Tennis (singles)

You can choose moderate or vigorous intensity activities, or a mix of both each week. Activities can be considered vigorous, moderate, or light in intensity. This depends on the extent to which they make you breathe harder and your heart beat faster.

Only moderate and vigorous intensity activities count toward meeting your physical activity needs. With vigorous activities, you get similar health benefits in half the time it takes you with moderate ones. You can replace some or all of your moderate activity with vigorous activity. Although you are moving, light intensity activities do not increase your heart rate, so you should not count these towards meeting the physical activity recommendations. These activities include walking at a casual pace, such as while grocery shopping, and doing light household chores.

Why Is Physical Activity Important?

Regular physical activity can produce long-term health benefits. People of all ages, shapes, sizes, and abilities can benefit from being physically active. The more physical activity you do, the greater the health benefits.

Being physically active can help you

- Increase your chances of living longer
- Feel better about yourself
- Decrease your chances of becoming depressed
- Sleep well at night
- Move around more easily
- Have stronger muscles and bones
- Stay at or get to a healthy weight
- Be with friends or meet new people
- Enjoy yourself and have fun

When you are not physically active, you are more likely to

- Get heart disease

- Get type 2 diabetes

- Have high blood pressure

- Have high blood cholesterol

- Have a stroke

Physical activity and nutrition work together for better health. Being active increases the amount of calories burned. As people age, their metabolism slows, so maintaining energy balance requires moving more and eating less.

Types of Physical Activities

- **Aerobic activities** make you breathe harder and make your heart beat faster. Aerobic activities can be moderate or vigorous in their intensity. Vigorous activities take more effort than moderate ones. For moderate activities, you can talk while you do them, but you cannot sing. For vigorous activities, you can only say a few words without stopping to catch your breath.

- **Muscle-strengthening activities** make your muscles stronger. These include activities such as push-ups and lifting weights. It is important to work all the different parts of the body—your legs, hips, back, chest, stomach, shoulders, and arms.

- **Bone-strengthening activities** make your bones stronger. Bone-strengthening activities, such as jumping, are especially important for children and adolescents. These activities produce a force on the bones that promotes bone growth and strength.

- **Balance and stretching activities** enhance physical stability and flexibility, which reduces risk of injuries. Examples are gentle stretching, dancing, yoga, martial arts, and tai chi.

How Much Physical Activity Is Needed?

Physical activity is important for everyone, but how much you need depends on your age.

Adult (18 to 64 Years of Age)

Adults should do at least 2 hours and 30 minutes each week of aerobic physical activity at a moderate level or 1 hour and 15 minutes each week of aerobic physical activity at a vigorous level. Being active 5 or more hours each week can provide even more health benefits. Spreading aerobic activity out over at least 3 days a week is best. Also, each activity should be done for at least 10 minutes at a time. Adults should also do strengthening activities, such as push-ups, sit-ups and lifting weights, at least 2 days a week.

Children and Adolescents (6 to 17 Years of Age)

Children and adolescents should do 60 minutes or more of physical activity each day. Most of the 60 minutes should be either moderate- or vigorous-intensity aerobic physical activity, and it should include vigorous-intensity physical activity at least 3 days a week. As part of their 60 or more minutes of daily physical activity, children and adolescents should include muscle-strengthening activities, such as climbing, at least 3 days a week and bone-strengthening activities, such as jumping, at least 3 days a week. Children and adolescents are often active in short bursts of time rather than for sustained periods of time, and these short bursts can add up to meet physical activity needs. Physical activities for children and adolescents should be developmentally appropriate, fun, and offer variety.

Young Children (2 to 5 Years of Age)

There is not a specific recommendation for the number of minutes young children should be active each day. Children between the ages of two and five should play actively several times each day. Their activity may happen in short bursts of time and not be all at once. Physical activities for young children should be developmentally appropriate, fun, and offer variety.

Physical activity is generally safe for everyone. The health benefits you gain from being active are far greater than the chances of getting hurt. Here are some things you can do to stay safe while you are active:

- If you have not been active in a while, start slowly and build up.

- Learn about the types and amounts of activity that are right for you.

- Choose activities that are appropriate for your fitness level.

- Build up the time you spend before switching to activities that take more effort.

- Use the right safety gear and sports equipment.

- Choose a safe place to do your activity.

- See a healthcare provider if you have a health problem.

How Many Calories Does Physical Activity Use (Burn)?

A 154-pound man who is 5' 10" will use up (burn) about the number of calories listed doing each activity below. Those who weigh more will use more calories; those who weigh less will use fewer calories. The calorie values listed include both calories used by the activity and the calories used for normal body functioning during the activity time.

Table 8.1. Calories and Physical Activity

	Approximate Calories Used (Burned) by a 154-Pound Man	
MODERATE physical activities:	**In 1 hour**	**In 30 minutes**
Hiking	370	185
Light gardening/yard work	330	165
Dancing	330	165
Golf (walking and carrying clubs)	330	165
Bicycling (less than 10 mph)	290	145
Walking (3.5 mph)	280	140
Weight training (general light workout)	220	110
Stretching	180	90
VIGOROUS physical activities:	**In 1 hour**	**In 30 minutes**
Running/ jogging (5 mph)	590	295
Bicycling (more than 10 mph)	590	295
Swimming (slow freestyle laps)	510	255
Aerobics	480	240
Walking (4.5 mph)	460	230
Heavy yard work (chopping wood)	440	220
Weight lifting (vigorous effort)	440	220
Basketball (vigorous)	440	220

Tips for Increasing Physical Activity
Make Physical Activity a Regular Part of the Day

Choose activities that you enjoy and can do regularly. Fitting activity into a daily routine can be easy, such as taking a brisk 10-minute walk to and from the parking lot, bus stop, or subway station. Or, join an exercise class. Keep it interesting by trying something different on alternate days. Every little bit adds up, and doing something is better than doing nothing.

Make sure to do at least 10 minutes of activity at a time, shorter bursts of activity will not have the same health benefits. For example, walking the dog for 10 minutes before and after work or adding a 10-minute walk at lunchtime can add to your weekly goal. Mix it up. Swim, take a yoga class, garden, or lift weights. To be ready anytime, keep some comfortable clothes and a pair of walking or running shoes in the car and at the office.

More Ways to Increase Physical Activity
At Home

- Join a walking group in the neighborhood or at the local shopping mall. Recruit a partner for support and encouragement.

- Push the baby in a stroller.

- Get the whole family involved—enjoy an afternoon bike ride with your kids.

- Walk up and down the soccer or softball field sidelines while watching the kids play.

- Walk the dog—do not just watch the dog walk.

- Clean the house, or wash the car.

- Walk, skate, or cycle more, and drive less.

- Do stretches, exercises, or pedal a stationary bike while watching television.

- Mow the lawn with a push mower.

- Plant and care for a vegetable or flower garden.

- Play with the kids—tumble in the leaves, build a snowman, splash in a puddle, or dance to your favorite music.

- Exercise to a workout video.

At Work

- Get off the bus or subway 1 stop early, and walk or skate the rest of the way.

- Replace a coffee break with a brisk 10-minute walk. Ask a friend to go with you.

- Take part in an exercise program at work or a nearby gym.

- Join the office softball team or walking group.

At Play

- Walk, jog, skate, or cycle.

- Swim or do water aerobics.

- Take a class in martial arts, dance, or yoga.

- Golf (pull a cart or carry your clubs).

- Canoe, row, or kayak.

- Play racquetball, tennis, or squash.

- Ski cross-country or downhill.

- Play basketball, softball, or soccer.

- Handcycle, or play wheelchair sports.

- Take a nature walk.

- Most importantly, have fun while being active.

Section 8.2

The Benefits of Physical Activity

This section includes text excerpted from "Benefits of Exercise," MedlinePlus, National Institutes of Health (NIH), August 30, 2017.

We have all heard it many times before—regular exercise is good for you, and it can help you lose weight. But if you are like many Americans, you are busy, you have a sedentary job, and you have not yet changed your exercise habits. The good news is that it is never too late to start. You can start slowly and find ways to fit more physical activity into your life. To get the most benefit, you should try to get the recommended amount of exercise for your age. If you can do it, the payoff is that you will feel better, help prevent or control many diseases, and likely even live longer.

What Are the Health Benefits of Exercise?

Regular exercise and physical activity may:

- **Help you control your weight.** Along with diet, exercise plays an important role in controlling your weight and preventing obesity. To maintain your weight, the calories you eat and drink must equal the energy you burn. To lose weight, you must use more calories than you eat and drink.

- **Reduce your risk of heart diseases.** Exercise strengthens your heart and improves your circulation. The increased blood flow raises the oxygen levels in your body. This helps lower your risk of heart diseases, such as high cholesterol, coronary artery disease, and heart attack. Regular exercise can also lower your blood pressure and triglyceride levels.

- **Help your body manage blood sugar and insulin levels.** Exercise can lower your blood sugar level and help your insulin work better. This can cut down your risk for metabolic syndrome and type 2 diabetes. And if you already have one of those diseases, exercise can help you to manage it.

- **Help you quit smoking.** Exercise may make it easier to quit smoking by reducing your cravings and withdrawal symptoms. It can also help limit the weight you might gain when you stop smoking.

139

- **Improve your mental health and mood.** During exercise, your body releases chemicals that can improve your mood and make you feel more relaxed. This can help you deal with stress and reduce your risk of depression.

- **Help keep your thinking, learning, and judgment skills sharp as you age.** Exercise stimulates your body to release proteins and other chemicals that improve the structure and function of your brain.

- **Strengthen your bones and muscles.** Regular exercise can help kids and teens build strong bones. Later in life, it can also slow the loss of bone density that comes with age. Doing muscle-strengthening activities can help you increase or maintain your muscle mass and strength.

- **Reduce your risk of some cancers,** including colon, breast, uterine, and lung cancer.

- **Reduce your risk of falls.** For older adults, research shows that doing balance and muscle-strengthening activities in addition to moderate-intensity aerobic activity can help reduce your risk of falling.

- **Improve your sleep.** Exercise can help you to fall asleep faster and stay asleep longer.

- **Improve your sexual health.** Regular exercise may lower the risk of erectile dysfunction (ED) in men. For those who already have ED, exercise may help improve their sexual function. In women, exercise may increase sexual arousal.

- **Increase your chances of living longer.** Studies show that physical activity can reduce your risk of dying early from the leading causes of death, such as heart disease and some cancers.

How Can I Make Exercise a Part of My Regular Routine?

- **Make everyday activities more active.** Even small changes can help. You can take the stairs instead of the elevator. Walk down the hall to a coworker's office instead of sending an email. Wash the car yourself. Park further away from your destination.

- **Be active with friends and family.** Having a workout partner may make you more likely to enjoy exercise. You can also plan social activities that involve exercise. You might also consider joining an exercise group or class, such as a dance class, hiking club, or volleyball team.

- **Keep track of your progress.** Keeping a log of your activity or using a fitness tracker may help you set goals and stay motivated.

- **Make exercise more fun.** Try listening to music or watching television while you exercise. Also, mix things up a little bit; if you stick with just one type of exercise, you might get bored. Try doing a combination of activities.

- **Find activities that you can do even when the weather is bad.** You can walk in a mall, climb stairs, or work out in a gym even if the weather stops you from exercising outside.

Part Two

Leading Causes of
Death in Men

Chapter 9

Causes of Death: A Statistical Overview

Chapter Contents

Section 9.1—Leading Causes of Death in
the United States 146

Section 9.2—Cancer among Men: Some Statistics................... 151

Section 9.1

Leading Causes of Death in the United States

This section includes text excerpted from "Mortality in the United
States, 2017," Centers for Disease Control and Prevention (CDC),
November 29, 2018.

Data from the National Vital Statistics System

- Life expectancy for the U.S. population declined to 78.6 years in
  2017.

- The age-adjusted death rate increased by 0.4 percent from 728.8
  deaths per 100,000 individuals of the standard population in
  2016 to 731.9 in 2017.

- Age-specific death rates increased from 2016 to 2017 for the age
  groups 25–34, 35–44, and 85 and older, and rates decreased for
  the age group 45 to 54.

- The 10 leading causes of death in 2017 remained the same as in
  2016.

- The infant mortality rate of 579.3 infant deaths per 100,000 live
  births in 2017 was not significantly different from the 2016 rate.

- The 10 leading causes of infant death in 2017 remained the
  same as in 2016, although 4 causes changed ranks.

This report presents the final 2017 U.S. mortality data on deaths
and death rates by demographic and medical characteristics. These
data provide information on mortality patterns among U.S. residents
by variables, such as sex, race and ethnicity, and cause of death. Life
expectancy estimates, age-specific death rates, age-adjusted death
rates by race and ethnicity and sex, the 10 leading causes of death,
and the 10 leading causes of infant death were analyzed by comparing
2017 and 2016 final data.

How Long Can We Expect to Live?

In 2017, life expectancy at birth was 78.6 years for the total U.S.
population—a decrease from 78.7 years in 2016 (Figure 9.1). For males,
life expectancy changed from 76.2 years in 2016 to 76.1 years in 2017.
For females, life expectancy remained the same at 81.1 years.

Life expectancy for females was consistently higher than it was for males. In 2017, the difference in life expectancy between females and males increased 0.1 year from 4.9 years in 2016 to 5 years in 2017.

In 2017, life expectancy at the age of 65 for the total population was 19.5 years, an increase of 0.1 year from 2016. Life expectancy at the age of 65 was 20.6 years for females and 18.1 years for males, both unchanged from 2016. The difference in life expectancy at the age of 65 between females and males was 2.5 years, unchanged from 2016.

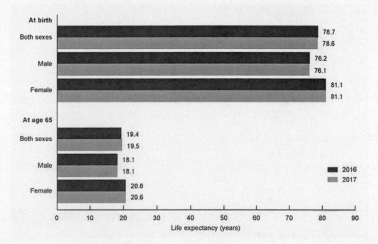

Figure 9.1. *Life Expectancy at Selected Ages, by Sex: The United States, 2016 and 2017* (Source: National Center for Health Statistics (NCHS), National Vital Statistics System (NVSS), Mortality.)

Notes: Life expectancies for 2016 were revised using updated Medicare data; therefore, figures may differ from those previously published.

What Are the Age-Adjusted Death Rates for Race–Ethnicity–Sex Groups?

The age-adjusted death rate for the total population increased 0.4 percent from 728.8 per 100,000 individuals of the standard population in 2016 to 731.9 in 2017 (Figure 9.2). Age-adjusted death rates increased in 2017 from 2016 for non-Hispanic White males (0.6%) and non-Hispanic White females (0.9%). The age-adjusted death rate decreased for non-Hispanic Black females (0.8%). Rates did not change significantly for non-Hispanic Black males, Hispanic males, and Hispanic females from 2016 to 2017.

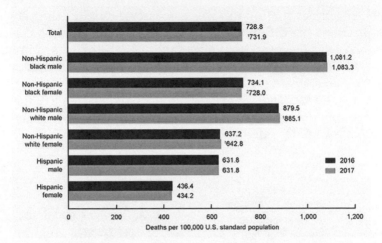

Figure 9.2. *Age-Adjusted Death Rates, by Race and Ethnicity and Sex: The United States, 2016 and 2017* (Source: National Center for Health Statistics (NCHS), National Vital Statistics System (NVSS), Mortality.)

[1] *Statistically significant increase in age-adjusted death rate from 2016 to 2017 (p < 0.05).*
[2] *Statistically significant decrease in age-adjusted death rate from 2016 to 2017 (p < 0.05).*

Did Age-Specific Death Rates Change among Those Aged 15 Years and Over?

Death rates increased significantly between 2016 and 2017 for the age groups 25–34 (2.9%), 35–44 (1.6%), and 85 and older (1.4%) (Figure 9.3).

The death rate decreased significantly for the age group 45–54 (1.0%).

Rates for other age groups did not change significantly between 2016 and 2017.

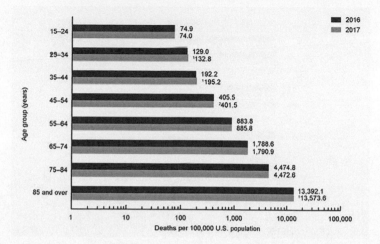

Figure 9.3. *Death Rates for Ages 15 Years and Over: United States, 2016 and 2017* (Source: National Center for Health Statistics (NCHS), National Vital Statistics System (NVSS), Mortality.)

[1] *Statistically significant increase in age-specific death rate from 2016 to 2017 (p < 0.05).*
[2] *Statistically significant decrease in age-specific death rate from 2016 to 2017 (p < 0.05).*

What Are the Leading Causes of Death?

In 2017, the 10 leading causes of death (heart disease, cancer, unintentional injuries, chronic lower respiratory diseases, stroke, Alzheimer disease, diabetes, influenza and pneumonia, kidney disease, and suicide) remained the same as in 2016. Causes of death are ranked according to number of deaths. The 10 leading causes accounted for 74.0 percent of all deaths in the United States in 2017.

From 2016 to 2017, age-adjusted death rates increased for 7 of the 10 leading causes of death and decreased for 1 leading cause (Figure 9.4). The rate increased 4.2 percent for unintentional injuries, 0.7 percent for chronic lower respiratory diseases, 0.8 percent for stroke, 2.3 percent for Alzheimer disease, 2.4 percent for diabetes, 5.9 percent for influenza and pneumonia, and 3.7 percent for suicide. The rate decreased 2.1 percent for cancer. Rates for heart disease and kidney disease did not change significantly.

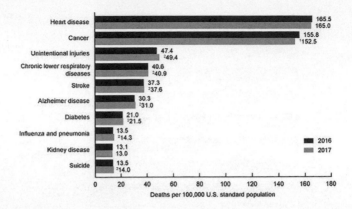

Figure 9.4. *Age-Adjusted Death Rates for the 10 Leading Causes of Death: the United States, 2016 and 2017* (Source: National Center for Health Statistics (NCHS), National Vital Statistics System (NVSS), Mortality.)

[1] *Statistically significant decrease in age-adjusted death rate from 2016 to 2017 (p < 0.05).*
[2] *Statistically significant increase in age-adjusted death rate from 2016 to 2017 (p < 0.05).*
Note: *A total of 2,813,503 resident deaths were registered in the United States in 2017. The 10 leading causes accounted for 74.0 percent of all deaths in the United States in 2017. Causes of death are ranked according to number of deaths. Rankings for 2016 data are not shown. Data table for figure 9.4 includes the number of deaths for leading causes.*

Section 9.2

Cancer among Men: Some Statistics

This section contains text excerpted from the following sources: Text in this section begins with excerpts from "Cancer," MedlinePlus, National Institutes of Health (NIH), May 18, 2017; Text beginning with the heading "Fast Facts about Cancer and Men" is excerpted from "Cancer and Men," Centers for Disease Control and Prevention (CDC), June 5, 2018.

Cancer begins in your cells, which are the building blocks of your body. Normally, your body forms new cells as you need them, replacing old cells that die. Sometimes this process goes wrong. New cells grow even when you do not need them, and old cells do not die when they should. These extra cells can form a mass called a "tumor." Tumors can be benign or malignant. Benign tumors are not cancerous, while malignant ones are. Cells from malignant tumors can invade nearby tissues. They can also break away and spread to other parts of the body.

Cancer is not just one disease but many diseases. There are more than 100 different types of cancer. Most cancers are named for where they start. For example, lung cancer starts in the lung, and breast cancer starts in the breast. The spread of cancer from one part of the body to another is called "metastasis." Symptoms and treatment depend on the cancer type and how advanced it is. Most treatment plans may include surgery, radiation, and/or chemotherapy. Some may involve hormone therapy, immunotherapy or other types of biologic therapy, or stem cell transplantation.

Fast Facts about Cancer and Men

The most common kinds of cancer among men in the United States are skin cancer, prostate cancer, lung cancer, and colorectal cancer.

Most prostate cancers grow slowly, and do not cause any health problems in men who have them. Treatment can cause serious side effects. Talk to your doctor before you decide to get tested or treated for prostate cancer.

A human papillomavirus (HPV) vaccine is recommended routinely for boys at 11 or 12 years of age to prevent anal cancer and genital warts. The vaccine also is recommended for all teenage boys and men through the age of 21, any man who has sex with men through the age of 26, and men with compromised immune systems (including those

151

resulted from human immunodeficiency virus (HIV)) through the age of 26, if they did not receive all doses of the vaccine when they were younger.

Tips for Lowering Your Cancer Risk

Every year, more than 300,000 men in the United States lose their lives to cancer. You can lower your cancer risk in several ways.

- Do not smoke, and avoid secondhand smoke.
- Stay up-to-date on screening tests for colorectal and lung cancer.
- Protect your skin from the sun when outdoors, and avoid indoor tanning.
- Make healthy choices, such as staying active, keeping a healthy weight, and limiting how much alcohol you drink.

Chapter 10

Alzheimer Disease

What Is Alzheimer Disease?

- The most common type of dementia

- A progressive disease, beginning with mild memory loss that possibly leads to loss of the ability to carry on a conversation and respond to the environment

- Involves the parts of the brain that control thought, memory, and language

- Can seriously affect a person's ability to carry out daily activities

Although scientists are learning more every day, right now, they still do not know what causes Alzheimer disease.

Who Has Alzheimer Disease

- In 2014, as many as five million Americans were living with Alzheimer disease.

- The symptoms of the disease can first appear after the age of 60 and the risk increases with age.

- Younger people may get Alzheimer disease, but it is less common.

This chapter includes text excerpted from "Alzheimer Disease," Centers for Disease Control and Prevention (CDC), October 1, 2018.

- The number of people living with the disease doubles every 5 years beyond the age of 65.

- This number is projected to nearly triple to 14 million people by 2060.

What Is Known about Alzheimer Disease?

Scientists do not yet fully understand what causes Alzheimer disease. There probably is not one single cause, but several factors that affect each person differently.

- Age is the best-known risk factor for Alzheimer disease.

- Family history—researchers believe that genetics may play a role in developing Alzheimer disease.

- Changes in the brain can begin years before the first symptoms appear.

- Researchers are studying whether education, diet, and environment play a role in developing Alzheimer disease.

- Scientists are finding more evidence that some of the risk factors for heart disease and stroke, such as high blood pressure and high cholesterol, may also increase the risk of Alzheimer disease.

- There is growing evidence that physical, mental, and social activities may reduce the risk of Alzheimer disease.

How Do I Know If It Is Alzheimer Disease?

Alzheimer disease is not a normal part of aging.

Memory problems are typically one of the first warning signs of cognitive loss.

According to the National Institute on Aging, in addition to memory problems, someone with Alzheimer disease may experience one or more of the following signs:

- Memory loss that disrupts daily life, such as getting lost in a familiar place or repeating questions

- Trouble handling money and paying bills

- Difficulty completing familiar tasks at home, at work, or at leisure

- Decreased or poor judgment

- Misplacing things and being unable to retrace steps to find them
- Changes in mood, personality, or behavior

If you or someone you know has several or even most of the signs listed above, it does not mean that you or they have Alzheimer disease. It is important to consult a healthcare provider when you or someone you know has concerns about memory loss, thinking skills, or behavioral changes.

- Some causes for symptoms, such as depression and drug interactions, are reversible. However, they can be serious and should be identified and treated by a healthcare provider as soon as possible.
- Early and accurate diagnosis provides opportunities for you and your family to consider or review financial planning, develop advance directives, enroll in clinical trials, and anticipate care needs.

How Is Alzheimer Disease Treated?

Medical management can improve the quality of life for individuals living with Alzheimer disease and their caregivers. There is currently no known cure for Alzheimer disease.

Treatment addresses several different areas:

- Helping people maintain mental function
- Managing behavioral symptoms
- Slowing or delaying the symptoms of the disease

Support for Family and Friends

Currently, many people living with Alzheimer disease are cared for at home by family members.

Caregiving can have positive aspects for the caregiver, as well as the person being cared for. It may bring personal fulfillment to the caregiver, such as satisfaction from helping a family member or friend, and lead to the development of new skills and improved family relationships.

Although most people willingly provide care to their loved ones and friends, caring for a person with Alzheimer disease at home can be a difficult task and might become overwhelming at times. Each day brings new challenges as the caregiver copes with changing levels of ability and new patterns of behavior. As the disease gets worse, people living with Alzheimer disease often need more intensive care.

What Is the Burden of Alzheimer Disease in the United States?

Alzheimer disease is:

- 1 of the top 10 leading causes of death in the United States
- The 6th leading cause of death among U.S. adults
- The 5th leading cause of death among adults 65 years of age or older

In 2014, an estimated 5 million Americans 65 years of age or older had Alzheimer disease. This number is projected to nearly triple to 14 million people by 2060.

In 2010, the costs of treating Alzheimer disease were projected to fall between $159 and $215 billion. By 2040, these costs are projected to jump to between $379 and more than $500 billion annually.

Death rates for Alzheimer disease are increasing, unlike heart disease and cancer death rates, which are on the decline. Dementia, including Alzheimer disease, has been shown to be underreported in death certificates; therefore, the proportion of older people who die from Alzheimer may be considerably higher.

Chapter 11

Chronic Liver Disease

Chapter Contents

Section 11.1—Viral Hepatitis.. 158

Section 11.2—Cirrhosis 159

Section 11.1

Viral Hepatitis

This section includes text excerpted from "What Is
Viral Hepatitis?" National Institute of Diabetes and Digestive and
Kidney Diseases (NIDDK), May 2017.

Your liver is one of the largest and most important organs in your body. You have only one liver. It is the size of a football and weighs about three pounds in the average-size person. It is reddish-brown. Your liver is located on the right side of your abdomen behind your lower ribs, and your ribs help to protect your liver.*

* Excerpted from "Viral Hepatitis and Liver Disease," U.S. Department of Veterans Affairs (VA), January 10, 2019.

Viral hepatitis is an infection that causes liver inflammation and damage. Inflammation is swelling that occurs when tissues of the body become injured or infected. Inflammation can damage organs. Researchers have discovered several different viruses that cause hepatitis, including hepatitis A, B, C, D, and E.

Hepatitis A and hepatitis E typically spread through contact with food or water that has been contaminated by an infected person's stool. People may also get hepatitis E by eating undercooked pork, deer, or shellfish.

Hepatitis B, hepatitis C, and hepatitis D spread through contact with an infected person's blood. Hepatitis B and D may also spread through contact with other bodily fluids. This contact can occur in many ways, including sharing drug needles or having unprotected sex.

The hepatitis A and E viruses typically cause only acute, or short-term, infections. In an acute infection, your body is able to fight off the infection, and the virus goes away.

The hepatitis B, C, and D viruses can cause acute and chronic, or long-lasting, infections. Chronic hepatitis occurs when your body is not able to fight off the hepatitis virus, and the virus does not go away. Chronic hepatitis can lead to complications, such as cirrhosis, liver failure, and liver cancer. Early diagnosis and treatment of chronic hepatitis can prevent or lower your chances of developing these complications.

When doctors cannot find the cause of a person's hepatitis, they may call this condition "non-A–E hepatitis" or "hepatitis X." Experts think that unknown viruses other than hepatitis A, B, C, D, and E may cause some cases of hepatitis. Researchers are working to identify these viruses.

Although non-A–E hepatitis is most often acute, it can become chronic.

Section 11.2

Cirrhosis

This section includes text excerpted from "Cirrhosis: A Patient's Guide," U.S. Department of Veterans Affairs (VA), October 29, 2018.

What Is Cirrhosis?

When something attacks and damages the liver, liver cells are killed and scar tissue is formed. This scarring process is called "fibrosis," and it happens little by little over many years. When the whole liver is scarred, it shrinks and gets hard. This is called "cirrhosis," and usually this damage cannot be undone.

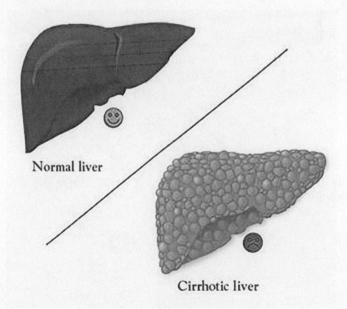

Normal liver

Cirrhotic liver

Figure 11.1. *Normal Liver and Cirrhotic Liver*

Any illness that affects the liver over a long period of time may lead to fibrosis and, eventually, cirrhosis. Heavy drinking and viruses (such as hepatitis C or hepatitis B) are common causes of cirrhosis. However, there are other causes as well. Cirrhosis may be caused by a buildup of fat in the liver of people who are overweight or have diabetes. Some people inherit genes for certain conditions that cause liver disease, such as genes that will cause iron buildup in the liver. In other diseases, bile collects in the liver and causes damage that can lead to cirrhosis. Other causes include certain prescribed and over-the-counter (OTC) medicines, environmental poisons, and autoimmune hepatitis, a condition in which a person's own immune system attacks the liver as if it were a foreign body.

What Happens When You Have Cirrhosis

Because the liver becomes lumpy and stiff in cirrhosis, blood cannot flow through it easily, so pressure builds up in the vein that brings blood to the liver. This vein is called the "portal vein." When pressure is high in the portal vein, the condition is called "portal hypertension." In order to relieve this pressure, the blood passes through other veins. Some of these veins, called "varices," can be found in the pipe that carries food from your mouth to your stomach (the esophagus) or in your stomach itself.

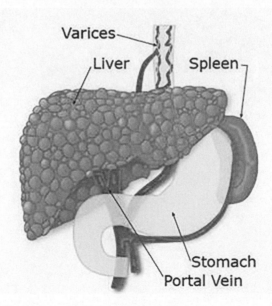

Figure 11.2. *Cirrhotic Live Detail*

When you have cirrhosis, the high pressure in the portal vein backs up into another organ called the "spleen," which gets big and destroys more platelets than usual. Platelets are blood particles that help with blood clotting.

When you have cirrhosis, entrance of blood to the liver is blocked and substances, such as ammonia that would normally be cleaned by the liver, escape into the general circulation. Aside from the problems with liver blood flow, when cirrhosis is advanced, there are not enough healthy worker cells to get all the work done, so these cells cannot make the good substances such as albumin and clotting factors that the liver normally makes.

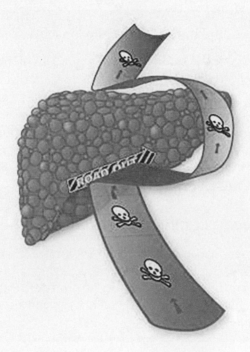

Figure 11.3. *Liver Cirrhosis*

Liver cancer, called "hepatocellular carcinoma" (HCC), can also occur in cirrhosis when some of the sick liver cells start to multiply out of control.

What Are the Symptoms of Cirrhosis?

At first, you may have no symptoms at all (this is called "compensated cirrhosis"). In fact, a person may live many years with cirrhosis without being aware that her or his liver is scarred. This is because the pressure in the portal vein is not yet too high, and there are still enough healthy liver cells to keep up with the body's needs.

But if nothing is done about the cause of cirrhosis (if you continue to drink, for example) or if your hepatitis is not treated, the pressure in the portal vein gets higher and the few remaining worker cells get overwhelmed.

Then, you may notice symptoms such as low energy, poor appetite, weight loss, or loss of muscle mass. You can also develop the following serious problems:

1. Internal bleeding from large blood vessels in the esophagus, called "bleeding varices"

2. A buildup of fluid in the belly, called "ascites"

3. Confusion from the buildup of toxins in the blood, called "encephalopathy"

4. Yellowing of the eyes and skin, called "jaundice"

As mentioned earlier, another serious complication of cirrhosis is liver cancer, which may occur in the compensated or decompensated stage. There may be no signs of liver cancer until the cancer has grown very large and causes pain.

What Is Decompensated Cirrhosis?

If you experience any of the serious problems described below, your disease has progressed from compensated cirrhosis to decompensated cirrhosis. You are then at risk of dying from life-threatening complications of liver disease unless your sick liver can be replaced with a healthy liver (liver transplant).

Bleeding Varices

Large blood vessels (varices) in the food tube get bigger and bigger over time and can burst open. When this happens, you may vomit blood or notice that your stool is black and tarry. If either of these things happens, you should go to the emergency room immediately to get help and stop the bleeding.

The risk of bleeding from varices can be reduced by taking special blood pressure medicines (called "beta-blockers") or by a special procedure in which tiny rubber bands are tied around the varices.

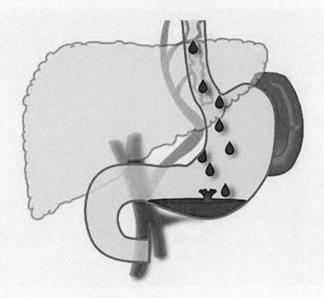

Figure 11.4. *Internal Bleeding*

Ascites

Another problem caused by high pressure in the veins of the liver is ascites. Fluid leaks out into the belly, and it begins to fill it up. This can make the abdomen enlarge like a balloon filled with water. The legs can get swollen too. This can be very uncomfortable. Eating can be a problem because there is less room for food. Even breathing can be a problem, especially when you are lying down. But the most dangerous problem associated with ascites is infection, which can be life-threatening. Ascites may go away with a low-salt diet and with diuretics (water pills) ordered by your provider. But sometimes, a provider must actually drain the fluid from the belly using a special kind of needle.

Encephalopathy

A liver that is working poorly may not be able to get rid of toxic substances, such as ammonia (which comes from the intestines), and it may allow these substances to go into the brain and cause confusion.

Besides confusion, toxins in the brain cause changes in your sleep, your mood, your concentration, and your memory. If it gets really bad, these toxins can even cause a coma. These changes are all symptoms of hepatic encephalopathy. If you have encephalopathy, you may have problems driving, writing, calculating, and performing other activities of daily living. Signs of encephalopathy are trembling and hand "flapping."

Encephalopathy may occur when you have an infection or when you have internal bleeding, and it may also occur if you are constipated or take too many water pills or take tranquilizers or sleeping pills. Your doctor might recommend lactulose. Lactulose is a syrup that makes your bowels move more often (up to two or three times a day) and helps get rid of ammonia.

Jaundice

A liver that is working poorly cannot get rid of bilirubin, a substance that produces jaundice. Too much alcohol and some medicines can also lead to jaundice.

How Do You Know If You Have Cirrhosis?

Often, you cannot know whether you have cirrhosis until the disease is advanced. Only your healthcare provider can tell you if you have cirrhosis.

There are many signs of cirrhosis that your provider may find. You may have red palms or small spider-like veins on your face or your body. You may have developed fluid in your abdomen.

Your provider may do some blood tests that point to cirrhosis. Other tests can also give your provider a good idea of whether you have cirrhosis, such as an ultrasound, a computed tomography (CAT) scan, magnetic resonance imaging (MRI), or a liver-spleen scan.

Sometimes, you may need a liver biopsy. A liver biopsy shows how much scarring your liver has and will help your healthcare provider figure out what is causing the damage and how best to treat it.

What Will Your Healthcare Provider Do about Cirrhosis?

People with cirrhosis need to see a healthcare provider from time to time. If you have compensated cirrhosis, these visits may be scheduled every year or even as often as every three to six months. These visits will let your provider watch for the development of complications. The provider can order the screening tests that can catch these complications early. Then, they can be treated or even delayed.

If you have decompensated cirrhosis, you may need to see your provider more often so that the complications that have developed already can be managed well.

People with cirrhosis have to have an upper endoscopy from time to time. This is a test in which you swallow a thin tube with a camera so that your provider can look for varices in the esophagus (food tube) and the stomach. If you have no varices, the endoscopy will be repeated every few years to see whether they show up. If you have large varices, you will get treatment to reduce the chance of bleeding.

You also will have a blood test and an ultrasound (or sometimes a CAT scan or an MRI) to look for signs of liver cancer and to check for ascites. It is important for your healthcare provider to look for cancer on a regular basis. If the cancer is caught early, there are often ways to treat it. If fluid is found in your belly, medications (for example, water pills) and changes in your diet (like a low-salt diet) may help control this fluid. If these methods stop working, you can have a procedure called "paracentesis." This procedure is used when your belly gets large and hard, which may happen every so often. You will go to a special procedures department where a trained provider will empty your belly of fluid using a special needle.

If you have developed decompensated cirrhosis, your provider may discuss the need for you to be considered for a liver transplant. You will want a healthcare provider who really knows you and can help you to decide if a transplant is right for you. Your provider will help you find out if your body can tolerate this operation and if it can help you and your loved ones get ready for the transplant procedure.

What Can You Do about Your Cirrhosis?

The most important thing you can do is to stop harming your liver and stick to the treatment prescribed by your provider. The following checklists are guides to taking care of your liver and keeping you well.

Put a check in the boxes next to the statements that show what you have done or are going to do to take care of your liver.

___ I am not drinking alcohol or using street drugs.

___ I always take the medications that my provider has ordered for me. I know their names and what each medication is for.

___ I keep all of my medical appointments.

___ I tell my provider if I am taking over-the-counter or herbal medications.

___ I have been tested to see whether I need to get the hepatitis A and B vaccines (hepatitis A and B are viruses that attack the liver).

___ I have received the pneumonia vaccine, and I get my annual flu shot (people with cirrhosis are more likely to get infections).

___ I eat a well-balanced diet that is low in fat and includes enough protein.

___ I keep a healthy weight.

___ I make sure to have a balance of work, rest, and exercise in my life.

___ I cope well with stress (or I ask for guidance when I cannot cope).

___ I tell my healthcare provider if I am depressed.

___ I have never smoked cigarettes, I have quit smoking, or I have discussed quitting with my healthcare provider.

___ I have asked my healthcare provider whether I need a liver transplant.

Put a check in the boxes next to the actions you are careful about.

___ I know what my medications are and when I have to take them.

___ I do not take pain pills, such as ibuprofen (Motrin®, Advil®) or Naprosyn (Aleve®), especially if I have ascites.

___ I do not take too many Tylenol® (acetaminophen) pills, and I never take Tylenol with alcohol. I read the labels and know the contents of all my medicines.

___ I cut down on salt (sodium), read food labels, and avoid canned or prepared foods, especially if I have ascites.

___ I avoid sleeping pills or tranquilizers.

___ If my provider tells me to take lactulose, I take enough to move my bowels two or three times a day.

___ I never let myself get constipated. If it happens, I tell my healthcare provider.

Stop and think! Put a check in the boxes next to the things you always do when you see your healthcare provider.

___ I always bring a written list of my medicines and their doses.

___ I tell my healthcare provider if I have pain in my belly.

___ I tell my healthcare provider if I have fevers or chills.

___ I tell my healthcare provider if I have black or tarry stool.

___ I keep track of my weight and tell my healthcare provider if I am getting too heavy or too skinny.

___ I mention if my belly seems bigger or my ankles are swollen.

___ I tell my healthcare provider if I am sleeping during the day, if I am confused, or if I cannot focus or drive.

___ I tell my healthcare provider if I am constipated.

When to Go to the Emergency Room

Use the following guidelines to determine if you need to go to the emergency room.

Danger

- Go to the emergency room (or call 911, say you have cirrhosis, and tell them what is happening)

Bleeding

- My stools are black and tarry.
- I am vomiting blood.

Confusion

- My head is cloudy.
- I am so confused and sleepy I cannot do anything.

Fever

- I have a fever and I cannot stop shaking.

Jaundice

- My eyes are suddenly turning yellow.

What You and Your Provider Should Do to Take Good Care of Your Liver

You and your provider can do the following things to keep your liver as healthy as possible for as long as possible. (Use this list in discussion with your provider.)

- Schedule liver clinic visits every six months, or more often if you have decompensated cirrhosis.
- Have blood tests (to see how well the liver is working and to check for liver cancer) and an ultrasound (or CT or MRI) every 6 to 12 months.
- Have an endoscopy to screen for varices (repeated every few years if you have no varices or only small ones).

- Take medicines called "beta-blockers" when varices are large to reduce the chance of bleeding.

- Take medicines called "diuretics" (spironolactone alone or with furosemide) to decrease ascites, and have regular blood tests to check for kidney health.

- Talk about how much alcohol you are drinking at every clinic visit.

- Go over your medicine list at every clinic visit.

- Talk about whether and when a liver transplant workup should be started for you

- Discuss and update your Child-Pugh-Turcotte (CPT) score and your MELD score at each visit. These scores are ratings that tell how sick your liver is and how urgently you need a transplant.

Chapter 12

Chronic Obstructive Pulmonary Disease

What Is Chronic Obstructive Pulmonary Disease?

Chronic obstructive pulmonary disease, or COPD, refers to a group of diseases that cause airflow blockage and breathing-related problems. It includes emphysema and chronic bronchitis.

What Are the Symptoms of Chronic Obstructive Pulmonary Disease?

Symptoms of COPD include:

- Frequent coughing or wheezing
- Excess phlegm, mucus, or sputum production
- Shortness of breath
- Trouble taking a deep breath

Who Has Chronic Obstructive Pulmonary Disease?

Chronic lower respiratory disease, primarily COPD, was the third leading cause of death in the United States in 2014. Almost 15.7 million

This chapter includes text excerpted from "Basics about COPD," Centers for Disease Control and Prevention (CDC), June 5, 2018.

169

Americans (6.4%) reported that they have been diagnosed with COPD. More than 50 percent of adults with low pulmonary function were not aware that they had COPD, so the actual number may be higher. The following groups were more likely to report COPD in 2013.

- People between 65 to 74 years of age and those older than 75 years of age
- American Indians/Alaska Natives and multiracial non-Hispanics
- Women
- People who were unemployed, retired, or unable to work
- People with less than a high-school education
- People who were divorced, widowed, or separated
- Current or former smokers
- People with a history of asthma

What Causes Chronic Obstructive Pulmonary Disease

In the United States, tobacco smoke is a key factor in the development and progression of COPD. Exposure to air pollutants in the home and workplace, genetic factors, and respiratory infections also play a role. In the developing world, indoor air quality is thought to play a larger role than it does in the United States. People should try to avoid inhaling tobacco smoke, home and workplace air pollutants, and respiratory infections to prevent developing COPD. Early detection of COPD may change its course and progress.

What Are the Complications or Effects of Chronic Obstructive Pulmonary Disease?

Compared to adults without COPD, those with this disease are more likely to:

- Have activity limitations, such as difficulty walking or climbing stairs
- Be unable to work
- Need special equipment, such as portable oxygen tanks
- Not engage in social activities, such as eating out, going to places of worship, going to group events, or getting together with friends or neighbors

- Have increased confusion or memory loss

- Have more emergency room visits or overnight hospital stays

- Have other chronic diseases, such as arthritis, congestive heart failure, diabetes, coronary heart disease, stroke, or asthma

- Have depression or other mental or emotional conditions

- Report a fair or poor health status

How Is Chronic Obstructive Pulmonary Disease Treated?

Treatment of COPD requires a careful and thorough evaluation by a physician. COPD treatment can alleviate symptoms, decrease the frequency and severity of exacerbations, and increase exercise tolerance. Treatment options that your physician may consider include:

- **Quit smoking.** For people who smoke, the most important part of treatment is smoking cessation.

- **Avoid tobacco smoke and other air pollutants** at home and at work.

- **Ask your doctor about pulmonary rehabilitation,** which is a personalized treatment program that teaches COPD management strategies to improve quality of life. Programs may include plans that teach people how to breathe better and conserve their energy, as well as provide advice on food and exercise.

- **Take medication.** Symptoms such as coughing or wheezing can be treated with medication.

- **Avoid lung infections.** Lung infections can cause serious problems in people with COPD. Certain vaccines, such as flu and pneumococcal vaccines, are especially important for people with COPD. Respiratory infections should be treated with antibiotics, if appropriate.

- **Use supplemental oxygen.** Some people may need to use a portable oxygen tank if their blood oxygen levels are low.

the colon or
reaming tests

Chapter 13

Colorectal Cancer

The entire colon is about 5 feet (150 cm) long, and is divided into five major segments. The rectum is the last anatomic segment before the anus.

The ascending and descending colon are supported by peritoneal folds called "mesentery."

The right colon consists of the cecum, ascending colon, hepatic flexure and the right half of the transverse colon. The left colon consists of the left half of the transverse colon, splenic flexure, descending colon, and sigmoid.

What Is Colorectal Cancer?

Colorectal cancer is cancer that occurs in the colon or rectum. Sometimes, it is called "colon cancer" for short. The colon is the large intestine or large bowel. The rectum is the passageway that connects the colon to the anus.

Sometimes abnormal growths, called "polyps," form in the colon or rectum. Over time, some polyps may turn into cancer. Screening tests can find polyps, so they can be removed before turning into cancer.

This chapter contains text excerpted from the following sources: Text in this chapter begins with excerpts from "Anatomy of Colon and Rectum," National Cancer Institute (NCI), August 15, 2003. Reviewed June 2019; Text beginning with the heading "What Is Colorectal Cancer?" is excerpted from "What Is Colorectal Cancer?" Centers for Disease Control and Prevention (CDC), January 30, 2019.

Screening also helps find colorectal cancer at an early stage, when treatment works best.

What Are the Risk Factors for Colorectal Cancer?

Your risk of getting colorectal cancer increases as you get older. More than 90 percent of cases occur in people who are 50 years of age or older. Other risk factors include having:

- Inflammatory bowel disease (IBD), such as Crohn disease or ulcerative colitis
- A personal or family history of colorectal cancer or colorectal polyps
- A genetic syndrome, such as familial adenomatous polyposis (FAP) or hereditary nonpolyposis colorectal cancer (Lynch syndrome)

Lifestyle factors that may contribute to an increased risk of colorectal cancer include:

- Lack of regular physical activity
- A diet low in fruit and vegetables
- A low-fiber and high-fat diet, or a diet high in processed meats
- Overweight and obesity
- Alcohol consumption
- Tobacco use

What Can I Do to Reduce My Risk of Colorectal Cancer?

Overall, the most effective way to reduce your risk of colorectal cancer is to get screened for colorectal cancer routinely, beginning at the age of 50.

Almost all colorectal cancers begin as precancerous polyps in the colon or rectum. Such polyps can be present in the colon for years before invasive cancer develops. They may not cause any symptoms, especially early on. Colorectal cancer screening can find precancerous polyps, so they can be removed before they turn into cancer. In this way, colorectal cancer is prevented. Screening can also find colorectal cancer early, when there is a greater chance that treatment will be most effective and lead to a cure.

Diet

Research is underway to find out if changes to your diet can reduce your colorectal cancer risk. Medical experts often recommend a diet low in animal fats and high in fruits, vegetables, and whole grains to reduce the risk of other chronic diseases, such as coronary artery disease (CAD) and diabetes. This diet also may reduce the risk of colorectal cancer.

Aspirin

Researchers are looking at the role of some medicines and supplements in preventing colorectal cancer. The U.S. Preventive Services Task Force (USPSTF) found that taking low-dose aspirin can help prevent cardiovascular disease and colorectal cancer in some adults, depending on age and risk factors.

Healthy Choices

Some studies suggest that people may reduce their risk of developing colorectal cancer by increasing their physical activity, limiting their alcohol consumption, and avoiding tobacco.

What Are the Symptoms of Colorectal Cancer?

Colorectal polyps and colorectal cancer do not always cause symptoms, especially at first. Someone could have polyps or colorectal cancer and not know it. That is why getting screened regularly for colorectal cancer is so important.

If you have symptoms, they may include:

- Blood in or on your stool (bowel movement)
- Stomach pain, aches, or cramps that do not go away
- Losing weight and you do not know why

If you have any of these symptoms, talk to your doctor. They may be caused by something other than cancer. The only way to know what is causing them is to see your doctor.

What Should I Know about Screening?
What Is Colorectal Cancer Screening?

A screening test is used to look for a disease when a person does not have symptoms. (When a person has symptoms, diagnostic tests are used to find out the cause of the symptoms.)

Colorectal cancer almost always develops from precancerous polyps in the colon or rectum. Screening tests can find precancerous polyps, so that they can be removed before they turn into cancer. Screening tests can also find colorectal cancer early, when treatment works best.

Screening Guidelines

Regular screening, beginning at the age of 50, is the key to preventing colorectal cancer. The USPSTF recommends that adults between the ages 50 and 75 be screened for colorectal cancer. The USPSTF also recommends that adults between 76 and 85 years of age ask their doctor if they should be screened.

The USPSTF recommends several colorectal cancer screening strategies, including stool tests, flexible sigmoidoscopy, colonoscopy, and computed tomography (CT) colonography (virtual colonoscopy).

When Should I Begin to Get Screened?

You should begin screening for colorectal cancer soon after turning 50 years of age, then continue getting screened at regular intervals. However, you may need to be tested before reaching 50 years of age, or more often than other people, if:

- You or a close relative has had colorectal polyps or colorectal cancer.

- You have an inflammatory bowel disease, such as Crohn disease or ulcerative colitis.

- You have a genetic syndrome, such as FAP or Lynch syndrome.

If you think you are at an increased risk for colorectal cancer, speak with your doctor about:

- When to begin screening

- Which test is right for you

- How often to get tested

Insurance and Medicare Coverage

Most insurance plans and Medicare help pay for colorectal cancer screening for people who are 50 years of age or older. Colorectal cancer screening tests may be covered by your health insurance policy without a deductible or co-pay.

Colorectal Cancer Screening Tests

The U.S. Preventive Services Task Force recommends that adults between the ages of 50 and 75 be screened for colorectal cancer. The decision to be screened after the age of 75 should be made on an individual basis. If you are older than 75 years of age, ask your doctor if you should be screened. People at an increased risk of getting colorectal cancer should talk to their doctor about when to begin screening, which test is right for them, and how often to get tested.

Several screening tests can be used to find polyps or colorectal cancer. The USPSTF outlines the following colorectal cancer screening strategies. Talk to your doctor about which test is right for you.

Stool Tests

- The **guaiac-based fecal occult blood test (gFOBT)** uses the chemical guaiac to detect blood in the stool. It is done once a year. For this test, you receive a test kit from your healthcare provider. At home, you use a stick or brush to obtain a small amount of stool. You return the test kit to the doctor or a lab, where the stool samples are checked for the presence of blood.

- The **fecal immunochemical test (FIT)** uses antibodies to detect blood in the stool. It is also done once a year in the same way as a gFOBT.

- The **FIT-DNA test** (also referred to as the "stool DNA test") combines the FIT with a test that detects altered DNA in the stool. For this test, you collect an entire bowel movement and send it to a lab, where it is checked for cancer cells. It is done once every one or three years.

Flexible Sigmoidoscopy

For this test, the doctor puts a short, thin, flexible, lighted tube into your rectum. The doctor checks for polyps or cancer inside the rectum and lower third of the colon.

How often: Every 5 years, or every 10 years with a FIT every year.

Colonoscopy

This is similar to flexible sigmoidoscopy, except the doctor uses a longer, thin, flexible, lighted tube to check for polyps or cancer inside the rectum and the entire colon. During the test, the doctor can find and remove most polyps and some cancers. Colonoscopy also is used as a follow-up test if anything unusual is found during one of the other screening tests.

How often: Every 10 years (for people who do not have an increased risk of colorectal cancer).

Computed Tomography Colonography (Virtual Colonoscopy)

Computed tomography (CT) colonography, also called a "virtual colonoscopy," uses X-rays and computers to produce images of the entire colon, which are displayed on a computer screen for the doctor to analyze.

How often: Every 5 years.

How Do I Know Which Screening Test Is Right for Me?

There is no single "best test" for any person. Each test has advantages and disadvantages. Talk to your doctor about the pros and cons of each test, and how often to be tested. Which test to use depends on:

• Your preferences

• Your medical condition

• The likelihood that you will get the test

• The resources available for testing and follow-up

Questions to Ask Your Doctor about Colorectal Cancer
Ask Your Doctor

Do I need to get a screening test for colorectal cancer?

• What screening test(s) do you recommend for me? Why?

• How do I prepare? Do I need to change my diet or my usual medication before taking the test?

• What is involved in the test? Will it be uncomfortable or painful?

• Is there any risk involved?

• When and from whom will I get results?

If you are having a colonoscopy or sigmoidoscopy, you will want to know:

- Who will do the exam?
- Will I need someone with me?

If You Are at an Increased Risk

Some people are at an increased risk because they have inflammatory bowel disease; a personal or family history of colorectal polyps or colorectal cancer; or genetic syndromes, such as FAP or Lynch syndrome. These people may need to start screening earlier than the age of 50. If you believe you are at an increased risk, ask your doctor if you should begin screening earlier.

If You Are Having Symptoms

Tell your doctor if you have any of these symptoms:

- Blood in or on your stool (bowel movement)
- Stomach pain, aches, or cramps that do not go away
- Losing weight and you do not know why

These symptoms may be caused by something other than cancer, but the only way to know what is causing them is to speak with your doctor about them.

Chapter 14

Diabetes

Diabetes is a chronic (long-lasting) health condition that affects how your body turns food into energy.

Most of the food you eat is broken down into sugar (also called "glucose") and released into your bloodstream. When your blood sugar goes up, it signals your pancreas to release insulin. Insulin acts like a key to let the blood sugar into your body's cells for use as energy.

If you have diabetes, your body either does not make enough insulin or cannot use the insulin it makes as well as it should. When there is not enough insulin or cells stop responding to insulin, too much blood sugar stays in your bloodstream. Over time, that can cause serious health problems, such as heart disease, vision loss, and kidney disease.

There is not a cure yet for diabetes, but losing weight, eating healthy food, and being active can really help. Taking medicine as needed, getting diabetes self-management education and support, and keeping healthcare appointments can also reduce the impact of diabetes on your life.

Types of Diabetes

There are three main types of diabetes: type 1, type 2, and gestational diabetes (diabetes while pregnant).

This chapter includes text excerpted from "About Diabetes," Centers for Disease Control and Prevention (CDC), June 1, 2017.

Type 1 diabetes is thought to be caused by an autoimmune reaction (the body attacks itself by mistake) that stops your body from making insulin. About five percent of the people who have diabetes have type 1. Symptoms of type 1 diabetes often develop quickly. It is usually diagnosed in children, teens, and young adults. If you have type 1 diabetes, you will need to take insulin every day to survive. Nowadays, no one knows how to prevent type 1 diabetes.

With type 2 diabetes, your body does not use insulin well and cannot keep blood sugar at normal levels. About 90 percent of people with diabetes have type 2. It develops over many years and is usually diagnosed in adults (but it has been occurring more in children, teens, and young adults). You may not notice any symptoms, so it is important to get your blood sugar tested if you are at risk. Type 2 diabetes can be prevented or delayed with healthy lifestyle changes, such as losing weight, eating healthy food, and being active.

Prediabetes

In the United States, 84.1 million adults—more than 1 in 3—have prediabetes. What is more, 90 percent of them do not know they have it. With prediabetes, blood sugar levels are higher than normal but not high enough yet to be diagnosed as type 2 diabetes. Prediabetes raises your risk for type 2 diabetes, heart disease, and stroke. The good news is if you have prediabetes, a Centers for Disease Control and Prevention (CDC)-recognized lifestyle change program can help you take healthy steps to reverse it.

Who Is at Risk?
Prediabetes

You are at risk for developing prediabetes if you:

- Are overweight

- Are 45 years of age or older

- Have a parent, brother, or sister with type 2 diabetes

- Are physically active less than three times a week nine

- Are African American, Hispanic/Latinx American, American Indian, or Alaska Native.

You can prevent or reverse prediabetes with simple, proven lifestyle changes, such as losing weight if you are overweight, eating healthier, and getting regular physical activity.

Type 2 Diabetes

You are at risk for developing type 2 diabetes if you:

- Have prediabetes
- Are overweight
- Are 45 years of age or older
- Have a parent, brother, or sister with type 2 diabetes
- Are physically active less than three times a week
- Have ever had gestational diabetes (diabetes during pregnancy) or given birth to a baby who weighed more than nine pounds
- Are African American, Hispanic/Latinx American, American Indian, or Alaska Native.

You can prevent or delay type 2 diabetes with simple, proven lifestyle changes, such as losing weight if you are overweight, eating healthier, and getting regular physical activity.

Type 1 Diabetes

Type 1 diabetes is thought to be caused by an immune reaction. Risk factors for type 1 diabetes are not as clear as for prediabetes and type 2 diabetes. Known risk factors include:

- **Family history:** Having a parent, brother, or sister with type 1 diabetes
- **Age:** You can get type 1 diabetes at any age, but it is more likely to develop when you are a child, teen, or young adult.

In the United States, Whites are more likely to develop type 1 diabetes than African Americans and Hispanic/Latinx Americans.

Symptoms

If you have any of the following diabetes symptoms, see your doctor about getting your blood sugar tested.

- Urinate a lot, often at night
- Are very thirsty
- Lose weight without trying
- Are very hungry

- Have blurry vision

- Have numb or tingling hands or feet

- Feel very tired

- Have very dry skin

- Have sores that heal slowly

- Have more infections than usual

People who have type 1 diabetes may also have nausea, vomiting, or stomach pains. Type 1 diabetes symptoms can develop in just a few weeks or months, and they can be severe. Type 1 diabetes usually starts when you are a child, teen, or young adult but can happen at any age.

Type 2 diabetes symptoms often develop over several years and can go on for a long time without being noticed (sometimes there are not any noticeable symptoms at all). Type 2 diabetes usually starts when you are an adult, though more and more children, teens, and young adults are developing it. Because symptoms are hard to spot, it is important to know the risk factors for type 2 diabetes and visit your doctor if you have any of them.

Prediabetes: Your Chance to Prevent Type 2 Diabetes
What Is Prediabetes?

Prediabetes is a serious health condition where blood sugar levels are higher than normal, but they are not high enough yet to be diagnosed as type 2 diabetes. Approximately 84 million American adults— more than 1 out of 3—have prediabetes. Of those with prediabetes, 90 percent do not know they have it. Prediabetes puts you at an increased risk of developing type 2 diabetes, heart disease, and stroke.

The good news is that if you have prediabetes, the CDC-led National Diabetes Prevention Program can help you make lifestyle changes to prevent or delay type 2 diabetes and other serious health problems.

What Causes Prediabetes

Insulin is a hormone made by your pancreas that acts like a key to let blood sugar into cells for use as energy. If you have prediabetes, the cells in your body do not respond normally to insulin. Your pancreas makes more insulin to try to get cells to respond. Eventually, your pancreas cannot keep up, and your blood sugar rises, setting the stage for prediabetes—and type 2 diabetes down the road.

Signs and Symptoms

You can have prediabetes for years but have no clear symptoms, so it often goes undetected until serious health problems, such as type 2 diabetes, show up. It is important to talk to your doctor about getting your blood sugar tested if you have any of the risk factors for prediabetes, which include:

- Being overweight

- Being 45 years of age or older

- Having a parent, brother, or sister with type 2 diabetes

- Being physically active less than three times a week

- Ever having gestational diabetes (diabetes during pregnancy) or giving birth to a baby who weighed more than nine pounds

Race and ethnicity are also a factor: African Americans, Hispanic/ Latinx Americans, American Indians, Pacific Islanders, and some Asian Americans are at higher risk.

Simple Blood Sugar Test

You can get a simple blood sugar test to find out if you have prediabetes. Ask your doctor if you should be tested.

Preventing Type 2 Diabetes

If you have prediabetes, losing a small amount of weight if you are overweight and getting regular physical activity can lower your risk for developing type 2 diabetes. A small amount of weight loss means around 5 to 7 percent of your body weight, just 10 to 14 pounds for a 200-pound person. Regular physical activity means getting at least 150 minutes a week of brisk walking or a similar activity. That is just 30 minutes a day, 5 days a week.

A lifestyle change program offered through the CDC-led National Diabetes Prevention Program can help you make those changes—and make them stick. Through the program, you can lower your risk of developing type 2 diabetes by as much as 58 percent (71 percent if you are over the age of 60). Highlights include:

- Working with a trained coach to make realistic, lasting lifestyle changes

- Discovering how to eat healthy and how to add more physical activity into your day

- Finding out how to manage stress, stay motivated, and solve problems that can slow your progress

- Getting support from people with similar goals and challenges

Ask your doctor or nurse if there is a CDC-recognized National Diabetes Prevention Program offered in your community. The best time to prevent type 2 diabetes is now.

Type 1 Diabetes

Type 1 diabetes (previously called "insulin-dependent" or "juvenile diabetes") is usually diagnosed in children, teens, and young adults, but it can develop at any age.

If you have type 1 diabetes, your pancreas is not making insulin or is making very little. Insulin is a hormone that enables blood sugar to enter the cells in your body where it can be used for energy. Without insulin, blood sugar cannot get into cells and builds up in the bloodstream. High blood sugar is damaging to the body and causes many of the symptoms and complications of diabetes.

Type 1 diabetes is less common than type 2—about five percent of people with diabetes have type 1. Nowadays, no one knows how to prevent type 1 diabetes, but it can be managed by following your doctor's recommendations for living a healthy lifestyle, controlling your blood sugar, getting regular health checkups, and getting diabetes self-management education.

Causes

Type 1 diabetes is caused by an autoimmune reaction that destroys the cells in the pancreas that make insulin, called "beta cells." This process can go on for months or years before any symptoms appear.

Some people have certain genes (traits passed on from parent to child) that make them more likely to develop type 1 diabetes, though many will not go on to have type 1 diabetes even if they have the genes. Being exposed to a trigger in the environment, such as a virus, is also thought to play a part in developing type 1 diabetes. Diet and lifestyle habits do not cause type 1 diabetes.

Symptoms and Risk Factors

It can take months or years for enough beta cells to be destroyed before symptoms of type 1 diabetes are noticed. Type 1 diabetes symptoms can develop in just a few weeks or months. Once symptoms appear, they can be severe.

Some type 1 diabetes symptoms are similar to symptoms of other health conditions. Do not guess—if you think you could have type 1 diabetes, see your doctor right away to get your blood sugar tested. Untreated diabetes can lead to very serious—even fatal—health problems.

Risk factors for type 1 diabetes are not as clear as for prediabetes and type 2 diabetes, though family history is known to play a part.

Getting Tested

A simple blood test will let you know if you have diabetes. If you have gotten your blood sugar tested at a health fair or pharmacy, follow up at a clinic or doctor's office to make sure the results are accurate.

If your doctor thinks you have type 1 diabetes, your blood may also tested for autoantibodies (substances that indicate your body is attacking itself) that are often present with type 1 diabetes but not with type 2. You may have your urine tested for ketones (produced when your body burns fat for energy), which also indicate type 1 diabetes instead of type 2.

Management

Unlike many health conditions, diabetes is managed mostly by you, with support from your healthcare team (including your primary care doctor, foot doctor, dentist, eye doctor, registered dietitian nutritionist, diabetes educator, and pharmacist), family, teachers, and other important people in your life. Managing diabetes can be challenging, but everything you do to improve your health is worth it.

If you have type 1 diabetes, you will need to take insulin shots (or wear an insulin pump) every day to manage your blood sugar levels and get the energy your body needs. Insulin cannot be taken as a pill because the acid in your stomach would destroy it before it could get into your bloodstream. Your doctor will work with you to figure out the most effective type and dosage of insulin for you.

You will also need to check your blood sugar regularly. Ask your doctor how often you should check it and what your target blood sugar levels should be. Keeping your blood sugar levels as close to target as possible will help you prevent or delay diabetes-related complications.

Stress is a part of life, but it can make managing diabetes harder, including controlling your blood sugar levels and dealing with daily diabetes care. Regular physical activity, getting enough sleep, and relaxation exercises can help. Talk to your doctor and diabetes educator about these and other ways you can manage stress.

Healthy lifestyle habits are really important too, and include:

- Making healthy food choices

- Being physically active

- Controlling your blood pressure

- Controlling your cholesterol

Make regular appointments with your healthcare team to be sure you are on track with your treatment plan and to get help with new ideas and strategies if needed.

Whether you just got diagnosed with type 1 diabetes or have had it for some time, meeting with a diabetes educator is a great way to get support and guidance, including how to:

- Develop and stick to a healthy eating and activity plan

- Test your blood sugar and keep a record of the results

- Recognize the signs of high or low blood sugar and what to do about it

- Give yourself insulin by syringe, pen, or pump

- Monitor your feet, skin, and eyes to catch problems early

- Buy diabetes supplies and store them properly

- Manage stress and deal with daily diabetes care

Ask your doctor about diabetes self-management education and to recommend a diabetes educator.

Hypoglycemia

Hypoglycemia can happen quickly and needs to be treated icon immediately. It is most often caused by too much insulin, waiting too long for a meal or snack, not eating enough, or getting extra physical activity. Hypoglycemia symptoms are different from person to person; make sure you know your specific symptoms, which could include:

- Shakiness

- Nervousness or anxiety

- Sweating, chills, or clamminess

- Irritability or impatience

- Dizziness and difficulty concentrating

- Hunger or nausea

- Blurred vision

- Weakness or fatigue

- Anger, stubbornness, or sadness

If you have hypoglycemia several times a week, talk to your doctor to see if your treatment needs to be adjusted.

Type 2 Diabetes

More than 30 million Americans have diabetes (about 1 in 10), and 90 to 95 percent of them have type 2 diabetes. Type 2 diabetes most often develops in people over the age of 45, but more and more children, teens, and young adults are also developing it.

Causes

If you have type 2 diabetes, cells do not respond normally to insulin; this is called "insulin resistance." Your pancreas makes more insulin to try to get cells to respond. Eventually your pancreas cannot keep up, and your blood sugar rises, setting the stage for prediabetes and type 2 diabetes. High blood sugar is damaging to the body and can cause other serious health problems, such as heart disease, vision loss, and kidney disease.

Symptoms and Risk Factors

Type 2 diabetes symptoms often develop over several years and can go on for a long time without being noticed (sometimes there are not any noticeable symptoms at all). Because symptoms can be hard to spot, it is important to know the risk factors for type 2 diabetes and to see your doctor to get your blood sugar tested if you have any of them.

Getting Tested

A simple blood test will let you know if you have diabetes. If you have gotten your blood sugar tested at a health fair or pharmacy, follow up at a clinic or doctor's office to make sure the results are accurate.

Management

Unlike many health conditions, diabetes is managed mostly by you, with support from your healthcare team (including your primary care doctor, foot doctor, dentist, eye doctor, registered dietitian nutritionist, diabetes educator, and pharmacist), family, and other important people in your life. Managing diabetes can be challenging, but everything you do to improve your health is worth it.

You may be able to manage your type 2 diabetes with healthy eating and being active, or your doctor may prescribe insulin, other injectable medications, or oral diabetes medicines to help control your blood sugar and avoid complications. You will still need to eat healthy and be active if you take insulin or other medicines. It is also important to keep your blood pressure and cholesterol under control and get necessary screening tests.

You will need to check your blood sugar regularly. Ask your doctor how often you should check it and what your target blood sugar levels should be. Keeping your blood sugar levels as close to target as possible will help you prevent or delay diabetes-related complications.

Stress is a part of life, but it can make managing diabetes harder, including controlling your blood sugar levels and dealing with daily diabetes care. Regular physical activity, getting enough sleep, and relaxation exercises can help. Talk to your doctor and diabetes educator about these and other ways you can manage stress.

Make regular appointments with your healthcare team to be sure you are on track with your treatment plan and to get help with new ideas and strategies if needed.

Whether you just got diagnosed with diabetes or have had it for some time, meeting with a diabetes educator is a great way to get support and guidance, including how to:

- Develop a healthy eating and activity plan

- Test your blood sugar and keep a record of the results

- Recognize the signs of high or low blood sugar and what to do about it

- If needed, give yourself insulin by syringe, pen, or pump

- Monitor your feet, skin, and eyes to catch problems early
- Buy diabetes supplies and store them properly
- Manage stress and deal with daily diabetes care

Ask your doctor about diabetes self-management education and to recommend a diabetes educator.

Type 2 Diabetes and Youth

Childhood obesity rates are rising, and so are the rates of type 2 diabetes in youth. More than 75 percent of children with type 2 diabetes have a close relative who has it too. But, it is not always because family members are related; it can also be because they share certain habits that can increase their risk. Parents can help prevent or delay type 2 diabetes by developing a healthy lifestyle plan for the whole family that includes:

- Drinking more water and fewer sugary drinks
- Eating more fruits and vegetables
- Making favorite foods healthier
- Making physical activity more fun

Healthy changes become habits more easily when everyone makes them together.

Getting Tested

You will need to get your blood sugar tested to find out for sure if you have prediabetes or type 1, type 2, or gestational diabetes. Testing is simple, and results are usually available quickly.

Type 1 Diabetes, Type 2 Diabetes, and Prediabetes

Your doctor will have you take one or more of the following blood tests to confirm the diagnosis:

A1C Test

This measures your average blood sugar level over the past 2 or 3 months. An A1C below 5.7 percent is normal, between 5.7 and 6.4 percent indicates you have prediabetes, and 6.5 percent or higher indicates you have diabetes.

Fasting Blood Sugar Test

This measures your blood sugar after an overnight fast (not eating). A fasting blood sugar level of 99 mg/dL or lower is normal, 100 to 125 mg/dL indicates you have prediabetes, and 126 mg/dL or higher indicates you have diabetes.

Glucose Tolerance Test

This measures your blood sugar before and after you drink a liquid that contains glucose. You will fast overnight before the test and have your blood drawn to determine your fasting blood sugar level. Then, you will drink the liquid and have your blood sugar level checked 1 hour, 2 hours, and possibly 3 hours afterward. At 2 hours, a blood sugar level of 140 mg/dL or lower is considered normal, 140 to 199 mg/dL indicates you have prediabetes, and 200 mg/dL or higher indicates you have diabetes.

Random Blood Sugar Test

This measures your blood sugar at the time you are tested. You can take this test at any time and do not need to fast first. A blood sugar level of 200 mg/dL or higher indicates you have diabetes.

Table 14.1. Basic Diabetes

Result*	A1C Test	Fasting Blood Sugar Test	Glucose Tolerance Test	Random Blood Sugar Test
Diabetes	6.5 percent or above	126 mg/dL or above	200 mg/dL or above	200 mg/dL or above
Prediabetes	5.7 to 6.4 percent	100 to 125 mg/dL	140 to 199 mg/dL	N/A
Normal	Below 5.7 percent	99 mg/dL or below	140 mg/dL or below	N/A

(Source: American Diabetes Association (ADA).)
* Results for gestational diabetes can differ. Ask your healthcare provider what your results mean if you are being tested for gestational diabetes.

If your doctor thinks you have type 1 diabetes, your blood may also tested for autoantibodies (substances that indicate your body is attacking itself) that are often present in type 1 diabetes but not in type 2 diabetes. You may have your urine tested for ketones, which also indicate type 1 diabetes instead of type 2 diabetes.

Glucose Screening Test

This measures your blood sugar at the time you are tested. You will drink a liquid that contains glucose, and then 1 hour later your blood will be drawn to check your blood sugar level. A normal result is 140 mg/dL or lower. If your level is higher than 140 mg/dL, you will need to take a glucose tolerance test.

Glucose Tolerance Test

This measures your blood sugar before and after you drink a liquid that contains glucose. You will fast overnight before the test and have your blood drawn to determine your fasting blood sugar level. Then, you will drink the liquid and have your blood sugar level checked 1 hour, 2 hours, and possibly 3 hours afterward. Results can differ depending on the size of the glucose drink and how often your blood sugar is tested. Ask your doctor what your test results mean.

What Is Next?

If your test results show that you have prediabetes, ask your doctor or nurse if there is a lifestyle change program offered through the CDC-led National Diabetes Prevention Program in your community. Having prediabetes puts you at a greater risk for developing type 2 diabetes, but participating in the program can lower your risk by as much as 58 percent (71 percent if you are over the age of 60).

If your test results show that you have type 1, type 2, or gestational diabetes, talk with your doctor or nurse about a detailed treatment plan—including diabetes self-management education—and specific steps you need to take to be your healthiest.

Diabetes Quick Facts
The Big Picture

- More than 30 million people in the United States have diabetes, and 1 in 4 of them do not know they have it.

- More than 84 million U.S. adults—over a third—have prediabetes, and 90 percent of them do not know they have it.

- Diabetes is the seventh leading cause of death in the United States (and maybe underreported).

- Type 2 diabetes accounts for about 90 to 95 percent of all diagnosed cases of diabetes; type 1 diabetes accounts for about 5 percent.

- In the last 20 years, the number of adults diagnosed with diabetes has more than tripled as the American population has aged and become more overweight or obese.

Risk

- You are at risk for developing prediabetes or type 2 diabetes if you:

  - Are overweight

  - Are 45 years of age or older

  - Have a parent, brother, or sister with type 2 diabetes

  - Are physically active less than three times a week

- African Americans, Hispanic/Latinx Americans, American Indians/Alaska Natives, Pacific Islanders, and some Asian Americans are at a higher risk for prediabetes and type 2 diabetes.

- American Indians/Alaska Natives are twice as likely as Whites to have diabetes.

- During their lifetime, half of all Hispanic men and women and non-Hispanic black women are predicted to develop diabetes.

- Type 1 diabetes is thought to be caused by an immune reaction. Known risk factors for type 1 diabetes include:

  - Family history (having a parent, brother, sister with type 1 diabetes)

  - Age (it is more likely to develop in children, teens, and young adults)

- In the United States, Whites are more likely to develop type 1 diabetes than African Americans and Hispanic/Latinx Americans.

Complications

- People with diabetes are twice as likely to have heart disease or a stroke as people without diabetes—and at an earlier age.

- Diabetes is the leading cause of chronic kidney disease, lower-limb amputations, and adult-onset blindness in the United States.

- Smokers are 30 to 40 percent more likely to develop type 2 diabetes than nonsmokers.

- People with diabetes who smoke are more likely to develop serious related health problems, including heart and kidney disease.

- In about 2 out of 3 American Indians/Alaska Natives with kidney failure, diabetes is the cause.

Cost

- Medical costs and lost work and wages for people with diagnosed diabetes total $327 billion yearly.

- Medical costs for people with diabetes are twice as high as for people who do not have diabetes.

Monitoring Your Blood Sugar

Regular blood sugar monitoring is the most important thing you can do to manage type 1 or type 2 diabetes. You will be able to see what makes your numbers go up or down, such as eating different foods, taking your medicine, or being physically active. With this information, you can work with your healthcare team to make decisions about your best diabetes care plan. These decisions can help delay or prevent diabetes complications, such as heart attack, stroke, kidney disease, blindness, and amputation. Your doctor will tell you when and how often to check your blood sugar levels.

Most blood sugar meters allow you to save your results, and you can use an app on your cell phone to track your levels. If you do not have a smartphone, keep a written daily record. You should bring your meter, phone, or paper record with you each time you visit your healthcare provider.

How to Use a Blood Sugar Meter

There are different kinds of meters, but most of them work the same way. Ask your healthcare team to show you the benefits of each. In addition to you, have someone else learn how to use your meter in case you are sick and cannot check your blood sugar yourself.

Below are some tips for how to use a blood sugar meter.

1. Make sure the meter is clean and ready to use.

2. After removing a test strip, immediately close the test strip container tightly. Test strips can be damaged if they are exposed to moisture.

3. Wash your hands with soap and warm water. Dry well. Massage your hand to get blood into your finger. Do not use alcohol because it dries the skin too much.

4. Use a lancet to prick your finger. Squeezing from the base of the finger, gently place a small amount of blood onto the test strip. Place the strip in the meter.

5. After a few seconds, the reading will appear. Track and record your results. Add notes about anything that might have made the reading out of your target range, such as food, activity, etc.

6. Properly dispose the lancet and strip in a trash container.

7. Do not share blood sugar monitoring equipment, such as lancets, with anyone, even other family members.

8. Store test strips in the container provided. Do not expose them to moisture, extreme heat, or cold temperatures.

Recommended Target Ranges

The following standard recommendations are from the American Diabetes Association (ADA) for people who have diagnosed diabetes and are not pregnant. Work with your doctor to identify your personal blood sugar goals based on your age, health, diabetes treatment, and whether you have type 1 or type 2 diabetes.

ADA targets for Blood Sugar Your doctor's targets for you may differ	My Goals	My Results
Before meals: 80 to 130 mg/dl	_____ to _____	_____ to _____ Date: _____ Time: _____ Note: _____
1-2 hours after meals: Below 180 mg/dl	_____ to _____	_____ to _____ Date: _____ Time: _____ Note: _____

Figure 14.1. *ADA Target Ranges for Blood Sugar*

Your range may be different if you have other health conditions or if your blood sugar is often low or high. Always follow your doctor's recommendations.

Getting an A1C Test

Make sure to get an A1C test at least twice a year. Some people may need to have the test more often, so follow your doctor's advice.

A1C results tell you your average blood sugar level over three months. A1C results may be different in people with hemoglobin problems, such as sickle cell anemia. Work with your doctor to decide the best A1C goal for you. Follow your doctor's advice and recommendations.

Your A1C result will be reported in two ways:

- A1C as a percentage

- Estimated average glucose (eAG), in the same kind of numbers as your day-to-day blood sugar readings

If after taking this test your results are too high or too low, your diabetes care plan may need to be adjusted. Below are ADA's standard target ranges:

ADA's Target	My Goal	My Results
A1C: below 7%		
eAG: below 154 mg/dl		

Figure 14.2. *ADA Target Range*

Questions to Ask Your Doctor

When visiting your doctor, you might keep these questions in mind to ask during your appointment.

- What is my target blood sugar range?

- How often should I check my blood sugar?

- What do these numbers mean?

- Are there patterns that show I need to change my diabetes treatment?

- What changes need to be made to my diabetes care plan?

If you have other questions about your numbers or your ability to manage your diabetes, make sure to work closely with your doctor or healthcare team.

Chapter 15

Heart Disease

Chapter Contents

Section 15.1—Men and Heart Disease 200

Section 15.2—Heart Failure....................................... 202

Section 15.3—Coronary Artery Disease 215

Section 15.4—Heart Attack....................................... 217

Section 15.1

Men and Heart Disease

This section contains text excerpted from the following sources:
Text in this section begins with excerpts from "How the Heart
Works," National Heart, Lung, and Blood Institute (NHLBI), July
29, 2015. Reviewed June 2019; Text beginning with the heading
"Heart Disease Facts in Men" is excerpted from "Men and Heart
Disease Fact Sheet," Centers for Disease Control and Prevention
(CDC), August 23, 2017; Text under the heading "Prevention Tips"
is excerpted from "Heart Disease and Men," Centers for Disease
Control and Prevention (CDC), June 3, 2019.

Your heart is a muscular organ that pumps blood to your body.
Your heart is at the center of your circulatory system. This system
consists of a network of blood vessels, such as arteries, veins, and
capillaries. These blood vessels carry blood to and from all areas of
your body.

An electrical system controls your heart and uses electrical signals
to contract the heart's walls. When the walls contract, blood is pumped
into your circulatory system. Inlet and outlet valves in your heart
chambers ensure that blood flows in the right direction.

Your heart is vital to your health and nearly everything that goes
on in your body. Without the heart's pumping action, blood can't move
throughout your body.

Your blood carries the oxygen and nutrients that your organs need
to work well. Blood also carries carbon dioxide (a waste product) to
your lungs so you can breathe it out.

A healthy heart supplies your body with the right amount of blood
at the rate needed to work well. If disease or injury weakens your
heart, your body's organs won't receive enough blood to work normally.

Heart Disease Facts in Men

- Heart disease is the leading cause of death for men in the United
  States, killing 321,000 men in 2013—that is 1 in every 4 male
  deaths.

- Heart disease is the leading cause of death for men of most
  racial/ethnic groups in the United States, including African
  Americans, American Indians or Alaska Natives, Hispanics,
  and Whites. For Asian American or Pacific Islander men, heart
  disease is second only to cancer.

- About 8.5 percent of all White men, 7.9 percent of Black men, and 6.3 percent of Mexican American men have coronary heart disease (CHD).

- Half of the men who die suddenly of coronary heart disease have no previous symptoms. Even if you have no symptoms, you may still be at risk for heart disease.

- Between 70 and 89 percent of sudden cardiac events occur in men.

Risk Factors

High blood pressure, high low-density lipoprotein (LDL) cholesterol, and smoking are key risk factors for heart disease. About half of Americans (49%) have at least one of these three risk factors.

Several other medical conditions and lifestyle choices can also put people at a higher risk for heart disease, including:

- Diabetes

- Overweight and obesity

- Poor diet

- Physical inactivity

- Excessive alcohol use

Prevention Tips

- **Eat a healthy diet.** Choosing healthful meal and snack options can help you avoid heart disease and its complications. Be sure to eat plenty of fresh fruits and vegetables.

- **Maintain a healthy weight.** Being overweight or obese can increase your risk for heart disease.

- **Exercise regularly.** Physical activity can help you maintain a healthy weight and lower cholesterol and blood pressure. The U.S. Surgeon General, the nation's doctor, recommends adults engage in moderate-intensity exercise for 2 hours and 30 minutes every week.

- **Do not smoke.** Cigarette smoking greatly increases your risk for heart disease. So, if you do not smoke, do not start. If you do smoke, quitting will lower your risk for heart disease. Your doctor can suggest ways to help you quit.

- **Limit alcohol use.** Avoid drinking too much alcohol, which causes high blood pressure.

Section 15.2

Heart Failure

This section includes text excerpted from "Heart Failure," National Heart, Lung, and Blood Institute (NHLBI), October 9, 2018.

What Is Heart Failure?

Heart failure is a condition in which the heart cannot pump enough blood to meet the body's needs. In some cases, the heart cannot fill with enough blood. In other cases, the heart cannot pump blood to the rest of the body with enough force. Some people have both problems.

The term "heart failure" does not mean that your heart has stopped or is about to stop working. However, heart failure is a serious condition that requires medical care.

Causes of Heart Failure

Conditions that damage or overwork the heart muscle can cause heart failure. Over time, the heart weakens. It is not able to fill with and/or pump blood as well as it should. As the heart weakens, certain proteins and substances might be released into the blood. These substances have a toxic effect on the heart and blood flow, and they worsen heart failure.

Causes of heart failure includes the following:

Ischemic Heart Disease

Ischemic heart disease is a condition in which a waxy substance called "plaque" builds up inside the coronary arteries. These arteries supply oxygen-rich blood to your heart muscle.

Plaque narrows the arteries and reduces blood flow to your heart muscle. The buildup of plaque also makes it more likely that blood clots will form in your arteries. Blood clots can partially or completely block blood flow. Ischemic heart disease can lead to chest pain or discomfort called "angina," a heart attack, and heart damage.

Diabetes

Diabetes is a disease in which the body's blood glucose (sugar) level is too high. The body normally breaks down food into glucose and then carries it to cells throughout the body. The cells use a hormone called "insulin" to turn the glucose into energy.

In diabetes, the body does not make enough insulin or does not use its insulin properly. Over time, high blood sugar levels can damage and weaken the heart muscle and the blood vessels around the heart, leading to heart failure.

High Blood Pressure

Blood pressure is the force of blood pushing against the walls of the arteries. If this pressure rises and stays high over time, it can weaken your heart and lead to plaque buildup.

Blood pressure is considered high if it stays at or above 140/90 mmHg over time. (The mmHg is millimeters of mercury—the units used to measure blood pressure.) If you have diabetes or chronic kidney disease (CKD), high blood pressure is defined as 130/80 mmHg or higher.

Other Heart Conditions or Diseases

Other conditions and diseases also can lead to heart failure, such as:

- Arrhythmia happens when a problem occurs with the rate or rhythm of the heartbeat.

- Cardiomyopathy happens when the heart muscle becomes enlarged, thick, or rigid.

- Congenital heart defects are problems with the heart's structure are present at birth.

- Heart valve disease occurs if one or more of your heart valves does not work properly, which can be present at birth or caused by infection, other heart conditions, and age.

Other Factors

Other factors also can injure the heart muscle and lead to heart failure. Examples include:

- Alcohol abuse or cocaine and other illegal drug use

- Human immunodeficiency virus/acquired immunodeficiency syndrome (HIV/AIDS)

- Thyroid disorders (having either too much or too little thyroid hormone in the body)

- Too much vitamin E

- Treatments for cancer, such as radiation and chemotherapy

Risk Factors of Heart Failure

About 5.7 million people in the United States have heart failure. The number of people who have this condition is growing.

Heart failure is more common in:

- People who are 65 years of age or older. Aging can weaken the heart muscle. Older people also may have had diseases for many years that led to heart failure. Heart failure is a leading cause of hospital stays among people on Medicare.

- Blacks are more likely to have heart failure than people of other races. They are also more likely to have symptoms at a younger age, have more hospital visits due to heart failure, and die from heart failure.

- People who are overweight. Excess weight puts strain on the heart. Being overweight also increases your risk of heart disease and type 2 diabetes. These diseases can lead to heart failure.

- People who have had a heart attack. Damage to the heart muscle from a heart attack can weaken the heart muscle.

Children who have congenital heart defects also can develop heart failure. These defects occur if the heart, heart valves, or blood vessels near the heart do not form correctly while the fetus develops in the womb. Congenital heart defects can make the heart work harder. This weakens the heart muscle, which can lead to heart failure. Children do not have the same symptoms of heart failure or get the same treatments as adults.

Screening and Prevention of Heart Failure

You can take steps to prevent heart failure. The sooner you start, the better your chances of preventing or delaying the condition.

For People Who Have Healthy Hearts

If you have a healthy heart, you can take action to prevent heart disease and heart failure. To reduce your risk of heart disease:

- Avoid using illegal drugs.
- Adopt heart-healthy lifestyle habits.

For People Who Are at High Risk for Heart Failure

Even if you are at high risk for heart failure, you can take steps to reduce your risk. People at high risk include those who have ischemic heart disease, high blood pressure, or diabetes.

- Follow all of the steps listed above. Talk with your doctor about what types and amounts of physical activity are safe for you.
- Treat and control any conditions that can cause heart failure. Take medicines as your doctor prescribes.
- Avoid drinking alcohol.
- See your doctor for ongoing care.

For People Who Have Heart Damage but No Signs of Heart Failure

If you have heart damage but no signs of heart failure, you can still reduce your risk of developing the condition. In addition to the steps above, take your medicines as prescribed to reduce your heart's workload.

Signs, Symptoms, and Complications of Heart Failure

The most common signs and symptoms of heart failure are:

- Shortness of breath or trouble breathing
- Fatigue (tiredness)
- Swelling in the ankles, feet, legs, abdomen, and veins in the neck

All of these symptoms are the result of fluid buildup in your body. When symptoms start, you may feel tired and short of breath after routine physical effort, such as climbing stairs.

As your heart grows weaker, symptoms get worse. You may begin to feel tired and short of breath after getting dressed or walking across the room. Some people have shortness of breath while lying flat.

Fluid buildup from heart failure also causes weight gain, frequent urination, and a cough that is worse at night and when you are lying down. This cough may be a sign of acute pulmonary edema. This is a condition in which too much fluid builds up in your lungs. The condition requires emergency treatment.

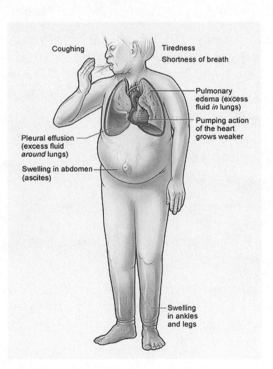

Figure 15.1. *Heart Failure Signs and Symptoms.*

Diagnosis of Heart Failure

Your doctor will diagnose heart failure based on your medical and family histories, a physical exam, and test results. The signs and symptoms of heart failure also are common in other conditions. Thus, your doctor will take these steps:

- Find out whether you have a disease or condition that can cause heart failure, such as ischemic heart disease, high blood pressure, or diabetes.

- Rule out other causes of your symptoms.

- Find any damage to your heart and check how well your heart pumps blood.

Early diagnosis and treatment can help people who have heart failure live longer, more active lives.

Medical and Family Histories

Your doctor will ask whether you or others in your family have or have had a disease or condition that can cause heart failure.

Your doctor also will ask about your symptoms. She or he will want to know which symptoms you have, when they occur, how long you have had them, and how severe they are. Your answers will help show whether and how much your symptoms limit your daily routine.

Physical Exam

During the physical exam, your doctor will:

- Listen to your heart for sounds that are not normal

- Listen to your lungs for the sounds of extra fluid buildup

- Look for swelling in your ankles, feet, legs, abdomen, and the veins in your neck

Diagnostic Tests

No single test can diagnose heart failure. If you have signs and symptoms of heart failure, your doctor may recommend one or more tests.

Your doctor also may refer you to a cardiologist. A cardiologist is a doctor who specializes in diagnosing and treating heart diseases and conditions.

Electrocardiogram

An electrocardiogram (EKG) is a simple, painless test that detects and records the heart's electrical activity. The test shows how fast your heart is beating and its rhythm (steady or irregular). An EKG also records the strength and timing of electrical signals as they pass through your heart.

An electrocardiogram may show whether the walls in your heart's pumping chambers are thicker than normal. Thicker walls can make it harder for your heart to pump blood. An EKG also can show signs of a previous or current heart attack.

Chest X-Ray

A chest X-ray takes pictures of the structures inside your chest, such as your heart, lungs, and blood vessels. This test can show whether your heart is enlarged, you have fluid in your lungs, or you have lung disease.

Brain Natriuretic Peptide Blood Test

This test checks the level of a hormone in your blood called "brain natriuretic peptide" (BNP). The level of this hormone rises during heart failure.

Echocardiography

Echocardiography (echo) uses sound waves to create a moving picture of your heart. The test shows the size and shape of your heart and how well your heart chambers and valves work.

An echo also can identify areas of poor blood flow to the heart, areas of heart muscle that are not contracting normally, and heart muscle damage caused by lack of blood flow.

An echo might be done before and after a stress test. A stress echo can show how well blood is flowing through your heart. The test also can show how well your heart pumps blood when it beats.

Doppler Ultrasound

A Doppler ultrasound uses sound waves to measure the speed and direction of blood flow. This test often is done with an echo to give a more complete picture of blood flow to the heart and lungs.

Doctors often use Doppler ultrasound to help diagnose right-side heart failure.

Holter Monitor

A Holter monitor records your heart's electrical activity for a full 24- or 48-hour period, while you go about your normal daily routine.

You wear small patches called "electrodes" on your chest. Wires connect the patches to a small, portable recorder. The recorder can be clipped to a belt, kept in a pocket, or hung around your neck.

Nuclear Heart Scan

A nuclear heart scan shows how well blood is flowing through your heart and how much blood is reaching your heart muscle.

During a nuclear heart scan, a safe, radioactive substance called a "tracer" is injected into your bloodstream through a vein. The tracer travels to your heart and releases energy. Special cameras outside of your body detect the energy and use it to create pictures of your heart.

A nuclear heart scan can show where the heart muscle is healthy and where it is damaged.

A positron emission tomography (PET) scan is a type of nuclear heart scan. It shows the level of chemical activity in areas of your heart. This test can help your doctor see whether enough blood is flowing to these areas. A PET scan can show blood flow problems that other tests might not detect.

Cardiac Catheterization

During cardiac catheterization, a long, thin, flexible tube called a "catheter" is put into a blood vessel in your arm, groin (upper thigh), or neck and threaded to your heart. This allows your doctor to look inside your coronary (heart) arteries.

During this procedure, your doctor can check the pressure and blood flow in your heart chambers, collect blood samples, and use X-rays to look at your coronary arteries.

Coronary Angiography

Coronary angiography usually is done with cardiac catheterization. A dye that can be seen on an X-ray is injected into your bloodstream through the tip of the catheter.

The dye allows your doctor to see the flow of blood to your heart muscle. Angiography also shows how well your heart is pumping.

Stress Test

Some heart problems are easier to diagnose when your heart is working hard and beating fast. During stress testing, you exercise to make your heart work hard and beat fast.

You may walk or run on a treadmill or pedal a bicycle. If you cannot exercise, you may be given medicine to raise your heart rate.

Heart tests, such as nuclear heart scanning and an echo, often are done during stress testing.

Cardiac Magnetic Resonance Imaging

Cardiac magnetic resonance imaging (MRI) uses radio waves, magnets, and a computer to create pictures of your heart as it is beating. The test produces both still and moving pictures of your heart and major blood vessels.

A cardiac MRI can show whether parts of your heart are damaged. Doctors also have used MRI in research studies to find early signs of heart failure, even before symptoms appear.

Thyroid Function Tests

Thyroid function tests show how well your thyroid gland is working. These tests include blood tests, imaging tests, and tests to stimulate the thyroid. Having too much or too little thyroid hormone in the blood can lead to heart failure.

Treatment for Heart Failure

Early diagnosis and treatment can help people who have heart failure live longer, more active lives. Treatment for heart failure depends on the type and severity of the heart failure.

The goals of treatment for all stages of heart failure include:

- Treating the condition's underlying cause, such as ischemic heart disease, high blood pressure, or diabetes

- Reducing symptoms

- Stopping the heart failure from getting worse

- Increasing your lifespan and improving your quality of life

Treatments usually include heart-healthy lifestyle changes, medicines, and ongoing care. If you have severe heart failure, you also may need medical procedures or surgery.

Heart-Healthy Lifestyle Changes

Your doctor may recommend heart-healthy lifestyle changes if you have heart failure. Heart-healthy lifestyle changes include:

- Heart-healthy eating
- Aiming for a healthy weight
- Physical activity
- Quitting smoking

Medicines

Your doctor will prescribe medicines based on the type of heart failure you have, how severe it is, and your response to certain medicines. The following medicines are commonly used to treat heart failure:

- **Angiotensin-converting enzymes (ACE)** lower blood pressure and reduce strain on your heart. They also may reduce the risk of a future heart attack.

- **Aldosterone antagonists** trigger the body to remove excess sodium through urine. This lowers the volume of blood that the heart must pump.

- **Angiotensin receptor blockers (ARBs)** relax your blood vessels and lower blood pressure to decrease your heart's workload.

- **Beta-blockers** slow your heart rate and lower your blood pressure to decrease your heart's workload.

- **Digoxin** makes the heart beat stronger and pump more blood.

- **Diuretics** (fluid pills) help reduce fluid buildup in your lungs and swelling in your feet and ankles.

- **Isosorbide dinitrate/hydralazine hydrochloride** helps relax your blood vessels so your heart does not work as hard to pump blood. Studies have shown that this medicine can reduce the risk of death in Black individuals.

Take all medicines regularly, as your doctor prescribes. Do not change the amount of your medicine or skip a dose unless your doctor tells you to. You should still follow a heart-healthy lifestyle, even if you take medicines to treat your heart failure.

Ongoing Care

You should watch for signs that heart failure is getting worse. For example, weight gain may mean that fluids are building up in your body. Ask your doctor how often you should check your weight and when to report weight changes.

Getting medical care for other related conditions is important. If you have diabetes or high blood pressure, work with your healthcare team to control these conditions. Have your blood sugar level and blood pressure checked. Talk with your doctor about when you should have tests and how often to take measurements at home.

Try to avoid respiratory infections, such as the flu and pneumonia. Talk with your doctor or nurse about getting flu and pneumonia vaccines.

Many people who have severe heart failure may need treatment in a hospital from time to time. Your doctor may recommend oxygen therapy, which can be given in a hospital or at home.

Medical Procedures and Surgery

As heart failure worsens, lifestyle changes and medicines may no longer control your symptoms. You may need a medical procedure or surgery.

In heart failure, the right and left sides of the heart may no longer contract at the same time. This disrupts the heart's pumping. To correct this problem, your doctor might implant a cardiac resynchronization therapy (CRT) device (a type of pacemaker) near your heart. This device helps both sides of your heart contract at the same time, which can decrease heart failure symptoms.

Some people who have heart failure have very rapid, irregular heartbeats. Without treatment, these heartbeats can cause sudden cardiac arrest (SCA). Your doctor might implant an implantable cardioverter defibrillator (ICD) near your heart to solve this problem. An ICD checks your heart rate and uses electrical pulses to correct irregular heart rhythms.

People who have severe heart failure symptoms at rest, despite other treatments, may need:

- A **mechanical heart pump**, such as a left ventricular assist device (LVAD). This device helps pump blood from the heart to the rest of the body. You may use a heart pump until you have surgery or as a long-term treatment.

- **Heart transplant.** A heart transplant is an operation in which a person's diseased heart is replaced with a healthy heart from a deceased donor. Heart transplants are done as a lifesaving measure for end-stage heart failure when medical treatment and less drastic surgery have failed.

Living with Heart Failure

Nowadays, heart failure has no cure. You will likely have to take medicine and follow a treatment plan for the rest of your life.

Despite treatment, symptoms may get worse over time. You may not be able to do many of the things that you did before you had heart failure. However, if you take all the steps your doctor recommends, you can stay healthier longer.

Researchers also might find new treatments that can help you in the future.

Follow Your Treatment Plan

Treatment can relieve your symptoms and make daily activities easier. It also can reduce the chance that you will have to go to the hospital. Thus, it is important that you follow your treatment plan.

- Take your medicines as your doctor prescribes. If you have side effects from any of your medicines, tell your doctor. She or he might adjust the dose or type of medicine you take to relieve side effects.

- Make all of the lifestyle changes that your doctor recommends.

- Get advice from your doctor about how active you can and should be. This includes advice on daily activities, work, leisure time, sex, and exercise. Your level of activity will depend on the stage of your heart failure (how severe it is).

- Keep all of your medical appointments, including visits to the doctor and appointments to get tests and lab work. Your doctor needs the results of these tests to adjust your medicine doses and help you avoid harmful side effects.

Take Steps to Prevent Heart Failure from Getting Worse

Certain actions can worsen your heart failure, such as:

- Forgetting to take your medicines
- Not following your diet (for example, eating salty foods)
- Drinking alcohol

These actions can lead to a hospital stay. If you have trouble following your diet, talk with your doctor. She or he can help arrange for a dietitian to work with you. Avoid drinking alcohol.

213

People who have heart failure often have other serious conditions that require ongoing treatment. If you have other serious conditions, you are likely taking medicines for them, as well as for heart failure.

Taking more than one medicine raises the risk of side effects and other problems. Make sure your doctors and your pharmacist have a complete list of all of the medicines and over-the-counter (OTC) products that you are taking.

Tell your doctor right away about any problems with your medicines. Also, talk with your doctor before taking any new medicine prescribed by another doctor or any new OTC medicines or herbal supplements.

Try to avoid respiratory infections, such as the flu and pneumonia. Ask your doctor or nurse about getting flu and pneumonia vaccines.

Plan Ahead

If you have heart failure, it is important to know:

- When to seek help. Ask your doctor when to make an office visit or get emergency care.

- Phone numbers for your doctor and hospital

- Directions to your doctor's office and hospital and people who can take you there

- A list of medicines you are taking

Emotional Issues and Support

Living with heart failure may cause fear, anxiety, depression, and stress. Talk about how you feel with your healthcare team. Talking to a professional counselor also can help. If you are very depressed, your doctor may recommend medicines or other treatments that can improve your quality of life.

Joining a patient support group may help you adjust to living with heart failure. You can see how other people who have the same symptoms have coped with them. Talk with your doctor about local support groups or check with an area medical center.

Support from family and friends also can help relieve stress and anxiety. Let your loved ones know how you feel and what they can do to help you.

Section 15.3

Coronary Artery Disease

This section contains text excerpted from the following
sources: Text in this section begins with excerpts from "Coronary
Artery Disease," MedlinePlus, National Institutes of Health (NIH),
November 1, 2016; Text beginning with the heading "Diagnosing
Coronary Artery Disease" is excerpted from "Coronary Artery
Disease (CAD)," Centers for Disease Control and
Prevention (CDC), August 10, 2015. Reviewed June 2019.

Coronary artery disease (CAD) is the most common type of heart
disease. It is the leading cause of death in the United States in both
women and men.

Coronary artery disease occurs when the arteries that supply blood
to heart muscle become hardened and narrowed. This is due to the
buildup of cholesterol and other material, called "plaque," on their inner
walls. This buildup is called "atherosclerosis." As it grows, less blood
can flow through the arteries. As a result, the heart muscle cannot get
the blood or oxygen it needs. This can lead to chest pain (angina) or a
heart attack. Most heart attacks happen when a blood clot suddenly
cuts off the hearts' blood supply, causing permanent heart damage.

Diagnosing Coronary Artery Disease

To find out your risk for CAD, your healthcare team may measure
your blood pressure, cholesterol, and sugar levels. Being overweight,
physical inactivity, unhealthy eating, and smoking tobacco are risk
factors for CAD. A family history of heart disease also increases your
risk for CAD. If you are at a high risk for heart disease or already have
symptoms, your doctor can use several tests to diagnose CAD.

Table 15.1. Test for Diagnosing Coronary Artery Disease Test

Test	What It Does
Electrocardiogram (ECD or EKG)	Measures the electrical activity, rate, and regularity of your heartbeat.
Echocardiogram	Uses ultrasound (special sound wave) to create a picture of the heart.
Exercise stress test	Measures your heart rate while you walk on a treadmill. This helps to determine how well your heart is working when it has to pump more blood.

Table 15.1. Continued

Test	What It Does
Chest X-ray	Uses X-rays to create a picture of the heart, lungs, and other organs in the chest.
Cardiac catheterization	Checks the inside of your arteries for blockage by inserting a thin, flexible tube through an artery in the groin, arm, or neck to reach the heart. Healthcare professionals can measure blood pressure within the heart and the strength of blood flow through the heart's chambers as well as collect blood samples from the heart or inject dye into the arteries of the heart (coronary arteries).
Coronary angiogram	Monitors blockage and flow of blood through the coronary arteries. Uses X-rays to detect dye injected via cardiac catheterization.

Reducing Your Risk for Coronary Artery Disease

If you have CAD, your healthcare team may suggest the following steps to help lower your risk for heart attack or worsening heart disease:

- Lifestyle changes, such as eating a healthier (lower sodium, lower fat) diet, increasing physical activity, and quitting smoking

- Medications to treat the risk factors for CAD, such as high cholesterol, high blood pressure, an irregular heartbeat, and low blood flow

- Surgical procedures to help restore blood flow to the heart

Section 15.4

Heart Attack

This section includes text excerpted from "Heart Attack," National Heart, Lung, and Blood Institute (NHLBI), June 12, 2017.

What Is Heart Attack?

A heart attack happens when the flow of oxygen-rich blood to a section of heart muscle suddenly becomes blocked, and the heart cannot get oxygen. If blood flow is not restored quickly, the section of the heart muscle begins to die.

Heart attack treatment works best when it is given right after symptoms occur. If you think you or someone else is having a heart attack, even if you are not sure, call 911 right away.

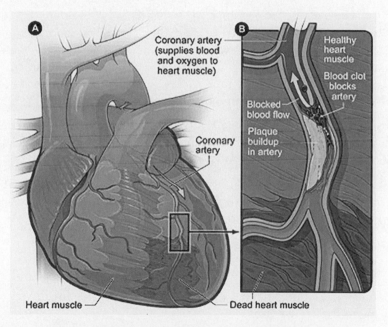

Figure 15.2. *Heart with Muscle Damage and a Blocked Artery*

Figure A is an overview of a heart and coronary artery showing damage (dead heart muscle) caused by a heart attack. Figure B is a cross-section of the coronary artery with plaque buildup and a blood clot.

A less common cause of heart attack is a severe spasm of a coronary artery. The spasm cuts off blood flow through the artery. Spasms can occur in coronary arteries that are not affected by atherosclerosis.

Heart attacks can be associated with or lead to severe health problems, such as heart failure and life-threatening arrhythmias.

Heart failure is a condition in which the heart cannot pump enough blood to meet the body's needs. Arrhythmias are irregular heartbeats. Ventricular fibrillation (VF) is a life-threatening arrhythmia that can cause death if it is not treated right away.

Do Not Wait—Get Help Quickly

Acting fast at the first sign of heart attack symptoms can save your life and limit damage to your heart. The treatment works best when it is given right after symptoms occur.

Many people are not sure what is wrong when they are having symptoms of a heart attack. Some of the most common warning symptoms of a heart attack for both men and women are:

- **Chest pain or discomfort.** Most heart attacks involve discomfort in the center or left side of the chest. The discomfort usually lasts more than a few minutes or goes away and comes back. It can feel like pressure, squeezing, fullness, or pain. It also can feel like heartburn or indigestion.

- **Upper body discomfort.** You may feel pain or discomfort in one or both arms, the back, shoulders, neck, jaw, or upper part of the stomach (above the belly button).

- **Shortness of breath.** This may be your only symptom or it may occur before or along with chest pain or discomfort. It can occur when you are resting or doing a little bit of physical activity.

Other possible symptoms of a heart attack include:

- Breaking out in a cold sweat

- Feeling unusually tired for no reason, sometimes for days (especially for women)

- Nausea (feeling sick to the stomach) and vomiting

- Light-headedness or sudden dizziness

- Any sudden, new symptom or a change in the pattern of symptoms you already have (for example, if your symptoms become stronger or last longer than usual)

Not all heart attacks begin with the sudden, crushing chest pain that often is shown on TV or in the movies or with other common symptoms, such as chest discomfort. The symptoms of a heart attack can vary from person to person. Some people can have few symptoms and are surprised to learn they have had a heart attack. If you have already had a heart attack, your symptoms may not be the same for another one.

Quick Action Can Save Your Life: Call 911

If you think you or someone else may be having heart attack symptoms or a heart attack, do not ignore it or feel embarrassed to call for help. **Call 911 for emergency medical care.** Acting fast can save your life.

Do not drive to the hospital or let someone else drive you. Call an ambulance so that medical personnel can begin lifesaving treatment on the way to the emergency room. Take a nitroglycerin pill if your doctor has prescribed this type of treatment.

Causes of Heart Attack
Coronary Heart Disease

A heart attack happens if the flow of oxygen-rich blood to a section of heart muscle suddenly becomes blocked, and the heart cannot get oxygen. Most heart attacks occur as a result of ischemic heart disease.

Ischemic heart disease is a condition in which a waxy substance called "plaque" builds up inside of the coronary arteries. These arteries supply oxygen-rich blood to your heart.

When plaque builds up in the arteries, the condition is called "atherosclerosis." The buildup of plaque occurs over many years.

Eventually, an area of plaque can rupture (break open) inside of an artery. This causes a blood clot to form on the plaque's surface. If the clot becomes large enough, it can mostly or completely block blood flow through a coronary artery.

If the blockage is not treated quickly, the portion of heart muscle fed by the artery begins to die. Healthy heart tissue is replaced with scar tissue. This heart damage may not be obvious, or it may cause severe or long-lasting problems.

Coronary Artery Spasm

A less common cause of heart attack is a severe spasm of a coronary artery. The spasm cuts off blood flow through the artery. Spasms can occur in coronary arteries that are not affected by atherosclerosis.

What causes a coronary artery to spasm is not always clear. A spasm may be related to:

- Taking certain drugs, such as cocaine

- Emotional stress or pain

- Exposure to extreme cold

- Cigarette smoking

Screening and Prevention of Heart Attack

Lowering your risk factors for ischemic heart disease can help you prevent a heart attack. Even if you already have heart disease, you still can take steps to lower your risk for a heart attack. These steps involve making heart-healthy lifestyle changes and getting ongoing medical care for related conditions that make a heart attack more likely. Talk to your doctor about whether you may benefit from aspirin primary prevention or from using aspirin to help prevent your first heart attack.

Heart-Healthy Lifestyle Changes

A heart-healthy lifestyle can help prevent a heart attack and includes heart-healthy eating, being physically active, quitting smoking, managing stress, and managing your weight.

Ongoing Care
Treat Related Conditions

Treating conditions that make a heart attack more likely also can help lower your risk for a heart attack. These conditions may include:

- **Diabetes (high blood sugar).** If you have diabetes, try to control your blood sugar level through diet and physical activity (as your doctor recommends). If needed, take medicine as prescribed.

- **High blood cholesterol.** Your doctor may prescribe a statin medicine to lower your cholesterol if diet and exercise are not enough.

- **High blood pressure.** Your doctor may prescribe medicine to keep your blood pressure under control.

- **Chronic kidney disease (CKD).** Your doctor may prescribe medicines to control your high blood pressure or high blood sugar levels.

- **Peripheral artery disease (PAD).** Your doctor may recommend surgery or procedures to unblock the affected arteries.

Have an Emergency Action Plan

Make sure that you have an emergency action plan in case you or someone in your family has a heart attack. This is very important if you are at a high risk for, or have already had, a heart attack.

Write down a list of medicines you are taking, medicines you are allergic to, your healthcare provider's phone numbers (both during and after office hours), and contact information for a friend or relative. Keep the list in a handy place to share in a medical emergency.

Talk with your doctor about the signs and symptoms of a heart attack, when you should call 911, and steps you can take while waiting for medical help to arrive.

Signs, Symptoms, and Complications of Heart Attack

Not all heart attacks begin with the sudden, crushing chest pain that often is shown on TV or in the movies. In one study, for example, one-third of the patients who had heart attacks had no chest pain. These patients were more likely to be older, female, or diabetic.

The symptoms of a heart attack can vary from person to person. Some people can have few symptoms and are surprised to learn they have had a heart attack. If you have already had a heart attack, your symptoms may not be the same for another one. It is important for you to know the most common symptoms of a heart attack and also remember these facts:

- Heart attacks can start slowly and cause only mild pain or discomfort. Symptoms can be mild or more intense and sudden. Symptoms also may come and go over several hours.

- People who have diabetes may have no symptoms or very mild ones.

- The most common symptom, in both men and women, is chest pain or discomfort.

- Women are somewhat more likely to have shortness of breath; nausea and vomiting; unusual tiredness (sometimes for days); and pain in the back, shoulders, and jaw.

Some people do not have symptoms at all. Heart attacks that occur without any symptoms or with very mild symptoms are called "silent heart attacks."

Most Common Symptoms

The most common warning symptoms of a heart attack for both men and women are:

- **Chest pain or discomfort.** Most heart attacks involve discomfort in the center or left side of the chest. The discomfort usually lasts for more than a few minutes or goes away and comes back. It can feel like pressure, squeezing, fullness, or pain. It also can feel like heartburn or indigestion. The feeling can be mild or severe.

- **Upper body discomfort.** You may feel pain or discomfort in one or both arms, the back, shoulders, neck, jaw, or upper part of the stomach (above the belly button).

- **Shortness of breath**. This maybe your only symptom, or it may occur before or along with chest pain or discomfort. It can occur when you are resting or doing a little bit of physical activity.

The symptoms of angina can be similar to the symptoms of a heart attack. Angina is chest pain that occurs in people who have ischemic heart disease, usually when they are active. Angina pain usually lasts for only a few minutes and goes away with rest.

Chest pain or discomfort that does not go away or changes from its usual pattern (for example, occurs more often or while you are resting) can be a sign of a heart attack.

All chest pain should be checked by a doctor.

Other Common Signs and Symptoms

Pay attention to these other possible symptoms of a heart attack:

- Breaking out in a cold sweat
- Feeling unusually tired for no reason, sometimes for days
- Nausea and vomiting
- Light-headedness or sudden dizziness

- Any sudden, new symptoms or a change in the pattern of symptoms you already have (for example, if your symptoms become stronger or last longer than usual)

Not everyone having a heart attack has typical symptoms. If you have already had a heart attack, your symptoms may not be the same for another one. However, some people may have a pattern of symptoms that recur.

The more signs and symptoms you have, the more likely it is that you are having a heart attack.

Quick Action Can Save Your Life: Call 911

The signs and symptoms of a heart attack can develop suddenly. However, they also can develop slowly—sometimes within hours, days, or weeks of a heart attack.

Any time you think you might be having heart attack symptoms or a heart attack, do not ignore it or feel embarrassed to call for help. Call 911 for emergency medical care, even if you are not sure whether you are having a heart attack. Here is why:

- Acting fast can save your life.

- An ambulance is the best and safest way to get to the hospital. Emergency medical services (EMS) personnel can check how you are doing and start lifesaving medicines and other treatments right away. People who arrive by ambulance often receive faster treatment at the hospital.

- The 911 operator or EMS technician can give you advice. You might be told to crush or chew an aspirin if you are not allergic, unless there is a medical reason for you not to take one. Aspirin taken during a heart attack can limit the damage to your heart and save your life.

Every minute matters. Never delay calling 911 to take aspirin or do anything else you think might help.

Diagnosis of Heart Attack

Your doctor will diagnose a heart attack based on your signs and symptoms, your medical and family histories, and test results.

Diagnostic Tests

Electrocardiogram

An electrocardiogram (EKG) is a simple, painless test that detects and records the heart's electrical activity. The test shows how fast the heart is beating and its rhythm (steady or irregular). An EKG also records the strength and timing of electrical signals as they pass through each part of the heart.

An EKG can show signs of heart damage due to ischemic heart disease and signs of a previous or current heart attack.

Blood Tests

During a heart attack, heart muscle cells die and release proteins into the bloodstream. Blood tests can measure the amount of these proteins in the bloodstream. Higher than normal levels of these proteins suggest a heart attack.

Commonly used blood tests include troponin tests, creatine kinase-MB (CK-MB) tests, and serum myoglobin tests. Blood tests often are repeated to check for changes over time.

Coronary Angiography

Coronary angiography is a test that uses dye and special X-rays to show the insides of your coronary arteries. This test often is done during a heart attack to help find blockages in the coronary arteries.

To get the dye into your coronary arteries, your doctor will use a procedure called "cardiac catheterization."

A thin, flexible tube called a "catheter" is put into a blood vessel in your arm, groin (upper thigh), or neck. The tube is threaded into your coronary arteries, and the dye is released into your bloodstream.

Special X-rays are taken while the dye is flowing through the coronary arteries. The dye lets your doctor study the flow of blood through the heart and blood vessels.

If your doctor finds a blockage, she or he may recommend a procedure called "percutaneous coronary intervention" (PCI), sometimes referred to as "coronary angioplasty." This procedure can help restore blood flow through a blocked artery. Sometimes, a small mesh tube called a "stent" is placed in the artery to help prevent blockages after the procedure.

Chapter 16

HIV and AIDS

What Is Human Immunodeficiency Virus/Acquired Immunodeficiency Syndrome?

HIV stands for human immunodeficiency virus. The abbreviation "HIV" can refer to the virus itself or to HIV infection.

AIDS stands for acquired immunodeficiency syndrome. Acquired immunodeficiency syndrome is the most advanced stage of HIV infection.

Human immunodeficiency virus attacks and destroys the infection-fighting CD4 cells of the immune system. The loss of CD4 cells makes it difficult for the body to fight infections and certain cancers. Without treatment, HIV can gradually destroy the immune system and advance to AIDS.

How Is Human Immunodeficiency Virus Spread?

HIV is spread through contact with certain body fluids from a person with HIV. These body fluids include:

- Blood
- Semen
- Pre-seminal fluid

This chapter includes text excerpted from "HIV/AIDS: The Basics," AIDS*info*, U.S. Department of Health and Human Services (HHS), November 6, 2018.

- Vaginal fluids
- Rectal fluids
- Breast milk

The spread of HIV from person to person is called "HIV transmission." The spread of HIV from a woman with HIV to her child during pregnancy, childbirth, or breastfeeding is called "mother-to-child transmission of HIV."

In the United States, HIV is spread mainly by:

- Having anal or vaginal sex with someone who has HIV without using a condom or taking medicines to prevent or treat HIV

- Sharing injection drug equipment ("works"), such as needles, with someone who has HIV

To reduce your risk of HIV infection, use condoms correctly every time you have sex, limit your number of sexual partners, and never share injection drug equipment. Also, talk to your healthcare provider about pre-exposure prophylaxis (PrEP). Pre-exposure prophylaxis is an HIV prevention option for people who do not have HIV but who are at a high risk of becoming infected with HIV. Pre-exposure prophylaxis involves taking a specific HIV medicine every day.

Mother-to-child transmission is the most common way that children get HIV. Human immunodeficiency virus medicines, given to women with HIV during pregnancy and childbirth and to their babies after birth, reduce the risk of mother-to-child transmission of HIV.

You cannot get HIV by shaking hands or hugging a person who has HIV. You also cannot get HIV from contact with objects, such as dishes, toilet seats, or doorknobs, used by a person with HIV. Human immunodeficiency virus is not spread through the air or in water or by mosquitoes, ticks, or other blood-sucking insects.

What Is the Treatment for Human Immunodeficiency Virus?

Antiretroviral therapy (ART) is the use of HIV medicines to treat HIV infection. People on ART take a combination of HIV medicines (called an "HIV regimen") every day. (HIV medicines are often called "antiretrovirals" or "ARVs.")

Antiretroviral therapy is recommended for everyone who has HIV. Antiretroviral therapy prevents HIV from multiplying and reduces the amount of HIV in the body (also called the "viral load"). Having less HIV in the body protects the immune system and prevents HIV infection from advancing to AIDS. Antiretroviral therapy cannot cure HIV, but HIV medicines help people with HIV live longer, healthier lives.

Antiretroviral therapy also reduces the risk of HIV transmission. A main goal of ART is to reduce a person's viral load to an undetectable level. An undetectable viral load means that the level of HIV in the blood is too low to be detected by a viral load test. People with HIV who maintain an undetectable viral load have effectively no risk of transmitting HIV to their HIV-negative partner through sex.

What Are the Symptoms of Human Immunodeficiency Virus/Acquired Immunodeficiency Syndrome?

Within two to four weeks after infection with HIV, some people may have flu-like symptoms, such as fever, chills, or rash. The symptoms may last for a few days to several weeks.

After this earliest stage of HIV infection, HIV continues to multiply but at very low levels. More severe symptoms of HIV infection, such as signs of opportunistic infections, generally do not appear for many years. (Opportunistic infections are infections and infection-related cancers that occur more frequently or are more severe in people with weakened immune systems than in people with healthy immune systems.)

Without treatment with HIV medicines, HIV infection usually advances to AIDS in 10 years or longer, though it may advance faster in some people.

Human immunodeficiency virus transmission is possible at any stage of HIV infection—even if a person with HIV has no symptoms of HIV.

How Is Acquired Immunodeficiency Syndrome Diagnosed?

Symptoms such as fever, weakness, and weight loss may be a sign that a person's HIV has advanced to AIDS. However, a diagnosis of AIDS is based on the following criteria:

- A drop in CD4 count to less than 200 cells/mm^3. A CD4 count measures the number of CD4 cells in a sample of blood.

- The presence of certain opportunistic infections

Although an AIDS diagnosis indicates severe damage to the immune system, HIV medicines can still help people at this stage of HIV infection.

Chapter 17

Influenza and Pneumonia

Chapter Contents

Section 17.1—Influenza 230
Section 17.2—Pneumonia 235

Section 17.1

Influenza

This section includes text excerpted from "Key Facts about
Influenza (Flu)," Centers for Disease Control and
Prevention (CDC), August 27, 2018.

What Is Influenza?

Influenza, also referred to as "flu," is a contagious respiratory illness caused by influenza viruses that infect the nose, throat, and
sometimes the lungs. It can cause mild to severe illness and, at times,
can lead to death. The best way to prevent flu is by getting a flu vaccine each year.

Flu Symptoms

Flu is different from a cold. As it usually comes on suddenly. People
who are sick with flu often feel some or all of these symptoms:

- Fever* or feeling feverish/chills
- Cough
- Sore throat
- Runny or stuffy nose
- Muscle or body aches
- Headaches
- Fatigue (tiredness)
- Some people may experience vomiting and diarrhea, though this
  is more common in children than adults.

* It is important to note that not everyone with flu will have a fever.

How Flu Spread?

Most experts believe that flu viruses spread mainly by tiny droplets
made when people with flu cough, sneeze, or talk. These droplets can
land in the mouths or noses of people who are nearby. Less often, a
person might get flu by touching a surface or object that has flu virus
on it and then touching their own mouth, nose, or eyes.

How Many People Get Sick with Flu Every Year?

A 2018 Centers for Disease Control and Prevention (CDC) study published in *Clinical Infectious Diseases (CID)* looked at the percentage of the U.S. population who were sickened by flu using 2 different methods and compared the findings. Both methods had similar findings, which suggested that on average, about 8 percent of the U.S. population gets sick from flu each season, with a range of between 3 percent and 11 percent, depending on the season.

Why Is the 3 to 11 Percent Estimate Different from the Previously Cited 5 Percent to 20 Percent Range?

The commonly cited 5 percent to 20 percent estimate was based on a study that examined both symptomatic and asymptomatic influenza illness, which means it also looked at people who may have had the flu but never knew it because they did not have any symptoms. The 3 percent to 11 percent range is an estimate of the proportion of people who have symptomatic flu illness.

Who Is Most Likely to Be Infected with Influenza?

The same *Clinical Infectious Diseases* study found that children are most likely to get sick from flu and that people 65 years of age and older are least likely to get sick from influenza. Median incidence values (or attack rate) by age group were 9.3 percent for children between 0 and 17 years of age, 8.8 percent for adults between 18 and 64 years of age, and 3.9 percent for adults 65 years of age and older. This means that children younger than 18 years of age are more than twice as likely to develop a symptomatic flu infection than adults 65 years of age and older.

How Is Seasonal Incidence of Influenza Estimated?

Influenza virus infection is so common that the number of people infected each season can only be estimated. These statistical estimations are based on the CDC-measured flu hospitalization rates that are adjusted to produce an estimate of the total number of influenza infections in the United States for a given flu season.

The estimates for the number of infections are then divided by the census population to estimate the seasonal incidence (or attack rate) of influenza.

Does Seasonal Incidence of Influenza Change Based on the Severity of Flu Season?

Yes. The proportion of people who get sick from flu varies. A paper published in CID found that between 3 percent and 11 percent of the U.S. population gets infected and develops flu symptoms each year. The 3 percent estimate is from the 2011 to 2012 season, which was an H1N1-predominant season classified as being of low severity. The estimated incidence of flu illness during 2 seasons was around 11 percent; 2012 to 2013 was an H3N2-predominant season classified as being of moderate severity, while 2014 to 2015 was an H3N2 predominant season classified as being of high severity.

Period of Contagiousness

You may be able to pass on flu to someone else before you know you are sick, as well as while you are sick.

- People with flu are most contagious in the first three to four days after their illness begins.

- Some otherwise healthy adults may be able to infect others beginning one day before symptoms develop and up to five to seven days after becoming sick.

- Some people, especially young children and people with weakened immune systems, might be able to infect others with flu viruses for an even longer time.

Onset of Symptoms

The time from when a person is exposed and infected with flu to when symptoms begin is about two days, but it can range from about one to four days.

Complications of Flu

Complications of flu can include bacterial pneumonia; ear infections; sinus infections; and the worsening of chronic medical conditions, such as congestive heart failure, asthma, or diabetes.

Table 17.1. Estimates of the Incidence of Symptomatic Influenza by Season and Age-Group, United States, 2010 to 2016

| Season | Predominant Virus(es) | Season Severity | Incidence, Percentage, by Age Group | | | | | |
			0 to 4 yrs	5 to 17 yrs	18 to 49 yrs	50 to 64 yrs	≥65 yrs	All Ages
2010-11	A/H3N2, A/H1N1pdm09	Moderate	14.1	8.4	5.3	8.1	4.3	6.8
2011-12	A/H3N2	Low	4.8	3.6	2.5	3.1	2.3	3
2012-13	A/H3N2	Moderate	18.6	12.7	8.9	14.3	9.9	11.3
2013-14	A/H1N1pdm09	Moderate	12.4	7.2	9.2	13	3.4	9
2014-15	A/H3N2	High	150	12.7	7.8	12.9	12.4	10.8
2015-16	A/H1N1pdm09	Moderate	11.1	7.4	7.1	11	3.5	7.6
Median			13.2	7.9	7.4	12	3.9	8.3

People at High Risk from Flu

Anyone can get flu (even healthy people), and serious problems related to flu can happen at any age. But, some people are at a high risk of developing serious flu-related complications if they get sick. This includes people 65 years of age and older, people of any age with certain chronic medical conditions (such as asthma, diabetes, or heart disease), pregnant women, and children younger than 5 years of age.

Preventing Seasonal Flu

The first and most important step in preventing flu is to get a flu vaccine each year. The flu vaccine has been shown to reduce flu-related illnesses and the risk of serious flu complications that can result in hospitalization or even death. The CDC also recommends everyday preventive actions (such as staying away from people who are sick, covering coughs and sneezes, and frequent handwashing) to help slow the spread of germs that cause respiratory (nose, throat, and lungs) illnesses, such as flu.

Diagnosing Flu

It is very difficult to distinguish flu from other viral or bacterial respiratory illnesses based on symptoms alone. There are tests available to diagnose flu.

Treating Flu

There are influenza antiviral drugs that can be used to treat flu illness.

Section 17.2

Pneumonia

This section includes text excerpted from "Pneumonia," National Heart, Lung, and Blood Institute (NHLBI), September 26, 2016.

What Is Pneumonia?

Pneumonia is a bacterial, viral, or fungal infection of one or both sides of the lungs that causes the air sacs, or alveoli, of the lungs to fill up with fluid or pus. Symptoms can be mild or severe and may include a cough with phlegm (a slimy substance), fever, chills, and trouble breathing. Many factors affect how serious pneumonia is, such as the type of germ causing the lung infection, your age, and your overall health. Pneumonia tends to be more serious for children under the age of 5; adults over the age of 65; people with certain conditions, such as heart failure, diabetes, or chronic obstructive pulmonary disease (COPD); or people who have weak immune systems due to human immunodeficiency virus (HIV)/acquired immunodeficiency syndrome (AIDS), chemotherapy (a treatment for cancer), or organ or blood and marrow stem cell transplant procedures.

To diagnose pneumonia, your doctor will review your medical history, perform a physical exam, and order diagnostic tests. This information can help your doctor determine what type of pneumonia you have. If your doctor suspects you got your infection while in a hospital, you may be diagnosed with hospital-acquired pneumonia. If you have been on a ventilator to help you breathe, you may have ventilator-associated pneumonia. The most common form of pneumonia is community-acquired pneumonia, which is when you get an infection outside of a hospital.

Treatment depends on whether bacteria, viruses, or fungi are causing your pneumonia. If bacteria are causing your pneumonia, you usually are treated at home with oral antibiotics. Most people respond quickly to treatment. If your symptoms worsen, you should see a doctor right away. If you have severe symptoms or underlying health problems, you may need to be treated in a hospital. It may take several weeks to recover from pneumonia.

Causes of Pneumonia

Bacteria, viruses, and fungi infections can cause pneumonia. These infections cause inflammation in the air sacs, or alveoli, of the lungs. This inflammation causes the air sacs to fill with fluid and pus.

235

Bacteria

Bacteria are the most common cause of pneumonia in adults. Many types of bacteria can cause bacterial pneumonia. *Streptococcus pneumoniae* or *pneumococcus* bacteria are the most common cause of bacterial pneumonia in the United States.

If your pneumonia is caused by one of the following types of bacteria, it is called "atypical pneumonia."

- **Legionella pneumophila.** This type of pneumonia sometimes is called "Legionnaire's disease," and it has caused serious outbreaks. Outbreaks have been linked to exposure to cooling towers, whirlpool spas, and decorative fountains.

- **Mycoplasma pneumoniae.** This is a common type of pneumonia that usually affects people younger than 40 years of age. People who live or work in crowded places, such as schools, homeless shelters, and prisons, are at a higher risk for this type of pneumonia. It is usually mild and responds well to treatment with antibiotics. However, Mycoplasma pneumoniae can be very serious. It may be associated with a skin rash and hemolysis. This type of bacteria is a common cause of "walking pneumonia."

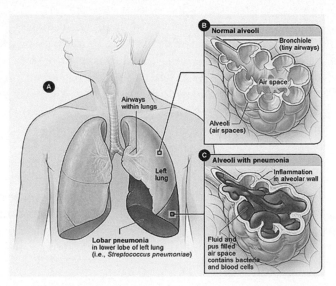

Figure 17.1. *Lobar Pneumonia*

This figure shows pneumonia affecting the single lower lobe of the left lung. Figure A shows the location of the lungs and airways in the body. Figure B shows normal alveoli. Figure C shows infected alveoli or air sacs.

- **Chlamydia pneumoniae.** This type of pneumonia can occur all year and often is mild. The infection is most common in people 65 to 79 years of age.

Bacterial pneumonia can occur on its own or develop after you have had a viral cold or the flu. Bacterial pneumonia often affects just one lobe, or area, of a lung. When this happens, the condition is called "lobar pneumonia."

Most of the time, the body filters bacteria out of the air that we breathe to protect the lungs from infection. Your immune system; the shape of your nose and throat; your ability to cough; and fine, hair-like structures called "cilia" help stop the germs from reaching your lungs.

Sometimes, bacteria manage to enter the lungs and cause infections. This is more likely to occur if:

- Your immune system is weak.

- A germ is very strong.

- Your body fails to filter out the bacteria from the air that you breathe. For example, if you cannot cough because you have had a stroke or are sedated, bacteria may remain in your airways.

When bacteria reach your lungs, your immune system goes into action. It sends many kinds of cells to attack the bacteria. These cells cause inflammation in alveoli and can cause these spaces to fill up with fluid and pus. This causes the symptoms of pneumonia.

Virus

Viruses that infect the respiratory tract may cause pneumonia. The influenza or flu virus is the most common cause of viral pneumonia in adults. Respiratory syncytial virus (RSV) is the most common cause of viral pneumonia in children younger than one year of age. Other viruses can cause pneumonia, such as the common cold virus known as "rhinovirus," "human parainfluenza virus" (HPIV), and "human metapneumovirus" (HMPV).

Most cases of viral pneumonia are mild. They get better in about one to three weeks without treatment. Some cases are more serious and may require treatment in a hospital. If you have viral pneumonia, you run the risk of getting bacterial pneumonia.

Fungi

Pneumocystis pneumonia is a serious fungal infection caused by *Pneumocystis jirovecii*. It occurs in people who have weak immune systems due to HIV/AIDS or the long-term use of medicines that suppress their immune systems, such as those used to treat cancer or as a part of organ or blood and marrow stem cell transplant procedures.

Other fungal infections also can lead to pneumonia. The following are three fungi that occur in the soil in some parts of the United States and can cause some people to get pneumonia.

- **Coccidioidomycosis.** This fungus is found in Southern California and the desert Southwest. It is the cause of valley fever.

- **Histoplasmosis.** This fungus is found in the Ohio and Mississippi River Valleys.

- **Cryptococcus.** This fungus is found throughout the United States in bird droppings and in soil contaminated with bird droppings.

Risk Factors of Pneumonia

Many factors, such as age, smoking, and other medical conditions, can increase your chances of getting pneumonia and having more severe pneumonia.

Age

Pneumonia can affect people of all ages. However, two age groups are at a greater risk of developing pneumonia and having more severe pneumonia:

- Infants who are two years of age or younger because their immune systems are still developing during the first few years of life.

- People who are 65 years of age or older because their immune systems begin to change as a normal part of aging.

Environment

Your risk for pneumonia may increase if you have been exposed to certain chemicals, pollutants, or toxic fumes.

Lifestyle Habits

Smoking cigarettes, excessive use of alcohol, or being undernourished also increases your risk for pneumonia.

Other Medical Conditions

Other conditions and factors also increase your risk for pneumonia. Your risk also goes up if you:

• Have trouble coughing because of a stroke or other condition, or have problems swallowing

• Cannot move around much or are sedated

• Recently had a cold or the flu

• Have a lung disease or other serious disease, including cystic fibrosis, asthma, chronic obstructive pulmonary disease (COPD), bronchiectasis, diabetes, heart failure, or sickle cell disease (SCD)

• Are in a hospital intensive-care unit (ICU), especially if you using a ventilator to help you breathe

• Have a weak or suppressed immune system due to HIV/AIDS, organ transplant or blood and marrow stem cell transplant, chemotherapy (a treatment for cancer), or long-term steroid use

Screening and Prevention of Pneumonia

Pneumonia can be very serious and even life-threatening. Vaccines can help prevent certain types of pneumonia. Good hygiene, quitting smoking, and keeping your immune system strong by exercising and healthy eating are other ways to prevent pneumonia.

Vaccines

Vaccines are available to prevent pneumonia caused by pneumococcal bacteria or the flu virus. Vaccines cannot prevent all cases of infection. However, compared to people who do not get vaccinated, those who are vaccinated and still get pneumonia tend to have:

• Milder infections

• Pneumonia that does not last as long

• Fewer serious complications

Pneumococcal Pneumonia Vaccines

Two vaccines are available to prevent pneumococcal pneumonia and potentially fatal complications, such as bacteremia and meningitis. Pneumococcal vaccines are particularly important for:

- Adults who are 65 years of age or older

- People who have chronic (ongoing) diseases, serious long-term health problems, or weak immune systems. For example, this may include people who have cancer, HIV/AIDS, asthma, sickle cell disease, or damaged or removed spleens.

- People who smoke

- Children who are younger than five years of age

- Children older than five years of age with certain medical conditions, such as heart or lung diseases or cancer

The Centers for Disease Control and Prevention (CDC) recommends that adults who are 65 years of age and older should have two pneumococcal vaccinations.

Influenza Vaccine

Because many people get pneumonia after having influenza or the flu, your yearly flu vaccine can help you and your family not get pneumonia. The flu vaccine is usually given in September through November before the months when influenza or the flu is most frequently spread.

Haemophilus Influenzae *Type B Vaccine*

Haemophilus influenzae type b (Hib) is a type of bacteria that can cause pneumonia and meningitis. The HIB vaccine is given to children to help prevent these infections. The vaccine is recommended for all children in the United States who are younger than five years of age. The vaccine often is given to infants starting at two months of age.

Other Ways to Help Prevent Pneumonia

You also can take the following steps to help prevent pneumonia:

- **Wash your hands** with soap and water or alcohol-based rubs to kill germs.

- **Do not smoke.** Smoking damages your lungs' ability to filter out and defend against germs.
- **Keep your immune system strong.** Get plenty of rest and physical activity, and follow a healthy diet.

Signs, Symptoms, and Complications of Pneumonia

The signs and symptoms of pneumonia vary from mild to severe. But some people are at risk for developing more severe pneumonia or potentially fatal complications.

Signs and Symptoms

See your doctor promptly if you have the following signs and symptoms:

- Have a high fever
- Have shaking chills
- Have a cough with phlegm (a slimy substance), which does not improve or worsens
- Develop shortness of breath with normal daily activities
- Have chest pain when you breathe or cough
- Feel suddenly worse after a cold or the flu

If you have pneumonia, you also may have other symptoms, including nausea (feeling sick to the stomach), vomiting, and diarrhea.

Symptoms may vary in certain populations. Newborns and infants may not show any signs of the infection. Or, they may vomit; have a fever and cough; or appear restless, sick, or tired and without energy.

Older adults and people who have serious illnesses or weak immune systems may have fewer and milder symptoms. They may even have a lower-than-normal temperature. If they already have a lung disease, it may get worse. Older adults who have pneumonia sometimes have sudden changes in mental awareness.

Complications

Often, people who have pneumonia can be successfully treated and do not have complications. Possible complications of pneumonia may include:

- **Bacteremia and septic shock.** Bacteremia is a serious complication in which bacteria from the initial site of infection spread into the blood. It may lead to septic shock, a potentially fatal complication.

- **Lung abscesses.** Lung abscesses usually are treated with antibiotics. Sometimes, surgery or drainage with a needle is needed to remove the pus.

- **Pleural effusions, empyema, and pleurisy.** These painful or even potentially fatal complications can occur if pneumonia is not treated. The pleura is a membrane that consists of two large, thin layers of tissue. One layer wraps around the outside of your lungs, and the other layer lines the inside of your chest cavity. Pleurisy is when the two layers of the pleura become irritated and inflamed, causing sharp pain each time you breathe in. The pleural space is a very thin space between the two pleura. Pleural effusions are the buildup of fluid in the pleural space. If the fluid becomes infected, it is called "empyema." If this happens, you may need to have the fluid drained through a chest tube or removed with surgery.

- **Renal failure**

- **Respiratory failure**

Diagnosis of Pneumonia

Sometimes, pneumonia is hard to diagnose because it may cause symptoms commonly seen in people with colds or the flu. You may not realize it is more serious until it lasts longer than these other conditions. Your doctor will diagnose pneumonia based on your medical history, a physical exam, and test results. Your doctor may be able to diagnose you with a certain type of pneumonia based on how you got your infection and the type of germ causing your infection.

Medical History

Your doctor will ask about your signs and symptoms and how and when they began. To find out whether you have bacterial, viral, or fungal pneumonia, your doctor also may ask about:

- Any recent traveling you have done
- Your hobbies
- Your exposure to animals

- Your exposure to sick people at home, school, or work

- Your past and current medical conditions, and whether any have gotten worse recently

- Any medicines you take

- Whether you smoke

- Whether you have had flu or pneumonia vaccinations

Physical Exam

Your doctor will listen to your lungs with a stethoscope. If you have pneumonia, your lungs may make crackling, bubbling, and rumbling sounds when you inhale. Your doctor also may hear wheezing. Your doctor may find it hard to hear sounds of breathing in some areas of your chest.

Diagnostic Tests

If your doctor thinks you have pneumonia, she or he may recommend one or more of the following tests.

- Chest X-ray to look for inflammation in your lungs. A chest X-ray is the best test for diagnosing pneumonia. However, this test will not tell your doctor what kind of germ is causing the pneumonia.

- Blood tests, such as a complete blood count (CBC), to see if your immune system is actively fighting an infection.

- Blood culture to find out whether you have a bacterial infection that has spread to your bloodstream. If so, your doctor can decide how to treat the infection.

Your doctor may recommend other tests if you are in the hospital, have serious symptoms, are older, or have other health problems.

- **Sputum test.** Your doctor may collect a sample of sputum (spit) or phlegm that was produced from one of your deep coughs and send the sample to the lab for testing. This may help your doctor find out if bacteria are causing your pneumonia. Then, she or he can plan your treatment.

- **Chest computed tomography (CT) scan** to see how much of your lungs is affected by your condition or to see if you have complications, such as lung abscesses or pleural effusions. A CT scan shows more detail than a chest X-ray.

- **Pleural fluid culture.** For this test, a fluid sample is taken from the pleural space. Doctors use a procedure called "thoracentesis" to collect the fluid sample. The fluid is studied for bacteria that may cause pneumonia.

- **Pulse oximetry.** For this test, a small sensor is attached to your finger or ear. The sensor uses light to estimate how much oxygen is in your blood. Pneumonia can keep your lungs from moving enough oxygen into your bloodstream. If you are very sick, your doctor may need to measure the level of oxygen in your blood using a blood sample. The sample is taken from an artery, usually in your wrist. This test is called an "arterial blood gas test."

- **Bronchoscopy** is a procedure used to look inside the lungs' airways. If you are in the hospital and treatment with antibiotics is not working well, your doctor may use this procedure. Your doctor passes a thin, flexible tube through your nose or mouth, down your throat, and into the airways. The tube has a light and small camera that allow your doctor to see your windpipe and airways and take pictures. Your doctor can see whether something is blocking your airways or whether another factor is contributing to your pneumonia. Your doctor may use this procedure to collect samples of fluid from the site of pneumonia (called "bronchoalveolar lavage" or "BAL") or to take small biopsies of lung tissue to help find the cause of your pneumonia.

Types of Pneumonia

Your doctor may also diagnose you with a certain type of pneumonia. Pneumonia is named for the way in which a person gets the infection or for the germ that causes the infection.

- **Community-acquired pneumonia (CAP).** CAP is the most common type of pneumonia and is usually caused by pneumococcus bacteria. Most cases occur during the winter. CAP occurs outside of hospitals and other healthcare settings. Most people get CAP by breathing in germs (especially while sleeping) that live in the mouth, nose, or throat.

- **Hospital-acquired pneumonia (HAP).** HAP is when people catch pneumonia during a hospital stay for another illness. HAP tends to be more serious than CAP because you are already sick. Also, hospitals tend to have more germs that are resistant to antibiotics that are used to treat bacterial pneumonia.

- **Ventilator-associated pneumonia (VAP).** VAP is when people who are on a ventilator machine to help them breathe get pneumonia.

- **Atypical pneumonia.** Atypical pneumonia is a type of CAP. It is caused by lung infections with less common bacteria than the pneumococcus bacteria that cause CAP. Atypical bacteria include Legionella pneumophila, Mycoplasma pneumoniae, or Chlamydia pneumoniae.

- **Aspiration pneumonia.** This type of pneumonia can occur if you inhale food, drink, vomit, or saliva from your mouth into your lungs. This may happen if something disturbs your normal gag reflex, such as a brain injury, swallowing problem, or excessive use of alcohol or drugs. Aspiration pneumonia can cause lung abscesses.

Treatment for Pneumonia

Treatment for pneumonia depends on the type of pneumonia you have, the germ causing your infection, and how severe your pneumonia is. Most people who have community-acquired pneumonia are treated at home. The goals of treatment are to cure the infection and prevent complications.

Bacterial Pneumonia

Bacterial pneumonia is treated with medicines called "antibiotics." You should take antibiotics as your doctor prescribes. You may start to feel better before you finish the medicine, but you should continue taking it as prescribed. If you stop too soon, the pneumonia may come back.

Most people begin to improve after one to three days of antibiotic treatment. This means that they should feel better and have fewer symptoms, such as cough and fever.

Viral Pneumonia

Antibiotics do not work when the cause of pneumonia is a virus. If you have viral pneumonia, your doctor may prescribe an antiviral medicine to treat it. Viral pneumonia usually improves in one to three weeks.

Treating Severe Symptoms

You may need to be treated in a hospital if:

- Your symptoms are severe.
- You are at risk for complications because of other health problems.

If the level of oxygen in your bloodstream is low, you may receive oxygen therapy. If you have bacterial pneumonia, your doctor may give you antibiotics through an intravenous (IV) line inserted into a vein.

General Treatment Advice and Follow-Up Care

If you have pneumonia, follow your treatment plan, take all medicines as prescribed, and get follow-up medical care.

Living with Pneumonia

If you have pneumonia, you can take steps to recover from the infection and prevent complications.

- Get plenty of rest.
- Follow your treatment plan as your doctor advises.
- Take all medicines as your doctor prescribes. If you are using antibiotics, continue to take the medicine until it is all gone. You may start to feel better before you finish the medicine, but you should continue to take it. If you stop too soon, the bacterial infection and your pneumonia may come back.
- Ask your doctor when you should schedule follow-up care. Your doctor may recommend a chest X-ray to make sure the infection is gone.

It may take time to recover from pneumonia. Some people feel better and are able to return to their normal routines within a week. For other people, it can take a month or more. Most people continue to feel tired for about a month. Talk with your doctor about when you can go back to your normal routine.

If you have pneumonia, limit contact with family and friends. Cover your nose and mouth while coughing or sneezing, get rid of used tissues right away, and wash your hands. These actions help keep the infection from spreading to other people.

Chapter 18

Kidney Disease

The kidneys are two bean-shaped organs, each about the size of a fist. They are located just below the rib cage, one on each side of your spine.

Healthy kidneys filter about a half cup of blood every minute, removing wastes and extra water to make urine. The urine flows from the kidneys to the bladder through two thin tubes of muscle called ureters, one on each side of your bladder. Your bladder stores urine. Your kidneys, ureters, and bladder are part of your urinary tract.

What Is Chronic Kidney Disease?

Chronic kidney disease (CKD) means that your kidneys are damaged and cannot filter blood the way they should. The disease is called "chronic" because the damage to your kidneys happens slowly over a long period of time. This damage can cause wastes to build up in your body. CKD can also cause other health problems.

The kidneys' main job is to filter extra water and wastes out of your blood to make urine. To keep your body working properly, the kidneys balance the salts and minerals—such as calcium, phosphorus, sodium,

This chapter contains text excerpted from the following sources: Text in this chapter begins with excerpts from "Your Kidneys and How They Work," National Institute of Diabetes and Digestive and Kidney Diseases (NIDDK), June 2018; Text beginning with the heading "What Is Chronic Kidney Disease?" is excerpted from "Chronic Kidney Disease (CKD)," National Institute of Diabetes and Digestive and Kidney Diseases (NIDDK), October 2016.

and potassium—that circulate in the blood. Your kidneys also make hormones that help control blood pressure, make red blood cells, and keep your bones strong.

Kidney disease often can get worse over time and may lead to kidney failure. If your kidneys fail, you will need dialysis or a kidney transplant to maintain your health.

The sooner you know you have kidney disease, the sooner you can make changes to protect your kidneys.

How Common Is Chronic Kidney Disease?

Chronic kidney disease is common among adults in the United States. More than 30 million American adults may have CKD.

Who Is More Likely to Develop Chronic Kidney Disease?

You are at risk for kidney disease if you have:

- **Diabetes.** Diabetes is the leading cause of CKD. High blood glucose, also called "blood sugar," from diabetes can damage the blood vessels in your kidneys. Almost one in three people with diabetes has CKD.

- **High blood pressure.** High blood pressure is the second leading cause of CKD. Similar to high blood glucose, high blood pressure also can damage the blood vessels in your kidneys. Almost one in five adults with high blood pressure has CKD.

- **Heart disease.** Research shows a link between kidney disease and heart disease. People with heart disease are at a higher risk for kidney disease, and people with kidney disease are at a higher risk for heart disease. Researchers are working to better understand the relationship between kidney disease and heart disease.

- **Family history of kidney failure.** If your mother, father, sister, or brother has kidney failure, you are at risk for CKD. Kidney disease tends to run in families. If you have kidney disease, encourage family members to get tested.

Your chances of having kidney disease increase with age. The longer you have had diabetes, high blood pressure, or heart disease, the more likely that you will have kidney disease.

African Americans, Hispanics, and American Indians tend to have a greater risk for CKD. The greater risk is due mostly to higher rates of diabetes and high blood pressure among these groups. Scientists are studying other possible reasons for this increased risk.

What Are the Symptoms of Chronic Kidney Disease?
Early Chronic Kidney Disease May Not Have Any Symptoms

You may wonder how you can have CKD and feel fine. Our kidneys have a greater capacity to do their job than is needed to keep us healthy. For example, you can donate one kidney and remain healthy. You can also have kidney damage without any symptoms because, despite the damage, your kidneys are still doing enough work to keep you feeling well. For many people, the only way to know if you have kidney disease is to get your kidneys checked with blood and urine tests.

As kidney disease gets worse, a person may have swelling, called "edema." Edema happens when the kidneys cannot get rid of extra fluid and salt. Edema can occur in the legs, feet, or ankles, and less often in the hands or face.

Symptoms of Advanced Chronic Kidney Disease

- Chest pain
- Dry skin
- Itching or numbness
- Feeling tired
- Headaches
- Increased or decreased urination
- Loss of appetite
- Muscle cramps
- Nausea
- Shortness of breath
- Sleep problems
- Trouble concentrating
- Vomiting
- Weight loss

People with CKD can also develop anemia, bone disease, and malnutrition.

Does Chronic Kidney Disease Cause Other Health Problems?

Kidney disease can lead to other health problems, such as heart disease. If you have kidney disease, it increases your chances of having a stroke or heart attack.

High blood pressure can be both a cause and a result of kidney disease. High blood pressure damages your kidneys, and damaged kidneys do not work as well to help control your blood pressure.

If you have CKD, you also have a higher chance of having a sudden change in kidney function caused by illness, injury, or certain medicines. This is called "acute kidney injury" (AKI).

How Can Chronic Kidney Disease Affect My Day-To-Day Life?

Many people are afraid to learn that they have kidney disease because they think that all kidney disease leads to dialysis. However, most people with kidney disease will not need dialysis. If you have kidney disease, you can continue to live a productive life, work, spend time with friends and family, stay physically active, and do other things you enjoy. You may need to change what you eat and add healthy habits to your daily routine to help you protect your kidneys.

Will My Kidneys Get Better?

Kidney disease is often progressive, which means that it gets worse over time. The damage to your kidneys causes scars and is permanent.

You can take steps to protect your kidneys, such as managing your blood pressure and your blood glucose, if you have diabetes.

What Happens If My Kidneys Fail?

Kidney failure means that your kidneys have lost most of their ability to function—less than 15 percent of normal kidney function. If you have kidney failure, you will need treatment to maintain your health.

Causes of Chronic Kidney Disease

Diabetes and high blood pressure are the most common causes of CKD. Your healthcare provider will look at your health history, and they may do tests to find out why you have kidney disease. The cause of your kidney disease may affect the type of treatment you receive.

Diabetes

Too much glucose, also called "sugar," in your blood damages your kidneys' filters. Over time, your kidneys can become so damaged that they no longer do a good job filtering wastes and extra fluid from your blood.

Often, the first sign of kidney disease from diabetes is protein in your urine. When the filters are damaged, a protein called "albumin," which you need to stay healthy, passes out of your blood and into your urine. A healthy kidney does not let albumin pass from the blood into the urine.

"Diabetic kidney disease" is the medical term for kidney disease caused by diabetes.

High Blood Pressure

High blood pressure can damage blood vessels in the kidneys so they do not work as well. If the blood vessels in your kidneys are damaged, your kidneys may not work as well to remove wastes and extra fluid from your body. Extra fluid in the blood vessels may then raise blood pressure even more, creating a dangerous cycle.

Other Causes of Kidney Disease

Other causes of kidney disease include:

- A genetic disorder that causes many cysts to grow in the kidneys, called "polycystic kidney disease" (PKD)

- An infection

- A drug that is toxic to the kidneys

- A disease that affects the entire body, such as diabetes or lupus. "Lupus nephritis" is the medical name for kidney disease caused by lupus

- IgA glomerulonephritis

- Disorders in which the body's immune system attacks its own cells and organs, such as Goodpasture syndrome

- Heavy metal poisoning, such as lead poisoning

- Rare genetic conditions, such as Alport syndrome

- Hemolytic uremic syndrome (HUS) in children

253

- Henoch-Schönlein purpura (HSP)

- Renal artery stenosis (RAS)

Tests and Diagnosis
How Can I Tell If I Have Kidney Disease?

Early kidney disease usually does not have any symptoms. Testing is the only way to know how well your kidneys are working. Get checked for kidney disease if you have:

- Diabetes

- High blood pressure

- Heart disease

- A family history of kidney failure

If you have diabetes, get checked every year. If you have high blood pressure, heart disease, or a family history of kidney failure, talk with your healthcare provider about how often you should get tested. The sooner you know you have kidney disease, the sooner you can get treatment to help protect your kidneys.

What Tests Do Doctors Use to Diagnose and Monitor Kidney Disease?

To check for kidney disease, healthcare providers use:

- A blood test that checks how well your kidneys are filtering your blood, called "glomerular filtration rate" (GFR)

- A urine test to check for albumin. Albumin is a protein that can pass into the urine when the kidneys are damaged.

If you have kidney disease, your healthcare provider will use the same two tests to help monitor your kidney disease and make sure your treatment plan is working.

Blood Test for Glomerular Filtration Rate

Your healthcare provider will use a blood test to check your kidney function. The results of the test mean the following:

- A GFR of 60 or more is in the normal range. Ask your healthcare provider when your GFR should be checked again.

- A GFR of less than 60 may mean you have kidney disease. Talk with your healthcare provider about how to keep your kidney health at this level.

- A GFR of 15 or less is called "kidney failure." Most people below this level need dialysis or a kidney transplant. Talk with your healthcare provider about your treatment options.

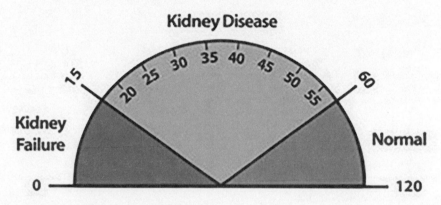

Figure 18.1. *Glomerular Filtration Rate*

GFR results show whether your kidneys are filtering at a normal level.

You cannot raise your GFR, but you can try to keep it from going lower.

Creatinine is a waste product from the normal breakdown of muscles in your body. Your kidneys remove creatinine from your blood. Providers use the amount of creatinine in your blood to estimate your GFR. As kidney disease gets worse, the level of creatinine goes up.

Urine Test for Albumin

If you are at risk for kidney disease, your provider may check your urine for albumin.

A healthy kidney does not let albumin pass into the urine. A damaged kidney lets some albumin pass into the urine. The less albumin in your urine, the better. Having albumin in the urine is called "albuminuria."

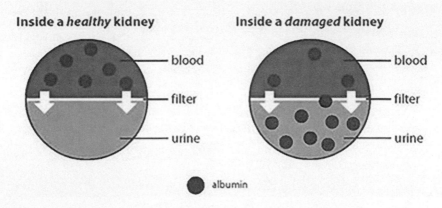

Figure 18.2. *Urine Test for Albumin*

A healthy kidney does not let albumin pass into the urine. A damaged kidney lets some albumin pass into the urine.

A healthcare provider can check for albumin in your urine in two ways:

Dipstick test for albumin. A provider uses a urine sample to look for albumin in your urine. You collect the urine sample in a container in a healthcare provider's office or lab. For the test, a provider places a strip of chemically treated paper, called a "dipstick," into the urine. The dipstick changes color if albumin is present in the urine.

Urine albumin-to-creatinine ratio (UACR). This test measures and compares the amount of albumin with the amount of creatinine in your urine sample. Providers use your UACR to estimate how much albumin would pass into your urine over 24 hours. A urine albumin result of

- 30 mg/g or less is normal
- More than 30 mg/g may be a sign of kidney disease

If you have albumin in your urine, your provider may want you to repeat the urine test one or two more times to confirm the results. Talk with your provider about what your specific numbers mean for you.

If you have kidney disease, measuring the albumin in your urine helps your provider know which treatment is best for you. A urine albumin level that stays the same or goes down may mean that treatments are working.

How Do I Know If My Kidney Disease Is Getting Worse?

You can keep track of your test results over time. You can tell that your treatments are working if your:

- GFR stays the same.

- Urine albumin stays the same or goes down.

Your healthcare provider will work with you to manage your kidney disease.

Managing Chronic Kidney Disease

If you have chronic kidney disease (CKD), you can take steps to protect your kidneys from more damage.

The sooner you know you have kidney disease, the better. The steps you take to protect your kidneys from damage also may help prevent heart disease and improve your health overall. Making these changes when you have no symptoms may be hard, but it is worthwhile.

Ten Ways to Manage Kidney Disease
Control Your Blood Pressure

The most important step you can take to treat kidney disease is to control your blood pressure. High blood pressure can damage your kidneys. You can protect your kidneys by keeping your blood pressure at or less than the goal set by your healthcare provider. For most people, the blood pressure goal is less than 140/90 mm Hg.

Work with your healthcare provider to develop a plan to meet your blood pressure goals. Steps you can take to meet your blood pressure goals may include eating heart-healthy and low-sodium meals, quitting smoking, being active, getting enough sleep, and taking your medicines as prescribed.

Meet Your Blood Glucose Goal If You Have Diabetes

To reach your blood glucose goal, check your blood glucose level regularly. Use the results to guide decisions about food, physical activity, and medicines. Ask your healthcare provider how often you should check your blood glucose level.

Your healthcare provider will also test your A1C. The A1C is a blood test that measures your average blood glucose level over the past three months. This test is different from the blood glucose checks you do regularly. The higher your A1C number, the higher your blood glucose levels have been during the past three months. Stay close to your daily blood glucose numbers to help you meet your A1C goal.

The A1C goal for many people with diabetes is below seven percent. Ask your healthcare provider what your goal should be. Reaching your goal numbers will help you protect your kidneys.

Work with Your Healthcare Team to Monitor Your Kidney Health

The tests that healthcare providers use to test for kidney disease can also be used to track changes to kidney function and damage. Kidney disease tends to get worse over time. Each time you get checked, ask your provider how the test results compare to the last results. Your goals will be to:

- Keep your GFR the same

- Keep your urine albumin the same or lower

Your healthcare provider will also check your blood pressure and, if you have diabetes, your A1C level to make sure you are meeting your blood pressure and blood glucose goals.

How Can I Prepare for Visits with My Healthcare Provider?

The more you plan for your visits, the more you will be able to learn about your health and treatment options.

Make a List of Questions

It is normal to have a lot of questions. Write down your questions as you think of them so that you can remember everything you want to ask when you see your healthcare provider. You may want to ask about what tests are being done, what test results mean, or the changes you need to make to your diet and medicines.

Sample Questions to Ask Your Provider for People with Kidney Disease
About Your Tests

- What is my GFR? What does that mean?

- Has my GFR changed since last time?

- What is my urine albumin? What does it mean?

- Has my urine albumin changed since the last time it was checked?

- Is my kidney disease getting worse?

- Is my blood pressure where it needs to be?

About Treatment and Self-Care

- What can I do to keep my disease from getting worse?

- Do any of my medicines or doses need to be changed?

- What time of day should I take each of my medicines?

- Do I need to change what I eat?

- Will you refer me to a dietitian for diet counseling?

- When will I need to see a nephrologist (kidney specialist)?

- Do I need to worry about dialysis or a kidney transplant?

- What do I need to do to protect my veins?

About Complications

- What other health problems may I face because of my kidney disease?

- Should I be looking for any symptoms? If so, what are they?

Bring a Friend or Relative with You for Support

A trusted friend or family member can take notes, ask questions you may not have thought of, offer support, and help remember what the provider said during the visit. Talk ahead of time about what you want to get out of the visit and the role you would like your friend or relative to play.

Who Is Part of My Healthcare Team?

The following healthcare providers may be part of the healthcare team involved in your treatment:

- **Primary care provider.** Your primary care provider (PCP)— doctor, nurse practitioner, or physician assistant—is the person you see for routine medical visits. Your PCP may monitor your kidney health and help you manage your diabetes and high blood pressure. A PCP also prescribes medicines and may refer you to specialists.

- **Nurse.** A nurse may help with your treatment and teach you about monitoring and treating kidney disease, as well as managing your health conditions. Some nurses specialize in kidney disease.

- **Registered dietitian.** A registered dietitian is a food and nutrition expert who helps people create a healthy eating plan when they have a health condition, such as kidney disease. Dietitians can help you by creating an eating plan based on how your kidneys are doing. "Renal dietitians" often work in dialysis centers and are specially trained to work with people with kidney failure.

- **Diabetes educator.** A diabetes educator teaches people with diabetes how to manage their disease and handle diabetes-related problems.

- **Pharmacist.** A pharmacist educates you about your medicines and fills your prescriptions. An important job for the pharmacist is to review all of your medicines, including over-the-counter (OTC) medicines, and supplements to avoid unsafe combinations and side effects.

- **Social worker.** When you are close to needing dialysis, you may have a chance to meet with a social worker. A dialysis social worker helps people and their families deal with the life changes and costs that come with having kidney disease and kidney failure. A dialysis social worker also can help people with kidney failure apply for help to cover treatment costs.

- **Nephrologist.** A nephrologist is a doctor who is a kidney specialist. Your PCP may refer you to a nephrologist if you have a complicated case of kidney disease, your kidney disease is quickly getting worse, or your kidney disease is advanced.

Take Medicines as Prescribed

Many people with CKD take medicines prescribed to lower blood pressure, control blood glucose, and lower cholesterol.

Two types of blood pressure medicines, angiotensin-converting enzyme (ACE) inhibitors and angiotensin II receptor blockers (ARBs), may slow kidney disease and delay kidney failure, even in people who do not have high blood pressure. The names of these medicines end in –pril or –sartan.

Many people need to take two or more medicines for their blood pressure. You may also need to take a diuretic, sometimes called a "water pill." The aim is to meet your blood pressure goal. These medicines may work better if you limit your salt intake.

Know That Your Medicines May Change over Time

Your healthcare provider may change your medicines as your kidney disease gets worse. Your kidneys do not filter as well as they did in the past, and this can cause an unsafe buildup of medicines in your blood. Some medicines can also harm your kidneys. As a result, your provider may tell you to:

- Take a medicine less often or take a smaller dose.
- Stop taking a medicine or switch to a different one.

Your pharmacist and healthcare provider need to know about all the medicines you take, including OTC medicines, vitamins, and supplements.

Be Careful about the Over-the-Counter Medicines You Take

If you take OTC or prescription medicines for headaches, pain, fever, or colds, you may be taking nonsteroidal anti-inflammatory drugs (NSAIDs). NSAIDs include commonly used pain relievers and cold medicines that can damage your kidneys and lead to acute kidney injury, especially in those with kidney disease, diabetes, and high blood pressure.

Ibuprofen and naproxen are NSAIDs. NSAIDs are sold under many different brand names, so ask your pharmacist or healthcare provider if the medicines you take are safe to use.

If you have been taking NSAIDs regularly to control chronic pain, you may want to ask your healthcare provider about other ways to treat pain, such as meditation or other relaxation techniques.

Tips for Managing Your Medicines

The next time you pick up a prescription or buy an OTC medicine or supplement, ask your pharmacist how the product may:

- Affect your kidneys
- Affect other medicines you take

Fill your prescriptions at only one pharmacy or pharmacy chain so your pharmacist can:

• Keep track of your medicines and supplements

• Check for harmful interactions

Keep track of your medicines and supplements:

• Keep an up-to-date list of your medicines and supplements in your wallet. Take your list with you, or bring all of your medicine bottles, to all healthcare visits.

Work with a Dietitian to Develop a Meal Plan

What you eat and drink can help you:

• Protect your kidneys

• Reach your blood pressure and blood glucose goals

• Prevent or delay health problems caused by kidney disease

As your kidney disease gets worse, you may need to make more changes to what you eat and drink.

A dietitian who knows about kidney disease can work with you to create a meal plan that includes foods that are healthy for you and that you enjoy eating. Cooking and preparing your food from scratch can help you eat healthier.

Nutrition counseling from a registered dietitian to help meet your medical or health goals is called "medical nutrition therapy" (MNT). If you have diabetes or kidney disease and a referral from your primary care provider, your health insurance may cover MNT. If you qualify for Medicare, MNT is covered.

Your healthcare provider may be able to refer you to a dietitian. You can also find a registered dietitian online through the Academy of Nutrition and Dietetics. Work closely with your dietitian to learn to eat right for CKD.

Make Physical Activity Part of Your Routine

Be active for 30 minutes or more on most days. Physical activity can help you reduce stress, manage your weight, and achieve your blood pressure and blood glucose goals. If you are not active now, ask your healthcare provider about the types and amounts of physical activity that are right for you.

Aim for a Healthy Weight

Being overweight makes your kidneys work harder and may damage your kidneys. The National Institutes of Health (NIH) Body Weight Planner is an online tool to help you tailor your calorie and physical activity plans to achieve and stay at a healthy weight.

Get Enough Sleep

Aim for seven to eight hours of sleep each night. Getting enough sleep is important to your overall physical and mental health, and it can help you meet your blood pressure and blood glucose goals. You can take steps to improve your sleep habits.

Stop Smoking

Cigarette smoking can make kidney damage worse. Quitting smoking may help you meet your blood pressure goals, which is good for your kidneys, and can lower your chances of having a heart attack or stroke.

Find Healthy Ways to Cope with Stress and Depression

Long-term stress can raise your blood pressure and your blood glucose and lead to depression. Some of the steps that you are taking to manage your kidney disease are also healthy ways to cope with stress. For example, physical activity and sleep help reduce stress. Listening to your favorite music, focusing on something calm or peaceful, or meditating may also help you.

Depression is common among people with a chronic, or long-term, illness. Depression can make it harder to manage your kidney disease. Ask for help if you feel down. Seek help from a mental-health professional. Talking with a support group, clergy member, friend, or family member who will listen to your feelings may help.

Eating Right

You may need to change what you eat to manage your CKD. Work with a registered dietitian to develop a meal plan that includes foods that you enjoy eating while maintaining your kidney health.

The steps below will help you eat right as you manage your kidney disease. The first three steps (one to three) are important for all people with kidney disease. The last two steps (four to five) may become important as your kidney function goes down.

The First Steps to Eating Right

Step 1: Choose and Prepare Foods with Less Salt and Sodium

Why? To help control your blood pressure. Your diet should contain less than 2,300 milligrams of sodium each day.

- Buy fresh food often. Sodium (a part of salt) is added to many prepared or packaged foods you buy at the supermarket or at restaurants.

- Cook foods from scratch instead of eating prepared foods, "fast" foods, frozen dinners, and canned foods that are higher in sodium. When you prepare your own food, you control what goes into it.

Nutrition Facts

Serving Size 1/4 Cup (30g)
Servings Per Container About 38

Amount Per Serving

Calories 200 Calories from Fat 150

	% Daily Value*
Total Fat 17g	**26%**
Saturated Fat 2.5g	**13%**
Trans Fat 0g	
Cholesterol 0mg	**0%**
Sodium 120mg	**5%**
Total Carbohydrate 7g	**2%**
Dietary Fiber 2g	**8%**
Sugars 1g	
Protein 5g	

Vitamin A 0%	Vitamin C 0%
Calcium 4%	Iron 8%

*Percent Daily Values are based on a 2,000 calorie diet.

Figure 18.3. *Nutrition Facts Label*

Look for sodium on the food label. A food label showing a Percent Daily Value of 5 percent or less is low sodium. Also, look for the amount of saturated and trans fats listed on the label.

- Use spices, herbs, and sodium-free seasonings in place of salt.

- Check for sodium on the Nutrition Facts label of food packages. A Daily Value of 20 percent or more means that the food is high in sodium.

- Try lower-sodium versions of frozen dinners and other convenience foods.

- Rinse canned vegetables, beans, meats, and fish with water before eating.

Look for food labels with words such as sodium-free or salt-free; or low, reduced, or no salt or sodium; or unsalted or lightly salted.

Step 2: Eat the Right Amount and the Right Types of Protein

Why? To help protect your kidneys. When your body uses protein, it produces waste. Your kidneys remove this waste. Eating more protein than you need may make your kidneys work harder.

- Eat small portions of protein foods.
- Protein is found in foods from plants and animals. Most people eat both types of protein. Talk to your dietitian about how to choose the right combination of protein foods for you.

Animal-Protein Foods

- Chicken
- Fish
- Meat
- Eggs
- Dairy

A cooked portion of chicken, fish, or meat is about 2 to 3 ounces or about the size of a deck of cards. A portion of dairy foods is ½ cup of milk or yogurt, or one slice of cheese.

Plant-Protein Foods

- Beans
- Nuts
- Grains

A portion of cooked beans is about ½ cup, and a portion of nuts is ¼ cup. A portion of bread is a single slice, and a portion of cooked rice or cooked noodles is ½ cup.

Step 3: Choose Foods That Are Healthy for Your Heart

Why? To help keep fat from building up in your blood vessels, heart, and kidneys. To help keep fat from building up in your blood vessels, heart, and kidneys.

- Grill, broil, bake, roast, or stir-fry foods instead of deep frying.
- Cook with nonstick cooking spray or a small amount of olive oil instead of butter.
- Trim fat from meat and remove skin from poultry before eating.
- Try to limit saturated and trans fats. Read the food label.

Heart-Healthy Foods

- Lean cuts of meat, such as loin or round
- Poultry without the skin
- Fish
- Beans
- Vegetables
- Fruits
- Low-fat or fat-free milk, yogurt, and cheese

Limit Alcohol

Drink alcohol only in moderation: no more than one drink per day if you are a woman, and no more than two if you are a man. Drinking too much alcohol can damage the liver, heart, and brain and cause serious health problems. Ask your healthcare provider how much alcohol you can drink safely.

The Next Steps to Eating Right

As your kidney function goes down, you may need to eat foods with less phosphorus and potassium. Your healthcare provider will use lab tests to check phosphorus and potassium levels in your blood, and you can work with your dietitian to adjust your meal plan.

Step 4: Choose Foods and Drinks with Less Phosphorus

Why? To help protect your bones and blood vessels. When you have CKD, phosphorus can build up in your blood. Too much phosphorus in your blood pulls calcium from your bones, making your bones thin, weak, and more likely to break. High levels of phosphorus in your blood can also cause itchy skin, and bone and joint pain.

- Many packaged foods have added phosphorus. Look for phosphorus—or for words with "PHOS"—on ingredient labels.

- Deli meats and some fresh meat and poultry can have added phosphorus. Ask the butcher to help you pick fresh meats without added phosphorus.

Table 18.1. Phosphorus in Foods

Foods Lower in Phosphorus	Foods Higher in Phosphorus
Fresh fruits and vegetables	Meat, poultry, fish
Breads, pasta, rice	Bran cereals and oatmeal
Rice milk (not enriched)	Dairy foods
Corn and rice cereals	Beans, lentils, nuts
Light-colored sodas/pop, such as lemon-lime or homemade iced tea	Dark-colored sodas/pop, fruit punch, some bottled or canned iced teas that have added phosphorus

Your healthcare provider may talk to you about taking a phosphate binder with meals to lower the amount of phosphorus in your blood. A phosphate binder is a medicine that acts like a sponge to soak up, or bind, phosphorus while it is in the stomach. Because it is bound, the phosphorus does not get into your blood. Instead, your body removes the phosphorus through your stool.

Step 5: Choose Foods with the Right Amount of Potassium

Why? To help your nerves and muscles work the right way. Problems can occur when blood potassium levels are too high or too low. Damaged kidneys allow potassium to build up in your blood, which can cause serious heart problems. Your food and drink choices can help you lower your potassium level, if needed.

- Salt substitutes can be very high in potassium. Read the ingredient label. Check with your provider about using salt substitutes.

- Drain canned fruits and vegetables before eating.

Table 18.2. Potassium in Foods

Foods Lower in Potassium	Foods Higher in Potassium
Apples, peaches	Oranges, bananas, and orange juice
Carrots, green beans	Potatoes, tomatoes
White bread and pasta	Brown and wild rice
White rice	Bran cereals
Rice milk (not enriched)	Dairy foods
Cooked rice and wheat cereals, grits	Whole-wheat bread and pasta
Apple, grape, or cranberry juice	Beans and nuts

Some medicines also can raise your potassium level. Your healthcare provider may adjust the medicines you take.

Preventing Chronic Kidney Disease

You are more likely to develop kidney disease if you have:

- Diabetes
- High blood pressure
- Heart disease
- A family history of kidney failure

What Can I Do to Keep My Kidneys Healthy?

You can protect your kidneys by preventing or managing health conditions that cause kidney damage, such as diabetes and high blood pressure. The steps described below may help keep your whole body healthy, including your kidneys.

During your next medical visit, you may want to ask your healthcare provider about your kidney health. Early kidney disease may not have any symptoms, so getting tested may be the only way to know your kidneys are healthy. Your healthcare provider will help decide how often you should be tested.

See a provider right away if you develop a urinary tract infection (UTI), which can cause kidney damage if left untreated.

Make Healthy Food Choices

Choose foods that are healthy for your heart and your entire body: fresh fruits, fresh or frozen vegetables, whole grains, and low-fat or fat-free dairy products. Eat healthy meals, and cut back on salt and added sugars. Aim for less than 2,300 milligrams of sodium each day. Try to have less than 10 percent of your daily calories come from added sugars.

Tips for Making Healthy Food Choices

- Cook with a mix of spices instead of salt.
- Choose veggie toppings, such as spinach, broccoli, and peppers, for your pizza.
- Try baking or broiling meat, chicken, and fish instead of frying.
- Serve foods without gravy or added fats.
- Try to choose foods with little or no added sugar.
- Gradually work your way down from whole milk to two percent milk until you are drinking and cooking with fat-free (skim) or low-fat milk and milk products.
- Eat foods made from whole grains—such as whole wheat, brown rice, oats, and whole-grain corn—every day. Use whole-grain bread for toast and sandwiches; substitute brown rice for white rice for home-cooked meals and when dining out.
- Read food labels. Choose foods low in saturated fats, trans fats, cholesterol, salt (sodium), and added sugars.
- Slow down at snack time. Eating a bag of low-fat popcorn takes longer than eating a slice of cake. Peel and eat an orange instead of drinking orange juice.
- Try keeping a written record of what you eat for a week. It can help you see when you tend to overeat or eat foods high in fat or calories.

Make Physical Activity Part of Your Routine

Be active for 30 minutes or more on most days. If you are not active now, ask your healthcare provider about the types and amounts of physical activity that are right for you.

Aim for a Healthy Weight

The NIH Body Weight Planner is an online tool to help you tailor your calorie and physical activity plans to achieve and stay at a healthy weight.

If you are overweight or have obesity, work with your healthcare provider or dietitian to create a realistic weight-loss plan.

Get Enough Sleep

Aim for 7 to 8 hours of sleep each night. If you have trouble sleeping, take steps to improve your sleep habits.

Stop Smoking

If you smoke or use other tobacco products, stop. Ask for help so you do not have to do it alone. You can start by calling the National Quitline at 800-QUITNOW or 800-784-8669.

Limit Alcohol

Drinking too much alcohol can increase your blood pressure and add extra calories, which can lead to weight gain. If you drink alcohol, limit yourself to one drink per day if you are a woman and two drinks per day if you are a man. One drink is:

- 12 ounces of beer

- 5 ounces of wine

- 1.5 ounces of liquor

Explore Stress-Reducing Activities

Learning how to manage stress, relax, and cope with problems can improve emotional and physical health. Physical activity can help reduce stress, as can mind and body practices, such as meditation, yoga, or tai chi.

Manage Diabetes, High Blood Pressure, and Heart Disease

If you have diabetes, high blood pressure, or heart disease, the best way to protect your kidneys from damage is to:

Keep blood glucose numbers close to your goal. Checking your blood glucose, or blood sugar, level is an important way to manage your diabetes. Your healthcare team may want you to test your blood glucose one or more times a day.

Keep your blood pressure numbers close to your goal. The blood pressure goal for most people with diabetes is below 140/90 mm Hg.

Take all your medicines as prescribed. Talk with your healthcare provider about certain blood pressure medicines, called "ACE inhibitors" and "ARBs," which may protect your kidneys. The names of these medicines end in –pril or –sartan.

Be careful about the daily use of over-the-counter pain medications. Regular use of NSAIDs, such as ibuprofen and naproxen, can damage your kidneys.

To help prevent heart attacks and stroke, keep your cholesterol levels in the target range. There are two kinds of cholesterol in your blood: low-density lipoprotein (LDL) and high-density lipoprotein (HDL). LDL, or "bad," cholesterol can build up and clog your blood vessels, which can cause a heart attack or stroke. HDL, or "good," cholesterol helps remove the bad cholesterol from your blood vessels. A cholesterol test also may measure another type of blood fat called "triglycerides."

Ask Your Healthcare Provider Questions

Ask your healthcare provider the following key questions about your kidney health during your next medical visit. The sooner you know you have kidney disease, the sooner you can get treatment to help protect your kidneys.

Key Questions for Your Healthcare Provider:

- What is my glomerular filtration rate?
- What is my urine albumin result?
- What is my blood pressure?
- What is my blood glucose (for people with diabetes)?
- How often should I get my kidneys checked?

Other important questions:

- What should I do to keep my kidneys healthy?
- Do I need to be taking different medicines?
- Should I be more physically active?
- What kind of physical activity can I do?
- What can I eat?
- Am I at a healthy weight?
- Do I need to talk with a dietitian to get help with meal planning?

- Should I be taking ACE inhibitors or ARBs for my kidneys?

- What happens if I have kidney disease?

What If My Kidneys Fail

Some people live with kidney disease for years and are able to maintain kidney function. Others progress quickly to kidney failure.

Kidney failure means that your kidneys have lost most of their ability to function—less than 15 percent of normal kidney function. If your kidney function drops to this level, you may have symptoms from the buildup of waste products and extra water in your body.

To replace your lost kidney function, you may have one of three treatment options:

- Hemodialysis

- Peritoneal dialysis

- Kidney transplant

End-stage renal disease (ESRD) is kidney failure that is treated by dialysis or kidney transplant.

Some people with kidney failure choose not to have dialysis or a transplant but continue to receive care from their healthcare team, take medicines, and monitor their diet and lifestyle choices.

Work with your healthcare team and family to consider your options, and choose a treatment that is right for you.

Chapter 19

Liver Cancer

What Is the Liver?

The liver is the largest organ in the human body, located on the upper right side of the body, behind the lower ribs. The liver does many jobs, including:

- Storing nutrients

- Removing waste products and worn-out cells from the blood

- Filtering and processing chemicals in food, alcohol, and medications

- Producing bile, a solution that helps digest fats and eliminates waste products

Liver Cancer Facts

Cancer is a disease in which cells in the body grow out of control. When cancer starts in the liver, it is called "liver cancer." Each year in the United States, about 33,000 people get liver cancer, and about 26,000 people die from the disease. The percentage of Americans who get liver cancer has been rising for several decades.

This chapter includes text excerpted from "Liver Cancer," Centers for Disease Control and Prevention (CDC), September 18, 2018.

What Causes Liver Cancer

Many liver cancer cases are related to hepatitis B virus or hepatitis C virus infections. Most people do not know they have the virus.

Other behaviors and conditions that increase risk for getting liver cancer are:

- Excessive alcohol use

- Cirrhosis (scarring of the liver, which can also be caused by hepatitis and alcohol use)

- Obesity

- Diabetes

- Having hemochromatosis, a condition where the body takes up and stores more iron than it needs

- Eating foods that have aflatoxin (a fungus that can grow on foods, such as grains and nuts, that have not been stored properly)

What Are the Symptoms of Liver Cancer?

In its early stages, liver cancer may not have symptoms that can be seen or felt. However, as the cancer grows larger, people may notice one or more of these common symptoms. It is important to remember that these symptoms could also be caused by other health conditions. If you have any of these symptoms, talk to your doctor.

Liver cancer symptoms may include:

- Discomfort in the upper abdomen, on the right side

- A swollen abdomen

- A hard lump on the right side of the abdomen, just below the rib cage

- Pain near the right shoulder blade or in the back

- Jaundice (yellowing of the skin and whites of the eyes)

- Easy bruising or bleeding

- Unusual tiredness

- Nausea and vomiting

- Loss of appetite

- Weight loss for no known reason

How Can I Reduce My Risk for Liver Cancer?

You can lower your risk of getting liver cancer in the following ways:

- Get vaccinated against hepatitis B. The hepatitis B vaccine is recommended for all infants at birth and for adults who may be at an increased risk.

- Get tested for hepatitis C, and get medical care if you have it.

- Avoid drinking too much alcohol.

Chapter 20

Lung Cancer

Your lungs are organs in your chest that allow your body to take in oxygen from the air. They also help remove carbon dioxide (a waste gas that can be toxic) from your body.

The lungs' intake of oxygen and removal of carbon dioxide is called gas exchange. Gas exchange is part of breathing. Breathing is a vital function of life; it helps your body work properly. Other organs and tissues also help make breathing possible.

What Is Lung Cancer?

Cancer is a disease in which cells in the body grow out of control. When cancer starts in the lungs, it is called "lung cancer."

Lung cancer begins in the lungs and may spread to lymph nodes or other organs in the body, such as the brain. Cancer from other organs also may spread to the lungs. When cancer cells spread from one organ to another, they are called "metastases."

Lung cancers usually are grouped into two main types called "small cell" and "nonsmall cell." These types of lung cancer grow differently and are treated differently. Nonsmall cell lung cancer is more common than small cell lung cancer.

This chapter contains text excerpted from the following sources: Text in this chapter begins with excerpts from "How the Lungs Work," National Heart, Lung, and Blood Institute (NHLBI), November 20, 2018; Text beginning with the heading "What Is Lung Cancer?" is excerpted from "What Is Lung Cancer?" Centers for Disease Control and Prevention (CDC), July 19, 2018.

What Are the Risk Factors for Lung Cancer?

Research has found several risk factors that may increase your chances of getting lung cancer.

Smoking

Cigarette smoking is the number 1 risk factor for lung cancer. In the United States, cigarette smoking is linked to about 80 to 90 percent of lung cancer deaths. Using other tobacco products, such as cigars or pipes, also increases the risk for lung cancer. Tobacco smoke is a toxic mix of more than 7,000 chemicals. Many are poisons. At least 70 are known to cause cancer in people or animals.

People who smoke cigarettes are 15 to 30 times more likely to get lung cancer or die from lung cancer than people who do not smoke. Even smoking a few cigarettes a day or smoking occasionally increases the risk of lung cancer. The more years a person smokes and the more cigarettes smoked each day, the higher the risk is.

People who quit smoking have a lower risk of lung cancer than if they had continued to smoke, but their risk is higher than the risk for people who never smoked. Quitting smoking at any age can lower the risk of lung cancer.

Cigarette smoking can cause cancer almost anywhere in the body. Cigarette smoking causes cancer of the mouth and throat, esophagus, stomach, colon, rectum, liver, pancreas, voicebox (larynx), trachea, bronchus, kidney and renal pelvis, urinary bladder, and cervix, and it causes acute myeloid leukemia (AML).

Secondhand Smoke

Smoke from other people's cigarettes, pipes, or cigars (secondhand smoke) also causes lung cancer. When a person breathes in secondhand smoke, it is like she or he is smoking. In the United States, 2 out of 5 adults who do not smoke and half of children are exposed to secondhand smoke, and about 7,300 people who never smoked die from lung cancer due to secondhand smoke every year.

Radon

Radon is a naturally occurring gas that comes from rocks and dirt, and it can get trapped in houses and buildings. It cannot be seen, tasted, or smelled. According to the U.S. Environmental Protection Agency (EPA), radon causes about 20,000 cases of lung cancer each year, making it the second leading cause of lung cancer. Nearly 1 out of every 15 homes in the United States is thought to have high radon levels. The EPA recommends testing homes for radon and using proven ways to lower high radon levels.

Other Substances

Examples of substances found at some workplaces that increase lung cancer risk include asbestos, arsenic, diesel exhaust, and some forms of silica and chromium. For many of these substances, the risk of getting lung cancer is even higher for those who smoke.

Personal or Family History of Lung Cancer

If you are a lung cancer survivor, there is a risk that you may develop another lung cancer, especially if you smoke. Your risk of lung cancer may be higher if your parents, brothers or sisters, or children have had lung cancer. This could be true because they also smoke, or they live or work in the same place where they are exposed to radon and other substances that can cause lung cancer.

Radiation Therapy to the Chest

Cancer survivors who had radiation therapy to the chest are at a higher risk of lung cancer.

Diet

Scientists are studying many different foods and dietary supplements to see whether they change the risk of getting lung cancer. There is much we still need to know. We do know that smokers who take beta-carotene supplements have an increased risk of lung cancer.

Also, arsenic in drinking water (primarily from private wells) can increase the risk of lung cancer.

What Are the Symptoms?

Different people have different symptoms for lung cancer. Some people have symptoms related to the lungs. Some people whose lung cancer has spread to other parts of the body (metastasized) have symptoms specific to that part of the body. Some people just have general symptoms of not feeling well. Most people with lung cancer do not have symptoms until the cancer is advanced. Lung cancer symptoms may include:

- Coughing that gets worse or does not go away
- Chest pain
- Shortness of breath
- Wheezing
- Coughing up blood
- Feeling very tired all the time
- Weight loss with no known cause

Other changes that can sometimes occur with lung cancer may include repeated bouts of pneumonia and swollen or enlarged lymph nodes (glands) inside the chest in the area between the lungs.

These symptoms can happen with other illnesses too. If you have some of these symptoms, talk to your doctor, who can help find the cause.

What Can I Do to Reduce My Risk

You can help lower your risk of lung cancer in the following ways:

- **Do not smoke.** Cigarette smoking causes about 80 to 90 percent of lung cancer deaths in the United States. The most important thing you can do to prevent lung cancer is to not start smoking or to quit if you smoke.

- **Avoid secondhand smoke.** Smoke from other people's cigarettes, cigars, or pipes is called "secondhand smoke." Make your home and car smoke-free.

- **Get your home tested for radon.** The U.S. Environmental Protection Agency recommends that all homes be tested for radon.

- **Be careful at work.** Health and safety guidelines in the workplace can help workers avoid carcinogens—things that can cause cancer.

Who Should Be Screened for Lung Cancer?

Screening means testing for a disease when there are no symptoms or history of that disease. Doctors recommend a screening test to find a disease early, when treatment may work better.

The only recommended screening test for lung cancer is low-dose computed tomography (also called a "low-dose CT scan," or "LDCT"). In this test, an X-ray machine scans the body and uses low doses of radiation to make detailed pictures of the lungs.

Who Should Be Screened?

The U.S. Preventive Services Task Force (USPSTF) recommends yearly lung cancer screening with low-dose computed tomography (LDCT) for people who:

- Have a history of heavy smoking

- Smoke now or have quit within the past 15 years

- Are between 55 and 80 years old

Heavy smoking means a smoking history of 30 pack years or more. A pack year is smoking an average of one pack of cigarettes per day for one year. For example, a person could have a 30 pack-year history by smoking 1 pack a day for 30 years or 2 packs a day for 15 years.

Risks of Screening

Lung cancer screening has at least three risks:

- A lung cancer screening test can suggest that a person has lung cancer when no cancer is present. This is called a "false-positive result." False-positive results can lead to follow-up tests and surgeries that are not needed and may have more risks.

- A lung cancer screening test can find cases of cancer that may never have caused a problem for the patient. This is called "overdiagnosis." Overdiagnosis can lead to treatment that is not needed.

- Radiation from repeated LDCT tests can cause cancer in otherwise healthy people.

That is why lung cancer screening is recommended only for adults who have no symptoms but are at high risk for developing the disease because of their smoking history and age.

If you are thinking about getting screened, talk to your doctor. If lung cancer screening is right for you, your doctor can refer you to a high-quality screening facility.

The best way to reduce your risk of lung cancer is to not smoke and to avoid secondhand smoke. Lung cancer screening is not a substitute for quitting smoking.

When Should Screening Stop?

The Task Force recommends that yearly lung cancer screening stop when the person being screened:

- Turns 81 years of age

- Has not smoked in 15 years

- Develops a health problem that makes her or him unwilling or unable to have surgery if lung cancer is found

How Is Lung Cancer Diagnosed and Treated?
Types of Lung Cancer

The two main types of lung cancer are small cell lung cancer and nonsmall cell lung cancer. These categories refer to what the cancer cells look like under a microscope. Nonsmall cell lung cancer is more common than small cell lung cancer.

Staging

If lung cancer is diagnosed, other tests are done to find out how far it has spread through the lungs, lymph nodes, and the rest of the body. This process is called "staging." The type and stage of lung cancer tells doctors what kind of treatment you need.

Types of Treatment

Lung cancer is treated in several ways, depending on the type of lung cancer and how far it has spread. People with nonsmall cell lung cancer can be treated with surgery, chemotherapy, radiation therapy, targeted therapy, or a combination of these treatments. People with small cell lung cancer are usually treated with radiation therapy and chemotherapy.

- **Surgery.** An operation where doctors cut out cancer tissue.

- **Chemotherapy.** Using special medicines to shrink or kill the cancer. The drugs can be pills you take or medicines given in your veins, or sometimes both.

- **Radiation therapy.** Using high-energy rays (similar to X-rays) to kill the cancer.

- **Targeted therapy.** Using drugs to block the growth and spread of cancer cells. The drugs can be pills you take or medicines given in your veins.

Doctors from different specialties often work together to treat lung cancer. Pulmonologists are doctors who are experts in diseases of the lungs. Surgeons are doctors who perform operations. Thoracic surgeons specialize in chest, heart, and lung surgery. Medical oncologists are doctors who treat cancer with medicines. Radiation oncologists are doctors who treat cancers with radiation.

Complementary and Alternative Medicine

Complementary and alternative medicine are medicines and health practices that are not standard cancer treatments.

- **Complementary medicine** is used in addition to standard treatments. Examples include acupuncture, dietary supplements, massage therapy, hypnosis, and meditation.

- **Alternative medicine** is used instead of standard treatments. Examples include special diets, megadose vitamins, herbal preparations, special teas, and magnet therapy.

Many kinds of complementary and alternative medicine have not been tested scientifically and may not be safe. Talk to your doctor about the risks and benefits before you start any kind of complementary or alternative medicine.

Which Treatment Is Right for Me?

Choosing the treatment that is right for you may be hard. Talk to your cancer doctor about the treatment options available for your type and stage of cancer. Your doctor can explain the risks and benefits of each treatment and their side effects. Side effects are how your body reacts to drugs or other treatments.

Sometimes people get an opinion from more than one cancer doctor. This is called a "second opinion." Getting a second opinion may help you choose the treatment that is right for you.

Living with Lung Cancer

When you have been diagnosed with cancer, you are considered a cancer survivor from that moment throughout the rest of your life.

Finding lung cancer earlier and making new treatments available are helping more lung cancer survivors live longer. The big challenge ahead is, "How do I live with lung cancer, as long and as best I can?" We offer some tips below.

It is important to get the treatment you need when you need it. You deserve timely and appropriate care for your lung cancer and its symptoms (including pain), as well as any side effects of treatment. Molecular testing (also called "tumor testing" or "biomarker testing") may help you make decisions about treatment.

Talk with your healthcare provider about how a survivorship care plan can help you coordinate your follow-up care to support your physical and emotional health.

Take steps to stay healthy. This can lower your risk of getting cancer again or having the cancer come back.

Some cancer survivors may blame themselves or feel that others blame them for having cancer. Lung cancer survivors may have these feelings of blame or stigma. You may find it helpful to talk about your experiences and feelings with a social worker or mental-health professional. You may also find it helpful to share your story with other cancer survivors or listen to their stories.

Chapter 21

Motor Vehicle Accidents

Chapter Contents

Section 21.1—Aggressive Driving.. 286

Section 21.2—Distracted Driving... 288

Section 21.3—Drowsy Driving 291

Section 21.4—Impaired Driving... 296

Section 21.5—Older Drivers.. 301

Section 21.1

Aggressive Driving

"Aggressive Driving,"
© 2016 Omnigraphics. Reviewed June 2019.

According to the National Highway Traffic Safety Administration (NHTSA), aggressive driving occurs when "an individual commits a combination of moving traffic offenses so as to endanger other persons or property." It can also be a single deliberate act that causes another driver to react defensively.

A related and more serious behavior, road rage, can be defined as an assault by the driver or passenger(s) of one motor vehicle on those in another vehicle—using the vehicle itself or any dangerous weapon—that is triggered by an incident on the roadway. While aggressive driving is treated as a traffic violation, road rage is an intentional disregard for the safety of others and is considered to be a criminal offense.

It is estimated that more than 1,500 people are killed each year in the United States as a result of aggressive-driving incidents. And men—particularly young men between the ages of 18 and 26—are three times more likely to be aggressive drivers than women, making this behavior a significant men's health issue.

Signs of Aggressive Driving

Aggressive driving involves a range of unlawful driving behaviors such as:

- **Speeding**: This includes actions like driving too fast for current conditions, driving above the posted speed limit, and racing.

- **Frequent lane changes**: Cutting between vehicles to move ahead of traffic, changing lanes without warning, improper passing, or any similar action can put both the driver and other motorists in danger.

- **Running a red light or stop sign**: Ignoring a stop light, entering an intersection on the yellow light, and not stopping at a stop sign are serious offenses that may cause injury to vehicle occupants and others.

- **Expressing frustration**: Condemning fellow motorists, either mentally or verbally, or making aggressive hand gestures to take out your frustration can result in violence or a crash.

- **Tailgating**: Following too closely to the vehicle ahead—especially in an aggressive manner—is one of the major causes of collisions and can result in serious injury or even death.

Other aggressive behaviors include driving recklessly; unnecessary use of the horn; excessive flashing of headlights at oncoming traffic; illegal driving on a sidewalk, median, road shoulder, or ditch; failing to yield right of way; and failing to obey traffic officers, traffic signs and control devices, or traffic laws concerning safety zones.

Avoiding Aggressive Driving

Avoid aggressive driving, as well as aggressive drivers, by following some simple measures, including:

- Drive within the posted speed limit.
- Make sure there is enough room when changing lanes or when entering traffic.
- Ensure a safe following distance between you and the vehicle ahead of you.
- Always signal before changing lanes or turning.
- To avoid traffic congestion, identify alternate routes.
- Opt for public transportation for some relief from sitting behind wheel.
- Pull over to get out of the way of an aggressive driver.
- Avoid conflict when possible. Be polite and avoid prolonged eye contact with an aggressive driver.
- Do not make offensive hand gestures, and ignore any made at you.
- Report dangerous aggressive drivers. If you are driving, either pull over to a safe spot to call the police or ask someone with you to make the call.

References

1. "Aggressive Driving," Arizona Department of Public Safety, n.d.
2. "Road Rage and Aggressive Driving," Washington State Patrol, n.d.

3. "Aggressive Driving," Insurance Information Institute, n.d.

4. "Aggressive Driving," National Highway Traffic Safety Administration (NHTSA), n.d.

5. Bierma, Paige. "Road Rage: When Stress Hits the Highway," HealthDay, Jan 20, 2016.

Section 21.2

Distracted Driving

This section includes text excerpted from "Distracted Driving," Centers for Disease Control and Prevention (CDC), June 9, 2017.

Each day in the United States, approximately 9 people are killed and more than 1,000 injured in crashes that are reported to involve a distracted driver.

Distracted driving is driving while doing another activity that takes your attention away from driving. Distracted driving can increase the chance of a motor vehicle crash.

What Are the Types of Distraction?

There are three main types of distraction:

- Visual: taking your eyes off the road

- Manual: taking your hands off the wheel

- Cognitive: taking your mind off of driving

Distracted Driving Activities

Anything that takes your attention away from driving can be a distraction. Sending a text message, talking on a cell phone, using a navigation system, and eating while driving are a few examples of distracted driving. Any of these distractions can endanger the driver and others.

Texting while driving is especially dangerous because it combines all three types of distraction. When you send or read a text message, you take your eyes off the road for about 5 seconds, long enough to cover the length a football field while driving at 55 mph.

How Big Is the Problem?
U.S. Deaths

In 2016, 3,450 people were killed in crashes involving a distracted driver.

U.S. Injuries

In 2015, 391,000 people were injured in motor vehicle crashes involving a distracted driver.

Table 21.1. U.S. Motor Vehicles and Injuries (2010 to 2015)

	2010	2011	2012	2013	2014	2015
Distracted Driving Deaths	3,092	3,331	3,328	3,154	3,179	3,477
All Motor Vehicle Deaths	32,999	32,479	33,782	32,894	32,744	35,092
Distracted Driving Injuries	416,000	387,000	421,000	424,000	431,000	391,000
All Motor Vehicle Injuries	2,239,000	2,217,000	2,362,000	2,313,000	2,338,000	2,443,000

Who Is Most at Risk?
Young Adult and Teen Drivers

- Drivers under the age of 20 have the highest proportion of distraction-related fatal crashes.

- In 2017, 9 percent of all teen motor vehicle crash deaths involved distracted driving.

- The Centers for Disease Control and Prevention (CDC) national Youth Risk Behavior Surveillance System (YRBSS) monitors health-risk behaviors among high school students, including texting or emailing while driving. The YRBSS findings include:

- In 2017, 42 percent of high school students who drove in the past 30 days reported sending a text or email while driving.

- Students who reported frequent texting while driving were:

  - Less likely to wear a seatbelt

  - More likely to ride with a driver who had been drinking

  - More likely to drink and drive

What Is Being Done to Prevent Distracted Driving?
States

- Many states are enacting laws—such as banning texting while driving, or using graduated driver licensing systems for teen drivers—to help raise awareness about the dangers of distracted driving and to help prevent it from occurring. However, the effectiveness of cell phone and texting laws on decreasing distracted driving-related crashes requires further study. The Insurance Institute for Highway Safety keeps track of distracted driving laws.

- As of March 2019, 16 states and the District of Columbia had banned drivers from hand-held phone use.

- As of March 2019, texting while driving is banned in 47 states and the District of Columbia. Two additional states ban texting while driving for new drivers.

- Some local governments also have bans on cell phone use and texting while driving.

Federal Government

- On September 30, 2009, President Obama issued an executive order prohibiting federal employees from texting while driving on government business or with government equipment.

- On September 17, 2010, the Federal Railroad Administration (FRA) banned cell phone and electronic device use of employees on the job.

- On October 27, 2010, the Federal Motor Carrier Safety Administration (FMCSA) enacted a ban that prohibits commercial vehicle drivers from texting while driving.

- In 2011, the Federal Motor Carrier Safety Administration and the Pipeline and Hazardous Materials Safety Administration (PHMSA) banned all hand-held cell phone use by commercial drivers and drivers carrying hazardous materials.

- From 2010 to 2013, the National Highway Traffic Safety Administration (NHTSA) evaluated the Distracted Driving Demonstration Projects. These projects increased police enforcement of distracted driving laws and increased awareness of distracted driving using radio advertisements, news stories, and similar media. After the projects were complete, observed driver cell phone use fell from 4.1 to 2.7 percent in California, 6.8 to 2.9 percent in Connecticut, 4.5 to 3.0 percent in Delaware, and 3.7 to 2.5 percent in New York.

- In April of 2014, the NHTSA began their annual "U Drive. U Text. U Pay." campaign to raise awareness of the dangers of distracted driving.

Section 21.3

Drowsy Driving

This section contains text excerpted from the following sources: Text in this section begins with excerpts from "Drowsy Driving," Centers for Disease Control and Prevention (CDC), March 21, 2017; Text beginning with the heading "Some Sleep Drugs Can Impair Driving" is excerpted from "Some Sleep Drugs Can Impair Driving," U.S. Food and Drug Administration (FDA), October 1, 2013. Reviewed June 2019.

Drowsy driving is a major problem in the United States. The risk, danger, and sometimes tragic results of drowsy driving are alarming. Drowsy driving is the dangerous combination of driving and sleepiness or fatigue. This usually happens when a driver has not slept enough, but it can also happen due to untreated sleep disorders, medications, drinking alcohol, and shift work.

The Impact of Drowsy Driving

Drowsy driving poses a serious risk not only for one's own health and safety, but also for the other people on the road.

The National Highway Traffic Safety Administration (NHTSA) estimates that between 2005 and 2009 drowsy driving was responsible for an annual average of:

- 83,000 crashes

- 37,000 injury crashes

- 886 fatal crashes (846 fatalities in 2014)

These estimates are conservative, though, and up to 6,000 fatal crashes each year maybe caused by drowsy drivers.

How Often Do Americans Fall Asleep While Driving?

Approximately 1 out of 25 adults 18 years of age and older surveyed reported that they had fallen asleep while driving in the past 30 days.

Individuals who snored or slept six hours or less per day were more likely to fall asleep while driving.

How Does Sleepiness Affect Driving?

Falling asleep at the wheel is very dangerous, but being sleepy affects your ability to drive safely even if you do not fall asleep. Drowsiness:

- Makes drivers less attentive

- Slows reaction time

- Affects a driver's ability to make decisions

The warning signs of drowsy driving include:

- Yawning or blinking frequently

- Difficulty remembering the past few miles driven

- Missing your exit

- Drifting from your lane

- Hitting a rumble strip

If you experience any of the warning signs of drowsy driving while driving, pull over to a safe place and take a 15 to 20 minute nap or change drivers. Simply turning up the radio or opening the window is not an effective ways to keep you alert.

Who Is More Likely to Drive Drowsy?

- Drivers who do not get enough sleep
- Commercial drivers who operate vehicles, such as tow trucks, tractor trailers, and buses
- Shift workers (work the night shift or long shifts)
- Drivers with untreated sleep disorders such as one where breathing repeatedly stops and starts (sleep apnea)
- Drivers who use medications that make them sleepy

How to Prevent Drowsy Driving

There are four things you should do before taking the wheel to prevent driving while drowsy.

1. Get enough sleep! Most adults need at least seven hours of sleep a day, while adolescents need at least eight hours.
2. Develop good sleeping habits such as sticking to a sleep schedule.
3. If you have a sleep disorder or have symptoms of a sleep disorder, such as snoring or feeling sleepy during the day, talk to your physician about treatment options.
4. Avoid drinking alcohol or taking medications that make you sleepy. Be sure to check the label on any medications or talk to your pharmacist.

Drowsy Driving Is Similar to Drunk Driving

Your body needs adequate sleep on a daily basis. The more hours of sleep you miss, the harder it is for you to think and perform as well as you would like. Lack of sleep can make you less alert and affect your coordination, judgment, and reaction time while driving. This is known as "cognitive impairment."

Studies have shown that going too long without sleep can impair your ability to drive the same way as drinking too much alcohol.

- Being awake for at least 18 hours is the same as someone having a blood content blood alcohol concentration (BAC) of 0.05 percent.

- Being awake for at least 24 hours is equal to having a blood alcohol content of 0.10 percent. This is higher than the legal limit (0.08% BAC) in all states.

Additionally, drowsiness increases the effect of even low amounts of alcohol.

Some Sleep Drugs Can Impair Driving

Many people take sedatives to help them sleep. The U.S. Food and Drug Administration (FDA) is reminding consumers that some drugs to treat insomnia could make them less able to perform activities for which they must be fully alert the next morning, including driving a car.

The FDA has informed manufacturers that the recommended dose should be lowered for sleep drugs approved for bedtime use that contain a medicine called "zolpidem." The FDA is also evaluating the risk of next-morning impairment in other insomnia medications.

People with insomnia have trouble falling or staying asleep. Zolpidem, which belongs to a class of medications called "sedative-hypnotics," is a common ingredient in widely prescribed sleep medications. Some sleep drugs contain an extended-release form of zolpidem that stays in the body longer than the regular form.

The FDA is particularly concerned about extended-release forms of zolpidem. They are sold as generic drugs and under the brand name "Ambien CR." New data show that in the morning after use, many people who take products containing extended-release zolpidem have drug levels that are high enough to impair driving and other activities. The FDA says that women are especially vulnerable because zolpidem is cleared from the body more slowly in women than in men.

The FDA also found that some medicines containing the immediate-release form of zolpidem can impair driving and other activities the next morning. They are marketed as generic drugs and under the following brand names:

- Ambien (oral tablet)

- Edluar (tablet placed under the tongue)

- Zolpimist (oral spray)

The FDA has informed the manufacturers of products containing zolpidem that the recommended dose for women for both immediate- and extended-release products should be lowered. The FDA is also suggesting a lower dose range for men.

Drowsiness is already listed as a side effect in the drug labels of insomnia drugs, along with warnings that patients may still feel drowsy the day after taking these products. However, people with high levels of zolpidem in their blood can be impaired even if they feel wide awake. "All insomnia drugs are potent medications, and they must be used carefully," says Russell Katz, M.D., director of The FDA's Division of Neurology Products (DNP.)

Recommended Doses

The FDA has informed manufacturers that changes to the dosage recommendations for the use of zolpidem products should be made:

* For women, dosing should be cut in half, from 10 mg to 5 mg for products containing the regular form of zolpidem (Ambien, Edluar, Zolpimist) and from 12.5 mg to 6.25 mg for zolpidem extended-release products (Ambien CR).

* For men, the lower dose of 5 mg for immediate-release zolpidem and 6.25 mg for extended-release should be considered.

Intermezzo, an approved drug containing zolpidem, is used when middle-of-the-night awakening is followed by difficulty returning to sleep and at least 4 hours remain available for sleep. The recommended dose for Intermezzo remains at 1.75 mg for women and 3.5 mg for men.

The FDA is evaluating the risk of next-day impairment with other insomnia drugs, both prescription and over-the-counter (OTC) drugs.

Most Widely Used Sleep Drug

Zolpidem—which has been on the market for nearly 20 years—is by far the most widely used active ingredient in prescription sleep medications, says Ronald Farkas, M.D., Ph.D., a medical team leader in FDA's neurology products division. About 9 million patients received products containing zolpidem from retail pharmacies in 2011.

The FDA's Adverse Event Reporting System (FAERS) has logged approximately 700 reports of zolpidem use and impaired driving ability and/or traffic accidents. However, the FDA cannot be certain that those incidents are conclusively linked to zolpidem. Many of those reports lacked important information, such as the dose of zolpidem and the time at which it was taken, the time of the accident, and whether alcohol or other drugs had also been used.

"We have had long standing concern about sleep medications and driving. However, only have data from clinical trials and specialized driving simulation studies become available that enabled the FDA to better establish the risk of driving impairment and to make new recommendations about dosing," Farkas says.

An Individual Decision

The FDA is urging healthcare professionals to caution patients who use these products about the risks of next-morning impairment and its effect on activities, such as driving, that require alertness.

The agency recommends that people who take sleep medications talk to their healthcare professional about ways to take the lowest effective dose. It should not be assumed that OTC sleep medicines are necessarily safer alternatives.

With zolpidem, Farkas notes that people must be aware of how this drug affects them personally. "Even with the new dosing recommendations, it is important to work with your healthcare professional to find the sleep medicine and dose that work best for you," he says.

Patients are asked to contact the FDA's MedWatch program if they suffer side effects from the use of zolpidem or another insomnia medication.

Section 21.4

Impaired Driving

This section includes text excerpted from "Impaired Driving: Get the Facts," Centers for Disease Control and Prevention (CDC), March 22, 2019.

Every day, 29 people in the United States die in motor vehicle crashes that involve an alcohol-impaired driver. This is one death every 50 minutes. The annual cost of alcohol-related crashes totals more than $44 billion. Thankfully, there are effective measures that can help prevent injuries and deaths from alcohol-impaired driving.

How Big Is the Problem?

- In 2016, 10,497 people died in alcohol-impaired driving crashes, accounting for 28 percent of all traffic-related deaths in the United States.

- Of the 1,233 traffic deaths among children ages between the ages of 0 and 14 in 2016, 214 (17%) involved an alcohol-impaired driver.

- In 2016, more than 1 million drivers were arrested for driving under the influence of alcohol or narcotics. That is 1 percent of the 111 million self-reported episodes of alcohol-impaired driving among U.S. adults each year (Figure 21.1).

- Drugs other than alcohol (legal and illegal) are involved in about 16 percent of motor vehicle crashes.

- Marijuana use is increasing and 13 percent of nighttime, weekend drivers have marijuana in their system.

- Marijuana users were about 25 percent more likely to be involved in a crash than drivers with no evidence of marijuana use, however other factors—such as age and sex—may account for the increased crash risk among marijuana users.

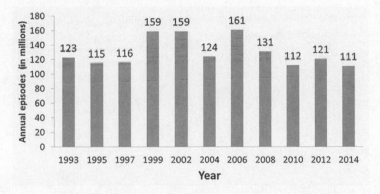

Figure 21.1. *Annual Self-Reported Alcohol-Impaired Driving Episodes among U.S. Adults, 1993 to 2014.* (Source: Centers for Disease Control and Prevention (CDC). Behavioral Risk Factor Surveillance System (BRFSS), 1993 to 2014.)

Note: The annual estimated alcohol-impaired driving episodes were calculated using BRFSS respondents' answers to this question: "During the past 30 days, how many times have you driven when you've had perhaps too much to drink?" Annual estimates per respondent were calculated by multiplying the reported episodes during the preceding 30 days by 12. These numbers were summed to obtain the annual national estimates.

Who Is Most at Risk?

Young people

- At all levels of blood alcohol concentration (BAC), the risk of being involved in a crash is greater for young people than for older people.

- Among drivers with BAC levels of 0.08 percent or higher involved in fatal crashes in 2016, nearly 3 in 10 were between 25 and 34 years of age (27%). The next 2 largest groups were between the ages of 21 and 24 (26%) and 35 to 44 (22%).

Motorcyclists

- Among motorcyclists killed in fatal crashes in 2016, 25 percent had BACs of 0.08 percent or greater.

- Motorcyclists between the ages of 35 and 39 have the highest percentage of deaths with BACs of 0.08 percent or greater (38% in 2016).

Done to Drivers with Prior Driving While Impaired Convictions

- Drivers with a BAC of 0.08 percent or higher involved in fatal crashes were 4.5 times more likely to have a prior conviction for driving while impaired than were drivers with no alcohol in their system (9% and 2%, respectively).

Blood Alcohol Concentration Effects

Information in this table shows the blood alcohol concentration level at which the effect usually is first observed.

How Can Deaths and Injuries from Impaired Driving Be Prevented?

Effective measures include:

- Actively enforcing existing 0.08 percent BAC laws, minimum legal drinking age laws, and zero tolerance laws for drivers younger than 21 years of age in all states

- Requiring ignition interlocks for all offenders, including first-time offenders

Table 21.2. Effects of Blood Alcohol Concentration (BAC)

Blood Alcohol Concentration *	Typical Effects	Predictable Effects on Driving
.02 percent about 2 alcoholic drinks**	• Some loss of judgment • Relaxation • Slight body warmth • Altered mood	• Decline in visual functions (rapid tracking of a moving target) • Decline in ability to perform two tasks at the same time (divided attention)
.05 percent about 3 alcoholic drinks**	• Exaggerated behavior • May have loss of small-muscle control (e.g., focusing your eyes) • Impaired judgment • Usually, good feeling • Lowered alertness • Release of inhibition	• Reduced coordination • Reduced ability to track moving objects • Difficulty steering • Reduced response to emergency driving situations
.08 percent about 4 alcoholic drinks**	• Muscle coordination becomes poor (e.g., balance, speech, vision, reaction time, and hearing) • Harder to detect danger • Judgment, self-control, reasoning, and memory are impaired	• Concentration • Short-term memory loss • Speed control • Reduced information processing capability (e.g., signal detection, visual search) • Impaired perception
.10 percent about 5 alcoholic drinks**	• Clear deterioration of reaction time and control • Slurred speech, poor coordination, and slowed thinking	• Reduced ability to maintain lane position and brake appropriately

Table 21.2. Continued

Blood Alcohol Concentration *	Typical Effects	Predictable Effects on Driving
.15 percent About 7 alcoholic drinks**	• Far less muscle control than normal • Vomiting may occur (unless this level is reached slowly or a person has developed a tolerance for alcohol) • Major loss of balance	• Substantial impairment in vehicle control, attention to driving task, and in necessary visual and auditory information processing

* Blood alcohol concentration measurement

The number of drinks listed represents the approximate amount of alcohol that a 160-pound man would need to drink in one hour to reach the listed BAC in each category.

** A standard drink size in the United States

A standard drink is equal to 14.0 grams (0.6 ounces) of pure alcohol. Generally, this amount of pure alcohol is found in:

• 12-ounces of beer (5% alcohol content)
• 8-ounces of malt liquor (7% alcohol content)
• 5-ounces of wine (12% alcohol content)
• 1.5-ounces or a "shot" of 80-proof (40% alcohol content) distilled spirits or liquor (e.g., gin, rum, vodka, whiskey)

- Using sobriety checkpoints

- Putting health promotion efforts into practice that influence economic, organizational, policy, and school/community action

- Using community-based approaches to alcohol control and DWI prevention

- Requiring mandatory substance abuse assessment and treatment, if needed, for DWI offenders

- Raising the unit price of alcohol by increasing taxes

What Safety Steps Can Individuals Take?

Whenever your social plans involve alcohol and/or drugs, make plans so that you do not have to drive while impaired. For example:

- Before drinking, designate a nondrinking driver when with a group.

- Do not let your friends drive impaired.

- If you have been drinking or using drugs, get a ride home, use a rideshare service or call a taxi.

- If you are hosting a party where alcohol will be served, remind your guests to plan ahead and designate their sober driver; offer alcohol-free beverages, and make sure all guests leave with a sober driver.

Section 21.5

Older Drivers

This section includes text excerpted from "Older Adult Drivers," Centers for Disease Control and Prevention (CDC), November 30, 2017.

In 2016, there were almost 42 million licensed drivers 65 years of age and older in the United States. Driving helps older adults stay mobile and independent. But the risk of being injured or killed in a motor vehicle crash increases as people age. Thankfully, there are steps that older adults can take to stay safer on the roads.

How Big Is the Problem?

In 2016, about 7,400 older adults 65 years of age and older were killed and more than 290,000 were treated in emergency departments for motor vehicle crash injuries. This amounts to 20 older adults killed and 794 injured in crashes on average every day. There were almost 42 million licensed older drivers in 2016, which is a 56 percent increase from 1999.

Who Is Most at Risk?

Involvement in fatal crashes, per mile traveled, begins increasing among drivers between the ages of 70 and 74 and are highest among drivers 85 years of age and older. This trend has been attributed more to an increased susceptibility to injury and medical complications among older drivers rather than an increased risk of crash involvement. Across all age groups, males have substantially higher death rates than females. Age-related declines in vision and cognitive functioning (ability to reason and remember), as well as physical changes, might affect some older adults' driving abilities.

How Can Older Driver Deaths and Injuries Be Prevented?

Older adults can take several steps to stay safe on the road.

Existing protective factors that might help improve older drivers' safety include:

High incidence of seat belt use. Among passenger vehicle occupants (drivers and passengers) killed in a crash, a higher proportion of older adults were wearing seat belts at the time of the crash 64 percent of those between the ages of 65 and 74 and 69 percent of those 75 years of age and older compared with younger adults who ranged from 37 percent (between the ages of 25 and 34) to 53 percent (between the ages of 55 and 64).

Tendency to drive when conditions are the safest. Older drivers tend to limit their driving during bad weather, at night, and on high-speed roads, in comparison with younger drivers.

Lower incidence of impaired driving. Older adult drivers are less likely to drink and drive than other adult drivers. In 2017, only 6 percent of drivers 75 years of age and older involved in fatal crashes had a blood alcohol concentration of 0.08 grams per deciliter (g/dL) or higher, compared with 27 percent of drivers ages 21 to 24 years. Overall, 20 percent of drivers, regardless of age, involved in fatal crashes had a BAC of 0.08 g/dL or higher.

Steps to Stay Safe on the Road

Older adults can take several steps to stay safe on the road:

- Older adults can use and download the Centers for Disease Control and Prevention (CDC) MyMobility Plan for tips and resources to make a plan to stay mobile and independent as they age. This planning tool helps older adults plan for mobility changes similar to the way that many plan financially for retirement. Older adults can take action now to prevent or reduce the effects of possible mobility changes, and stay safe and independent longer. In addition, older adults can review their medicines to reduce their risk of falls and car crashes.

- Follow a regular activity program to increase strength and flexibility.

- Ask your doctor or pharmacist to review medicines—both prescription and over-the-counter (OTC)—to reduce side effects and interactions.

- Have your eyes checked by an eye doctor at least once a year. Wear glasses and corrective lenses as required.

- Drive during daylight and in good weather.

- Find the safest route with well-lit streets, intersections with left turn arrows, and easy parking.

- Plan your route before you drive.

- Leave a large following distance behind the car in front of you.

- Avoid distractions in your car, such as listening to a loud radio, talking on your cell phone, texting, and eating.

- Always wear your seat belt and never drive impaired by alcohol or drugs/medicines.

- Consider potential alternatives to driving, such as riding with a friend, ride share services, or using public transit, which you can use to get around.

Chapter 22

Other Accidents and Injuries

Chapter Contents

Section 22.1—Falls 306

Section 22.2—Fire-Related Injuries... 309

Section 22.3—Occupational Injuries.. 319

Section 22.4—Poisoning 322

Section 22.5—Water-Related Accidents 325

Section 22.1

Falls

This section includes text excerpted from "Important
Facts about Falls," Centers for Disease Control and
Prevention (CDC), February 10, 2017.

Falls Are Serious and Costly

- One out of five falls causes a serious injury, such as broken
  bones or a head injury

- Each year, three million older people are treated in emergency
  departments (EDs) for fall injuries.

- Over 800,000 patients a year are hospitalized because of a fall
  injury, most often because of a head injury or hip fracture.

- Each year, at least 300,000 older people are hospitalized for hip
  fractures.

- More than 95 percent of hip fractures are caused by falling,
  usually by falling sideways.

- Falls are the most common cause of traumatic brain injuries (TBI).

- In 2015, the total medical costs for falls totaled more than $50
  billion. Medicare and Medicaid shouldered 75 percent of these
  costs.

What Can Happen after a Fall?

Many falls do not cause injuries. But, one out of five falls does cause
a serious injury, such as a broken bone or a head injury. These injuries
can make it hard for a person to get around, do everyday activities,
or live on their own.

- Falls can cause broken bones, such as wrist, arm, ankle, and hip
  fractures.

- Falls can cause head injuries. These can be very serious,
  especially if the person is taking certain medicines (such as
  blood thinners). An older person who falls and hits their head
  should see their doctor right away to make sure they do not have
  a brain injury.

- Many people who fall, even if they are not injured, become afraid of falling. This fear may cause a person to cut down on their everyday activities. When a person is less active, they become weaker and this increases their chances of falling.

What Conditions Make You More Likely to Fall

Research has identified many conditions that contribute to falling. These are called "risk factors." Many risk factors can be changed or modified to help prevent falls. They include:

- Lower body weakness

- Vitamin D deficiency (that is, not enough vitamin D in your system)

- Difficulties with walking and balance

- Use of medicines, such as tranquilizers, sedatives, or antidepressants. Even some over-the-counter (OTC) medicines can affect balance and how steady you are on your feet.

- Vision problems

- Foot pain or poor footwear

- Home hazards or dangers, such as:

  - Broken or uneven steps

  - Throw rugs or clutter that can be tripped over

Most falls are caused by a combination of risk factors. The more risk factors a person has, the greater their chances of falling.

Healthcare providers can help cut down a person's risk by reducing the fall risk factors listed above.

What You Can Do to Prevent Falls

Falls can be prevented. These are some simple things you can do to keep yourself from falling.

Talk to Your Doctor

- Ask your doctor or healthcare provider to evaluate your risk for falling, and talk with them about specific things you can do.

- Ask your doctor or pharmacist to review your medicines to see if any might make you dizzy or sleepy. This should include prescription medicines and over-the-counter medicines.

- Ask your doctor or healthcare provider about taking vitamin D supplements.

Do Strength and Balance Exercises

Do exercises that make your legs stronger and improve your balance. Tai chi is a good example of this kind of exercise.

Have Your Eyes Checked

Have your eyes checked by an eye doctor at least once a year, and be sure to update your eyeglasses if needed.

If you have bifocal or progressive lenses, you may want to get a pair of glasses with only your distance prescription for outdoor activities, such as walking. Sometimes, these types of lenses can make things seem closer or farther away than they really are.

Make Your Home Safer

Get rid of things you could trip over.

- Add grab bars inside and outside your tub or shower and next to the toilet.

- Put railings on both sides of stairs.

- Make sure your home has lots of light by adding more or brighter light bulbs.

Section 22.2

Fire-Related Injuries

This section includes text excerpted from "Civilian
Fire Injuries in Residential Buildings (2013-2015),"
U.S. Fire Administration (USFA), July 2017.

Fires can strike anywhere—in structures, buildings, automobiles, and the outdoors. Fires that affect our homes are often the most tragic and the most preventable. While the loss of our possessions can be upsetting, the physical injuries and psychological impacts that fires can inflict on our lives are often far more devastating. It is a sad fact that each year, over 70 percent of all civilian fire injuries occurred as a result of fires in residential buildings.

From 2013 to 2015, 76 percent of all civilian fire injuries occurred in residential buildings. This section focuses on the characteristics of these injuries as reported to the National Fire Incident Reporting System (NFIRS) from 2013 to 2015. NFIRS data is used for the analyses presented throughout this section.

By definition, civilian fire injuries involve people who are injured as a result of a fire and are not on active duty with a firefighting organization. These injuries generally occur from activities of fire control, escaping from the dangers of fire, or sleeping. Fires resulting in injuries are those fires where one or more injuries occur.

Annually, from 2013 to 2015, an estimated 12,000 civilian fire injuries resulted from an estimated 7,700 residential building fires resulting in injuries and 380,200 total residential building fires. On average, someone is injured in a residential building fire every 44 minutes. For the purpose of this section, the term "residential building fires resulting in injuries" is synonymous with "residential fires resulting in injuries" and the term "residential building fires" is synonymous with "residential fires." The term "residential fires resulting in injuries" is used throughout the body of this section; the findings, tables, charts, headings, and endnotes reflect the full category, "residential building fires resulting in injuries."

Civilian Fire Injuries in Residential Buildings (2013 to 2015)

Not all fires produce injuries. When civilian fire injuries were averaged over reported residential fires, the overall injury rate was nearly

3 civilian injuries per 100 residential fires (Table 22.1). Residential fires that resulted in injuries, however, had 130 injuries for every 100 fires. Of the residential fires resulting in injuries, 82 percent resulted in one civilian injury, 13 percent resulted in 2 civilian injuries, and 5 percent resulted in 3 or more civilian injuries.

Table 22.1. Civilian Injury Rates for Residential Building Fires per 100 Fires (2013 to 2015)

Injuries per 100 Injury-Producing Residential Building Fires	Injuries per 100 Residential Building Fires
129.8	2.6

(Source: National Fire Incident Reporting System (NFIRS))

When Residential Building Fires Resulting in Injuries Occur

Residential fires resulting in injuries follow a daily pattern. In addition—unlike fatal residential fires, which occurred most frequently late at night or in the very early morning hours—residential fires resulting in civilian injuries follow a pattern similar to that of all residential fires. As shown in figure 22.1, residential fires resulting in injuries occurred most frequently in the late afternoon and early evening hours, when many people are expected to be cooking dinner. The time period from 4 to 8 p.m. accounted for 23 percent of the residential fires resulting in injuries. Cooking was the primary cause (37%) for residential fires that resulted

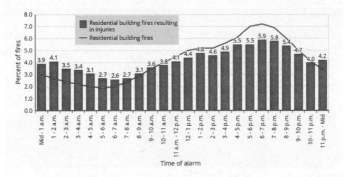

Figure 22.1. *Residential Building Fires Resulting in Injuries by Time of Alarm (2013 to 2015)* (Source: National Fire Incident Reporting System (NFIRS).)

Note: Total does not add up to 100 percent due to rounding.

in injuries. In general, residential fires resulting in injuries decreased to the lowest point of the day, between 5 and 8 a.m., and then steadily increased during the daytime hours until reaching the daily peak.

Residential fires resulting in injuries also follow a yearly pattern similar to that of all residential fires. In addition, residential fires resulting in injuries tend to follow a seasonal trend, with more fires taking place during the colder months than the warmer months (Figure 22.2.). January, peaking at 11 percent, had the highest incidence of residential fires resulting in injuries. June through September resulted in the least amount of residential fires resulting in injuries. This drop may be explained by a decrease in residential heating fires and their associated injuries during the warmer months. Similar to all fires in residential buildings, residential fires resulting in injuries occurred most often on Saturdays and Sundays (Figure 22.3.)

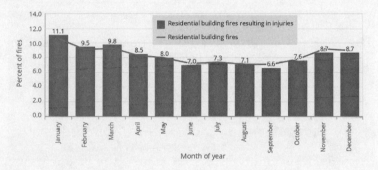

Figure 22.2. *Residential Building Fires Resulting in Injuries by Month (2013 to 2015)* (Source: National Fire Incident Reporting System (NFIRS).)

Note: Total does not add up to 100 percent due to rounding.

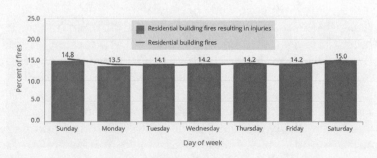

Figure 22.3. *Residential Building Fires Resulting in Injuries by Day of Week (2013 to 2015)* (Source: National Fire Incident Reporting System (NFIRS).)

Cause of Injury

The predominant cause of residential fire injuries, by far, involved exposure to fire products (80%), such as flame, heat, smoke, or gas (Figure 22.4.). The next two leading causes were exposure to toxic fumes other than smoke (8%) and other, unspecified causes (4%).

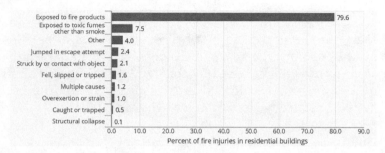

Figure 22.4. *Civilian Fire Injuries in Residential Buildings by Cause of Injury (2013 to 2015)* (Source: National Fire Incident Reporting System (NFIRS).)

Note: Percentages computed for only those injuries where causes were specified. The cause of injury was specified in 70 percent of reported injuries.

Primary Symptoms of Civilian Fire Injuries

Smoke inhalation and thermal burns were the primary symptoms of reported injuries, accounting for 78 percent of all injuries resulting from residential fires (Figure 22.5.). Smoke inhalation alone accounted for 41 percent of residential fire injuries.

Thermal burns (as opposed to scalds or chemical or electrical burns) accounted for another 24 percent, and burns combined with smoke inhalation accounted for an additional 13 percent. Breathing difficulty was reported for only 6 percent of injuries. Scalds (4%) and cuts or lacerations (3%) accounted for an even smaller proportion of the injuries. Thermal burns are caused by contact with flames, hot liquids, hot surfaces, and other sources of high heat. Of the thermal burns to the body, 71 percent were to the upper and lower extremities (56 percent and 15 percent, respectively.)

Of the smoke inhalation injuries, 70 percent were internal injuries, which are particularly critical, as they can lead to lung damage. The inflammation and damage caused by smoke inhalation to delicate breathing sacs in the lungs actually grow worse in the hours after the incident. A chest X-ray can look clear, and oxygen levels in the blood may appear normal in the first few hours after a fire. A day or two later, however, the victim can suddenly take a turn for the worse as the lungs become unable to properly exchange oxygen.

Based on the severity of the injury, 57 percent of the civilian fire injuries in residential fires were deemed minor. Only 14 percent of the injuries were considered serious or life-threatening.

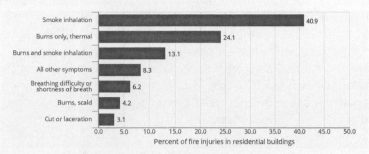

Figure 22.5. *Civilian Fire Injuries in Residential Buildings by Primary Symptoms (2013 to 2015)* (Source: National Fire Incident Reporting System (NFIRS).)

Notes: 1. Percentages computed for only those injuries where symptoms were specified. The primary symptoms were specified in 64 percent of reported injuries. 2. Total does not add up to 100 percent due to rounding.

Areas of the Body Affected

The body parts affected most by residential fire injuries (Figure 22.6.) included internal parts (32%) and the upper extremities (25%). As discussed, the types of injuries that affected most areas of the body consisted of smoke inhalation, thermal burns, or a combination of both.

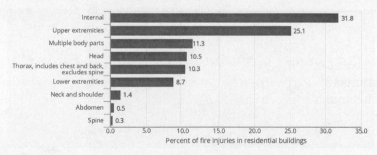

Figure 22.6. *Civilian fire injuries in residential buildings by part of body injured (2013 to 2015)* (Source: National Fire Incident Reporting System (NFIRS).)

Notes: 1. Percentages computed for only those injuries where part of body injured was specified. The part of body injured was specified in 58 percent of reported injuries. 2. Total does not add up to 100 percent due to rounding.

Factors Contributing to Civilian Fire Injuries

As shown in Figure 22.7 the most notable factors contributing to civilian fire injuries (outside of "other (unspecified) factors") involved escape (27%), fire pattern (24%), and equipment-related factors (17%). Escape factors include unfamiliarity with exits, excessive travel distance to the nearest clear exit, a choice of an inappropriate exit route, reentering the building, and clothing catching fire while escaping. Fire pattern factors involve such situations as exits are blocked by smoke and flame, vision is blocked or impaired by smoke, and civilians are trapped above or below the fire. Equipment-related problems include such factors as the improper use of cooking or heating equipment and the use of unvented heating equipment.

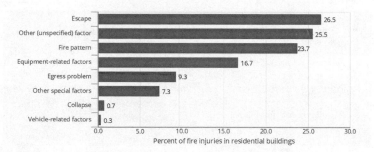

Figure 22.7. *Factors Contributing to Civilian Fire Injuries in Residential Buildings (2013 to 2015)* (Source: National Fire Incident Reporting System (NFIRS).)

Notes: 1. Includes incidents where factors contributing to injury were specified. Factors contributing to injury were specified in 30 percent of reported injuries.
2. As multiple factors contributing to injury may be noted for each injury, the total sums to more than 100 percent.

Human Factors Contributing to Civilian Fire Injuries

Human factors also play an important role in residential fire injuries. Table 22.2. shows that the leading human factor contributing to injuries was being "asleep" (52%). This is not unexpected, as the largest number of injuries occurred in bedrooms (34%). "Possibly impaired by alcohol" (17%) was the second leading human factor contributing to injuries. This was followed by "unattended or unsupervised" individuals (11%) and people with "physical disabilities" (also 11%).

Table 22.2. Residential Fire Injuries

Human Factors Contributing to Injury	Percent of Fire Injuries in Residential Buildings (Unknowns Apportioned)
Asleep	52.2
Possibly impaired by alcohol 17.4	17.4
Unattended or unsupervised	11.3
Physical disabilities	11.3
Possibly impaired by other drug or chemical	9.1
Possible intellectual disabilities	7.7
Unconscious	4.8
Physically restrained	0.7

(Source: National Fire Incident Reporting System (NFIRS).)

Causes of Residential Building Fires Resulting in Injuries

As shown in Figure 22.8 "cooking" (37%) was the leading cause of residential fires that resulted in injuries. "Other unintentional, careless" actions (9%) and "open flame" (9%) were the next leading causes. "Other unintentional, careless" actions include misuse of material or product, abandoned or discarded materials or products, and heat source too close to combustibles. "Open flame" includes torches, candles, matches, lighters, embers and the like. These two causes were followed by "electrical malfunction" (7%) and "appliances" (also 7%).

Civilian Activity When Injured

Most civilian fire injuries occurred when the victim was attempting to control the fire (35%), followed by attempting to escape (26%), and sleeping (11%), as shown in Figure 22.9. The USFA recommends leaving fighting a fire to trained firefighters and that efforts be focused on following a preset escape plan. To escape a fire, many civilians make the mistake of fleeing through the area where the fire is located. That area of a fire has tremendous heat, smoke, and a toxic atmosphere that can render a person unconscious. As a result, it is imperative that an escape plan be prepared and practiced. With a well-thought-out plan that includes multiple escape options, the chances of survival and escaping without injuries greatly increase. In addition, it has been demonstrated that people may not wake up from the smell of

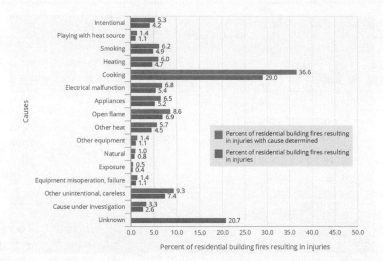

Figure 22.8. *Causes of Residential Building Fires Resulting in Injuries (2013 to 2015) (Source: National Fire Incident Reporting System (NFIRS).)*

Notes: 1. Causes are listed in order of the U.S. Fire Administration (USFA) Structure Fire Cause Hierarchy for ease of comparison of fire causes across different aspects of the fire problem. Fires are assigned to one of 16 cause groupings using a hierarchy of definitions, approximately as shown in the figure above. A fire is included in the highest category into which it fits. If it does not fit the top category, then the second one is considered, and if not that one, the third, and so on. For example, if the fire is judged to be intentionally set and a match was used to ignite it, it is classified as intentional and not open flame because intentional is higher in the hierarchy.
2. Fires caused by intentional actions include, but are not limited to, fires that are deemed to be arson. Intentional fires are those fires that are deliberately set and include fires that result from the deliberate misuse of a heat source and fires of an incendiary nature (arson) that require fire service intervention.

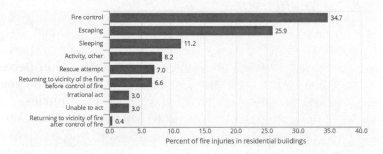

Figure 22.9. *Civilian Fire Injuries in Residential Buildings by Activity When Injured (2013 to 2015) (Source: National Fire Incident Reporting System (NFIRS).)*

Note: Percentages computed for only those injuries where activity information was available. The activity when injured was specified in 56 percent of reported injuries.

smoke while sleeping. Therefore, it is also vital that smoke alarms are installed in homes to alert sleeping people to the presence of fire.

Sex, Race, and Ethnicity of Civilian Fire Injuries

Males accounted for 54 percent, and females accounted for 46 percent of residential fire injuries. Figure 22.10 shows the percentage distribution of civilian fire injuries by race. Where racial information was provided, Whites constituted 62 percent of the injuries, followed by Blacks (30%); other, including multiracial (6%); Asians (1%); American Indians or Alaska Natives (less than 1%); and Native Hawaiians or other Pacific Islanders (also less than 1%).

The ethnicity element shows that 87 percent of the injuries occurred to non-Hispanics or non-Latinxs, compared to Hispanics or Latinxs (13%). Ethnicity was specified for 40 percent of reported injuries.

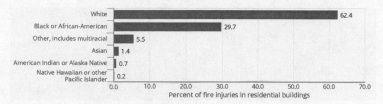

Figure 22.10. *Civilian Fire Injuries in Residential Buildings by Race (2013 to 2015)* (Source: National Fire Incident Reporting System (NFIRS).)

Notes: 1. Percentages computed for only those injuries where race information was available. Race was specified in 53 percent of reported injuries.
2. Total does not add up to 100 percent due to rounding.

Age of Civilians Injured and Activity When Injured

Civilians between the ages of 20 and 49 accounted for 46 percent of injuries in residential fires (Figure 22.11). An additional 17 percent of those with injuries were less than 20 years of age. Adults 50 years of age and older accounted for 38 percent of those with injuries.

With the exception of children 9 years of age or younger, the first reaction of civilians is either to try to control or escape the fire (Table 22.3). At the time of injury, for those 10 years of age and older, trying to control the fire and escaping were the two leading activities that resulted in injuries. Those between the ages of 10 and 69 primarily got injured trying to control the fire (38%), followed by trying to escape the fire (24%). Those 70 years of age and older primarily got injured trying to escape the fire (34%), followed by trying to control the fire (24%.)

For children between the ages of 0 and 9, escaping and sleeping were the two leading activities that resulted in injuries. Those between the ages of 0 and 9 primarily got injured when trying to escape the fire (37%), followed by sleeping (27%.)

The young and the very old are less likely to be as mobile or ready to act in a fire situation. Infants, young children, and older adults may require special provisions in a fire or emergency situation. Thus, it is not surprising that these individuals are less likely to attempt to control the fire.

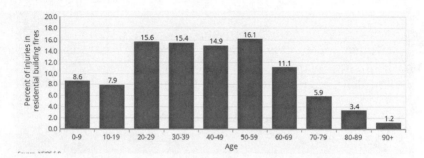

Figure 22.11. *Civilian Fire Injuries in Residential Buildings by Age Group (2013 to 2015)* (Source: National Fire Incident Reporting System (NFIRS).)

Notes: 1. Percentages computed for only those injuries where age was valid. A valid age was provided for nearly all (99.8 percent) reported injuries.
2. Total does not add up to 100 percent due to rounding.

Table 22.3. Leading Activities Resulting in Civilian Fire Injuries in Residential Buildings by Age Group (2013 to 2015).

| Age Group | Fire Control | Percent of Fire Injuries Where Age and Activity Reported (2013–2015) | |
		Escaping	Sleeping
0 to 9	8.8	37.2	27
10 to 19	37.8	28.3	8.8
20 to 29	42.1	22.1	9.1
30 to 39	40.9	22.4	9.2
40 to 49	38.4	22.9	9.4
50 to 59	35.7	24.5	10.9
60 to 69	29.4	27.8	11.9
70 to 79	26.3	34.3	12.4

Table 22.3. Continued

Age Group	Fire Control	Percent of Fire Injuries Where Age and Activity Reported (2013–2015)	
		Escaping	Sleeping
80 to 89	22.3	35.1	10.7
90+	20.5	31.3	10.7
Overall	34.7	25.9	11.2

(Source: National Fire Incident Reporting System (NFIRS).)

Section 22.3

Occupational Injuries

This section includes text excerpted from "News Release Bureau of Labor Statistics," U.S. Bureau of Labor Statistics (BLS), U.S. Department of Labor (DOL), December 18, 2018.

Type of Incident

Fatal falls were at their highest level in the 26-year history of the Census of Fatal Occupational Injuries (CFOI) accounting for 887 (17%) worker deaths. Transportation incidents remained the most frequent fatal event in 2017 with 2,077 (40%) occupational fatalities. Violence and other injuries by persons or animals decreased 7 percent in 2017, with homicides and suicides decreasing by 8 and 5 percent, respectively.

- Unintentional overdoses due to nonmedical use of drugs or alcohol while at work increased 25 percent from 217 in 2016 to 272 in 2017. This was the fifth consecutive year in which unintentional workplace overdose deaths have increased by at least 25 percent.

- Contact with objects and equipment incidents were down 9 percent (695 in 2017 from 761 in 2016), with caught in running equipment or machinery deaths down 26 percent (76 in 2017 from 103 in 2016).

- Fatal occupational injuries involving confined spaces rose 15 percent to 166 in 2017 from 144 in 2016.

- Crane-related workplace fatalities fell to their lowest level ever recorded in CFOI, 33 deaths in 2017.

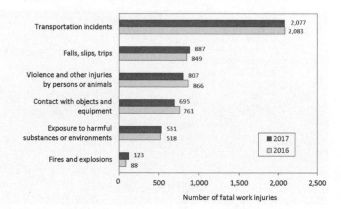

Figure 22.12. *Fatal Occupational Injuries by Major Event, 2016 to 2017*

Occupation

The transportation and material moving occupational group and the construction and extraction occupational group accounted for 47 percent of worker deaths in 2017. Within the occupational subgroup driver/sales workers and truck drivers, heavy and tractor-trailer truck drivers had the largest number of fatal occupational injuries with 840. This represented the highest value for heavy and tractor-trailer truck drivers since the occupational series began in 2003. Fishers and related fishing workers and logging workers had the highest published rates of fatal injury in 2017.

- Grounds maintenance workers (including first-line supervisors) incurred 244 fatalities in 2017. This was a small decrease from the 2016 figure (247) but was still the second-highest total since 2003. A total of 36 deaths were due to falls from trees, and another 35 were due to being struck by a falling tree or branch.

- There were 258 fatalities among farmers, ranchers, and other agricultural managers in 2017. Approximately 63 percent of these farmers were 65 years of age and older (162), with 48 being 80 years of age or older. Of the 258 deaths, 103 involved a farm tractor.

- Police and sheriff's patrol officers incurred 95 fatal occupational injuries in 2017, fewer than the 108 fatalities in 2016.

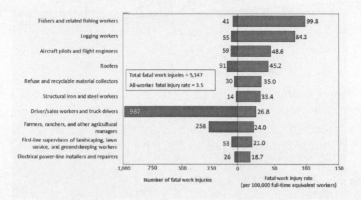

	Number of fatal work injuries	Fatal work injury rate
Fishers and related fishing workers	41	99.8
Logging workers	55	84.3
Aircraft pilots and flight engineers	59	48.6
Roofers	91	45.2
Refuse and recyclable material collectors	30	35.0
Structural iron and steel workers	14	33.4
Driver/sales workers and truck drivers	987	26.8
Farmers, ranchers, and other agricultural managers	258	24.0
First-line supervisors of landscaping, lawn service, and groundskeeping workers	53	21.0
Electrical power-line installers and repairers	26	18.7

Total fatal work injuries = 5,147
All-worker fatal injury rate = 3.5

Number of fatal work injuries

Fatal work injury rate
(per 100,000 full-time equivalent workers)

Figure 22.13. *Civilian Occupations with High Fatal Work Injury Rates, 2017*

Other Key Findings of the 2017 Census of Fatal Occupational Injuries

About 15 percent of the fatally-injured workers in 2017 were age 65 or over—a series high. In 1992, the first year CFOI published national data, that figure was 8 percent. These workers also had a higher fatality rate than other age groups in 2017.

- Fatalities incurred by non-Hispanic Black or African American workers and non-Hispanic Asian workers each decreased 10 percent from 2016 to 2017.

- Fatal occupational injuries in the private manufacturing industry and wholesale trade industry were the lowest since this series began in 2003.

- Workplace fatalities in the private mining, quarrying, and oil and gas extraction industry increased 26 percent to 112 in 2017 from a series low of 89 in 2016. Over 70 percent of these fatalities were incurred by workers in the oil and gas extraction industries.

- A total of 27 states had fewer fatal workplace injuries in 2017 than 2016, while 21 states and the District of Columbia had more; California and Maine had the same number as 2016. A total of 192 metropolitan statistical areas (MSAs) had 5 or more fatal work injuries in 2017.

Section 22.4

Poisoning

This section includes text excerpted from "Poisoning,"
Centers for Disease Control and Prevention (CDC),
November 24, 2015. Reviewed June 2019.

A poison is any substance, including medications, that is harmful to your body if too much is eaten, inhaled, injected, or absorbed through the skin. An unintentional poisoning occurs when a person taking or giving too much of a substance did not mean to cause harm.

Tips to Prevent Poisonings
Safety Tips for You, Your Family, and Friends

Unless noted, the safety tips below were adapted from the American Association of Poison Control Centers' (AAPCC) poison prevention tips for children and adults.

Drugs and Medicines

- Only take prescription medications that are prescribed to you by a healthcare professional. Misusing or abusing prescription or over-the-counter (OTC) medications is not a safe alternative to illicit substance abuse.

- Never take larger or more frequent doses of your medications, particularly prescription pain medications, to try to get faster or more powerful effects.

- Never share or sell your prescription drugs. Keep all prescription medicines (especially prescription painkillers, such as those containing methadone, hydrocodone, or oxycodone), over-the-counter medicines (including pain or fever relievers and cough and cold medicines), vitamins, and herbals in a safe place that can only be reached by people who take or give them.

- Follow directions on the label when you give or take medicines. Read all warning labels. Some medicines cannot be taken safely when you take other medicines or drink alcohol.

- Turn on a light when you give or take medicines at night so that you know you have the correct amount of the right medicine.

- Keep medicines in their original bottles or containers.

- Monitor the use of medicines prescribed for children and teenagers, such as medicines for attention deficit hyperactivity disorder, or ADHD.

- Dispose of unused, unneeded, or expired prescription drugs.

Household Chemicals and Carbon Monoxide

- Always read the label before using a product that may be poisonous.

- Keep chemical products in their original bottles or containers. Do not use food containers, such as cups, bottles, or jars, to store chemical products, such as cleaning solutions or beauty products.

- Never mix household products together. For example, mixing bleach and ammonia can result in toxic gases.

- Wear protective clothing (gloves, long sleeves, long pants, socks, shoes) if you spray pesticides or other chemicals.

- Turn on the fan and open windows when using chemical products, such as household cleaners.

Keep Young Children Safe from Poisoning

Be Prepared

Put the poison help number, 800-222-1222, on or near every home telephone and save it on your cell phone. The line is open 24 hours a day, 7 days a week.

Be Smart About Storage

- Store all medicines and household products up and away and out of sight in a cabinet where a child cannot reach them.

- When you are taking or giving medicines or are using household products:

  - Do not put your next dose on the counter or table where children can reach them—it only takes seconds for a child to get them.

  - If you have to do something else while taking medicine, such as answer the phone, take any young children with you.

323

- Secure the child safety cap completely every time you use a medicine.

- After using them, do not leave medicines or household products out. As soon as you are done with them, put them away and out of sight in a cabinet where a child cannot reach them.

- Be aware of any legal or illegal drugs that guests may bring into your home. Ask guests to store drugs where children cannot find them. Children can easily get into pillboxes, purses, backpacks, or coat pockets.

Other Tips

- Do not call medicine "candy."
- Identify poisonous plants in your house and yard, and place them out of reach of children or remove them.

What to Do If a Poisoning Occurs

- Remain calm.
- Call 911 if you have a poison emergency, and the victim has collapsed or is not breathing. If the victim is awake and alert, dial 800-222-1222. Try to have this information ready:

  - The victim's age and weight

  - The container or bottle of the poison if available

  - The time of the poison exposure

  - The address where the poisoning occurred

- Stay on the phone, and follow the instructions from the emergency operator or poison control center.

Poisoning Prevention in Your Community

National Poison Prevention Week occurs each year during the third week of March. It is a great time for communities to raise awareness about unintentional poisonings and to share prevention tips.

Section 22.5

Water-Related Accidents

This section includes text excerpted from "Water-Related Injuries,"
Centers for Disease Control and Prevention (CDC), May 2, 2016.

Every day, about 10 people die from unintentional drowning. Of
these, 2 will be children 14 years of age or younger. Drowning is the
fifth leading cause of unintentional injury death for people of all ages,
and the second leading cause of injury death for children between the
ages of 1 and 14.

In fact, more children between the ages of one and four die from
drowning than any other cause of death, except birth defects.

Unintentional Drowning: Get the Facts

How Big Is the Problem?

- From 2005 to 2014, there were an average of 3,536 fatal
  unintentional drownings (nonboating related) annually in
  the United States—about 10 deaths per day. An additional
  332 people died each year from drowning in boating-related
  incidents.

- About 1 in 5 people who die from drowning are children 14 years
  of age and younger. For every child who dies from drowning,
  another 5 receive emergency department care for nonfatal
  submersion injuries.

- More than 50 percent of drowning victims treated in emergency
  departments (EDs) require hospitalization or transfer for further
  care (compared with a hospitalization rate of about 6 percent
  for all unintentional injuries). These nonfatal drowning injuries
  can cause severe brain damage that may result in long-term
  disabilities, such as memory problems, learning disabilities, and
  permanent loss of basic functioning (e.g., permanent vegetative
  state).

Who Is Most at Risk?

- **Males:** Nearly 80 percent of people who die from drowning are
  male.

- **Children:** Children between the ages of 1 and 4 have the highest drowning rates. In 2014, among children between 1 and 4 years of age who died from an unintentional injury, one-third died from drowning. Among children between the ages of 1 and 4, most drownings occur in home swimming pools. Drowning is responsible for more deaths among children 1 to 4 years of age than any other cause except congenital anomalies (birth defects). Among those between the ages of 1 and 14, fatal drowning remains the second-leading cause of unintentional injury-related death behind motor vehicle crashes.

- **Minorities:** Between 1999 to 2010, the fatal unintentional drowning rate for African Americans was significantly higher than that of Whites across all ages. The disparity is widest among children 5 to 18 years of age. The disparity is most pronounced in swimming pools; African American children between the ages of 5 and 19 drown in swimming pools at rates 5.5 times higher than those of Whites. This disparity is greatest among those 11 to 12 years where African Americans drown in swimming pools at rates 10 times those of Whites.

Factors, such as access to swimming pools, the desire or lack of desire to learn how to swim, and choosing water-related recreational activities, may contribute to the racial differences in drowning rates. Available rates are based on population not on participation. If rates could be determined by actual participation in water-related activities, the disparity in minorities' drowning rates compared to Whites would be much greater.

What Factors Influence Drowning Risk

The main factors that affect drowning risk are lack of swimming ability, lack of barriers to prevent unsupervised water access, lack of close supervision while swimming, location, failure to wear life jackets, alcohol use, and seizure disorders.

- **Lack of swimming ability:** Many adults and children report that they cannot swim. Research has shown that participation in formal swimming lessons can reduce the risk of drowning among children one to four years of age.

- **Lack of barriers:** Barriers, such as pool fencing, prevent young children from gaining access to the pool area without caregivers' awareness. A 4-sided isolation fence (separating the pool area from the house and yard) reduces a child's risk of drowning 83 percent when compared to 3-sided property-line fencing.

- **Lack of close supervision:** Drowning can happen quickly and quietly anywhere there is water (such as in bathtubs, swimming pools, and buckets), and even in the presence of lifeguards.

- **Location:** People of different ages drown in different locations. For example, most children between the ages of 1 and 4 drown in home swimming pools. The percentage of drownings in natural water settings, including lakes, rivers, and oceans, increases with age. More than half of fatal and nonfatal drownings among those 15 years of age and older (57% and 57%, respectively) occurred in natural water settings.

- **Failure to wear life jackets:** In 2010, the U.S. Coast Guard received reports for 4,604 boating incidents; 3,153 boaters were reported injured, and 672 died. Most (72%) boating deaths that occurred during 2010 were caused by drowning, with 88 percent of victims not wearing life jackets.

- **Alcohol use:** Among adolescents and adults, alcohol use is involved in up to 70 percent of deaths associated with water recreation, almost a quarter of ED visits for drowning, and about 1 in 5 reported boating deaths. Alcohol influences balance, coordination, and judgment, and its effects are heightened by sun exposure and heat.

- **Seizure disorders:** For persons with seizure disorders, drowning is the most common cause of unintentional injury death, with the bathtub as the site of highest drowning risk.

What Has Research Found?

- **Swimming skills help.** Taking part in formal swimming lessons reduces the risk of drowning among children between the ages of one and four. However, many people do not have basic swimming skills. The Centers for Disease Control and Prevention (CDC) study about self-reported swimming ability found that:

  - Younger adults reported greater swimming ability than older adults.

  - Self-reported ability increased with level of education.

- Among racial groups, African Americans reported the most limited swimming ability.

- Men of all ages, races, and educational levels consistently reported greater swimming ability than women.

- **Seconds count—learn cardiopulmonary resuscitation (CPR).** CPR performed by bystanders has been shown to save lives and improve outcomes in drowning victims. The more quickly CPR is started, the better the chance of improved outcomes.

- **Life jackets can reduce risk.** Potentially, half of all boating deaths might be prevented with the use of life jackets.

Tips to Help You Stay Safe in the Water

- **Supervise when in or around water.** Designate a responsible adult to watch young children while in the bath and all children swimming or playing in or around water. Supervisors of preschool children should provide "touch supervision," being close enough to reach the child at all times. Because drowning occurs quickly and quietly, adults should not be involved in any other distracting activity (such as reading, playing cards, talking on the phone, or mowing the lawn) while supervising children, even if lifeguards are present.

- **Use the buddy system.** Always swim with a buddy. Select swimming sites that have lifeguards when possible.

- **Seizure disorder safety.** If you or a family member has a seizure disorder, provide one-on-one supervision around water, including swimming pools. Consider taking showers rather than using a bathtub for bathing. Wear life jackets when boating.

- **Learn to swim.** Formal swimming lessons can protect young children from drowning. However, even when children have had formal swimming lessons, constant, careful supervision when children are in the water and barriers, such as pool fencing to prevent unsupervised access, are still important.

- **Learn cardiopulmonary resuscitation.** In the time it takes for paramedics to arrive, your CPR skills could save someone's life.

- **Air-filled or foam toys are not safety devices.** Do not use air-filled or foam toys, such as "water wings," "noodles," or inner-tubes, instead of life jackets. These toys are not life jackets and are not designed to keep swimmers safe.

- **Avoid alcohol.** Avoid drinking alcohol before or during swimming, boating, or water skiing. Do not drink alcohol while supervising children.

- **Do not let swimmers hyperventilate before swimming underwater or try to hold their breath for long periods of time.** This can cause them to pass out (sometimes called "hypoxic blackout" or "shallow water blackout") and drown.

- **Know how to prevent recreational water illnesses**.

- **Know the local weather conditions and forecast before swimming or boating.** Strong winds and thunderstorms with lightning strikes are dangerous.

If you have a swimming pool at home:

- **Install four-sided fencing.** Install a four-sided pool fence that completely separates the pool area from the house and yard. The fence should be at least four feet high. Use self-closing and self-latching gates that open outward with latches that are out of reach of children. Also, consider additional barriers, such as automatic door locks and alarms, to prevent access or alert you if someone enters the pool area.

- **Clear the pool and deck of toys.** Remove floats, balls, and other toys from the pool and surrounding area immediately after use so children are not tempted to enter the pool area unsupervised.

If you are in and around natural water settings:

- **Use U.S. Coast Guard-approved life jackets.** This is important regardless of the distance to be traveled, the size of the boat, or the swimming ability of boaters; life jackets can reduce risk for weaker swimmers too.

- **Know the meaning of and obey warnings represented by colored beach flags.** These may vary from one beach to another.

329

- **Watch for dangerous waves and signs of rip currents.**
  Some examples are water that is discolored and choppy, foamy,
  or filled with debris and moving in a channel away from shore.

- **If you are caught in a rip current, swim parallel to shore.**
  Once free of the current, swim diagonally toward shore.

Chapter 23

Penile Cancer

General Information about Penile Cancer

Penile cancer is a disease in which malignant cells form in the tissues of the penis.

The penis is a rod-shaped male reproductive organ that passes sperm and urine from the body. It contains two types of erectile tissue (spongy tissue with blood vessels that fill with blood to make an erection):

- **Corpora cavernosa.** The two columns of erectile tissue that form most of the penis.

- **Corpus spongiosum.** The single column of erectile tissue that forms a small portion of the penis. The corpus spongiosum surrounds the urethra (the tube through which urine and sperm pass from the body).

The erectile tissue is wrapped in connective tissue and covered with skin. The glans (head of the penis) is covered with loose skin called the "foreskin."

This chapter includes text excerpted from "Penile Cancer Treatment (PDQ®)–Patient Version," National Cancer Institute (NCI), April 9, 2019.

Human Papillomavirus Infection and Penile Cancer Risks

Anything that increases your chance of getting a disease is called a "risk factor." Having a risk factor does not mean that you will get cancer; not having risk factors does not mean that you will not get cancer. Talk with your doctor if you think you may be at risk. Risk factors for penile cancer include the following:

Circumcision may help prevent infection with the human papillomavirus (HPV). A circumcision is an operation in which the doctor removes part or all of the foreskin from the penis. Many boys are circumcised shortly after birth. Men who were not circumcised at birth may have a higher risk of developing penile cancer.

Other risk factors for penile cancer include the following:

- Being 60 years of age or older

- Having phimosis (a condition in which the foreskin of the penis cannot be pulled back over the glans)

- Having poor personal hygiene

- Having many sexual partners

- Using tobacco products

Signs of Penile Cancer

These and other signs may be caused by penile cancer or by other conditions. Check with your doctor if you have any of the following:

- Redness, irritation, or a sore on the penis

- A lump on the penis

Diagnosis of Penile Cancer

The following tests and procedures may be used:

- **Physical exam and history:** An exam of the body to check general signs of health, including checking the penis for signs of disease, such as lumps or anything else that seems unusual. A history of the patient's health habits and past illnesses and treatments will also be taken.

- **Biopsy:** The removal of cells or tissues so they can be viewed under a microscope by a pathologist to check for signs of cancer.

The tissue sample is removed during one of the following procedures:

- **Incisional biopsy:** The removal of part of a lump or a sample of tissue that does not look normal.

- **Excisional biopsy:** The removal of an entire lump or area of tissue that does not look normal.

Factors Affecting Prognosis and Treatment Options

The prognosis (chance of recovery) and treatment options depend on the following:

- The stage of the cancer

- The location and size of the tumor

- Whether the cancer has just been diagnosed or has recurred (come back)

Stages of Penile Cancer

After penile cancer has been diagnosed, tests are done to find out if cancer cells have spread within the penis or to other parts of the body.

The process used to find out if cancer has spread within the penis or to other parts of the body is called "staging." The information gathered from the staging process determines the stage of the disease. It is important to know the stage in order to plan treatment.

The following tests and procedures may be used in the staging process:

- **Computed tomography (CT or CAT) scan:** A procedure that makes a series of detailed pictures of areas inside the body, such as the pelvis, taken from different angles. The pictures are made by a computer linked to an X-ray machine. A dye may be injected into a vein or swallowed to help the organs or tissues show up more clearly. This procedure is also called "computed tomography," "computerized tomography," or "computerized axial tomography."

- **Positron emission tomography (PET) scan:** A procedure to find malignant tumor cells in the body. A small amount of radioactive glucose (sugar) is injected into a vein. The PET scanner rotates around the body and makes a picture of where glucose is being used in the body. Malignant tumor cells show

333

up brighter in the picture because they are more active and take up more glucose than normal cells do. When this procedure is done at the same time as a CT scan, it is called a "PET/CT scan."

- **Magnetic resonance imaging (MRI):** A procedure that uses a magnet, radio waves, and a computer to make a series of detailed pictures of areas inside the body. A substance called "gadolinium" is injected into a vein. The gadolinium collects around the cancer cells so they show up brighter in the picture. This procedure is also called "nuclear magnetic resonance imaging" (NMRI).

- **Ultrasound exam:** A procedure in which high-energy sound waves (ultrasound) are bounced off internal tissues or organs and make echoes. The echoes form a picture of body tissues called a "sonogram."

- **Chest X-ray:** An X-ray of the organs and bones inside the chest. An X-ray is a type of energy beam that can go through the body and onto film, making a picture of areas inside the body.

- **Biopsy:** The removal of cells or tissues so they can be viewed under a microscope by a pathologist to check for signs of cancer. The tissue sample is removed during one of the following procedures:

  - **Sentinel lymph node biopsy:** The removal of the sentinel lymph node during surgery. The sentinel lymph node is the first lymph node in a group of lymph nodes to receive lymphatic drainage from the primary tumor. It is the first lymph node the cancer is likely to spread to from the primary tumor. A radioactive substance and/or blue dye is injected near the tumor. The substance or dye flows through the lymph ducts to the lymph nodes. The first lymph node to receive the substance or dye is removed. A pathologist views the tissue under a microscope to look for cancer cells. If cancer cells are not found, it may not be necessary to remove more lymph nodes. Sometimes, a sentinel lymph node is found in more than one group of nodes.

  - **Lymph node dissection:** A procedure to remove one or more lymph nodes in the groin during surgery. A sample of tissue is checked under a microscope for signs of cancer. This procedure is also called a "lymphadenectomy."

Ways Cancer Spreads

Cancer can spread through tissue, the lymph system, and the blood:

- **Tissue.** The cancer spreads from where it began by growing into nearby areas.

- **Lymph system.** The cancer spreads from where it began by getting into the lymph system. The cancer travels through the lymph vessels to other parts of the body.

- **Blood.** The cancer spreads from where it began by getting into the blood. The cancer travels through the blood vessels to other parts of the body.

Cancer may spread from where it began to other parts of the body. When cancer spreads to another part of the body, it is called "metastasis." Cancer cells break away from where they began (the primary tumor) and travel through the lymph system or blood.

- **Lymph system**. The cancer gets into the lymph system, travels through the lymph vessels, and forms a tumor (metastatic tumor) in another part of the body.

- **Blood.** The cancer gets into the blood, travels through the blood vessels, and forms a tumor (metastatic tumor) in another part of the body.

The metastatic tumor is the same type of cancer as the primary tumor. For example, if penile cancer spreads to the lung, the cancer cells in the lung are actually penile cancer cells. The disease is metastatic penile cancer, not lung cancer.

Stages of Penile Cancer
Stage 0

Stage 0 is divided into stages 0is and 0a.

- In stage 0is, abnormal cells are found on the surface of the skin of the penis. These abnormal cells form growths that may become cancer and spread into nearby normal tissue. Stage 0is is also called "carcinoma in situ" or "penile intraepithelial neoplasia."

- In stage 0a, squamous cell cancer that does not spread is found on the surface of the skin of the penis or on the underneath surface of the foreskin of the penis. Stage 0a is also called "noninvasive localized squamous cell carcinoma."

Stage I

In stage I, cancer has formed and spread to tissue just under the skin of the penis. Cancer has not spread to lymph vessels, blood vessels, or nerves. The cancer cells look more like normal cells under a microscope.

Stage II

Stage II is divided into stages IIA and IIB.
In stage IIA, cancer has spread:

* To tissue just under the skin of the penis. Cancer has spread to lymph vessels, blood vessels, and/or nerves.

* To tissue just under the skin of the penis. Under a microscope, the cancer cells look very abnormal or the cells are sarcomatoid.

* Into the corpus spongiosum (spongy erectile tissue in the shaft and glans that fills with blood to make an erection)

In stage IIB, cancer has spread:

* Through the layer of connective tissue that surrounds the corpus cavernosum and into the corpus cavernosum (spongy erectile tissue that runs along the shaft of the penis)

Stage III

Stage III is divided into stages IIIA and stage IIIB. Cancer is found in the penis.

* In stage IIIA, cancer has spread to one or two lymph nodes on one side of the groin.

* In stage IIIB, cancer has spread to three or more lymph nodes on one side of the groin or to lymph nodes on both sides of the groin.

Stage IV

In stage IV, cancer has spread:

* To tissues near the penis, such as the scrotum, prostate, or pubic bone, and may have spread to lymph nodes in the groin or pelvis

* To one or more lymph nodes in the pelvis, or cancer has spread through the outer covering of the lymph nodes to nearby tissue

- To lymph nodes outside the pelvis or to other parts of the body, such as the lung, liver, or bone

Recurrent Penile Cancer

Recurrent penile cancer is cancer that has recurred after it has been treated. The cancer may come back in the penis or in other parts of the body.

Treatment Options Overview
Types of Treatment for Penile Cancer

Different types of treatments are available for patients with penile cancer. Some treatments are standard (the currently used treatment), and some are being tested in clinical trials. A treatment clinical trial is a research study meant to help improve current treatments or obtain information on new treatments for patients with cancer. When clinical trials show that a new treatment is better than the standard treatment, the new treatment may become the standard treatment. Patients may want to think about taking part in a clinical trial. Some clinical trials are open only to patients who have not started treatment.

Types of Standard Treatments
Surgery

Surgery is the most common treatment for all stages of penile cancer. A doctor may remove the cancer using one of the following operations:

- **Mohs microsurgery.** A procedure in which the tumor is cut from the skin in thin layers. During the surgery, the edges of the tumor and each layer of tumor removed are viewed through a microscope to check for cancer cells. Layers continue to be removed until no more cancer cells are seen. This type of surgery removes as little normal tissue as possible and is often used to remove cancer on the skin. It is also called "Mohs surgery."

- **Laser surgery.** A surgical procedure that uses a laser beam (a narrow beam of intense light) as a knife to make bloodless cuts in tissue or to remove a surface lesion, such as a tumor.

- **Cryosurgery.** A treatment that uses an instrument to freeze and destroy abnormal tissue. This type of treatment is also called "cryotherapy."

- **Circumcision.** Surgery to remove part or all of the foreskin of the penis.

- **Wide local excision.** Surgery to remove only the cancer and some normal tissue around it.

- **Amputation of the penis.** Surgery to remove part or all of the penis. If part of the penis is removed, it is a partial penectomy. If all of the penis is removed, it is a total penectomy.

Lymph nodes in the groin may be taken out during surgery.

After the doctor removes all the cancer that can be seen at the time of the surgery, some patients may be given chemotherapy or radiation therapy after surgery to kill any cancer cells that are left. Treatment given after the surgery to lower the risk that the cancer will come back is called "adjuvant therapy."

Radiation Therapy

Radiation therapy is a cancer treatment that uses high-energy X-rays or other types of radiation to kill cancer cells or keep them from growing. There are two types of radiation therapy:

- **External radiation therapy** uses a machine outside the body to send radiation toward the cancer.

- **Internal radiation therapy** uses a radioactive substance sealed in needles, seeds, wires, or catheters that are placed directly into or near the cancer.

The way the radiation therapy is given depends on the type and stage of the cancer being treated. External and internal radiation therapy are used to treat penile cancer.

Chemotherapy

Chemotherapy is a cancer treatment that uses drugs to stop the growth of cancer cells, either by killing the cells or by stopping them from dividing. When chemotherapy is taken by mouth or injected into a vein or muscle, the drugs enter the bloodstream and can reach cancer cells throughout the body (systemic chemotherapy). When chemotherapy is placed directly onto the skin (topical chemotherapy) or into the cerebrospinal fluid; an organ; or a body cavity, such as the abdomen, the drugs mainly affect cancer cells in those areas (regional chemotherapy). The way the chemotherapy is given depends on the type and stage of the cancer being treated.

Topical chemotherapy may be used to treat stage 0 penile cancer.

Biologic Therapy

Biologic therapy is a treatment that uses the patient's immune system to fight cancer. Substances made by the body or made in a laboratory are used to boost, direct, or restore the body's natural defenses against cancer. This type of cancer treatment is also called "biotherapy" or "immunotherapy." Topical biologic therapy with imiquimod may be used to treat stage 0 penile cancer.

New Types of Treatment in Clinical Trials

This summary section describes treatments that are being studied in clinical trials. It may not mention every new treatment being studied.

Radiosensitizers

Radiosensitizers are drugs that make tumor cells more sensitive to radiation therapy. Combining radiation therapy with radiosensitizers helps kill more tumor cells.

Sentinel Lymph Node Biopsy Followed by Surgery

Sentinel lymph node biopsy is the removal of the sentinel lymph node during surgery. The sentinel lymph node is the first lymph node in a group of lymph nodes to receive lymphatic drainage from the primary tumor. It is the first lymph node the cancer is likely to spread to from the primary tumor. A radioactive substance and/or blue dye is injected near the tumor. The substance or dye flows through the lymph ducts to the lymph nodes. The first lymph node to receive the substance or dye is removed. A pathologist views the tissue under a microscope to look for cancer cells. If cancer cells are not found, it may not be necessary to remove more lymph nodes. Sometimes, a sentinel lymph node is found in more than one group of nodes. After the sentinel lymph node biopsy, the surgeon removes the cancer.

Side Effects of Penile Cancer Treatments

For information about side effects caused by treatment for cancer, visit the National Cancer Institute's website.

Patients may want to think about taking part in a clinical trial.

For some patients, taking part in a clinical trial may be the best treatment choice. Clinical trials are part of the cancer research process. Clinical trials are done to find out if new cancer treatments are safe and effective or better than the standard treatment.

Many of today's standard treatments for cancer are based on earlier clinical trials. Patients who take part in a clinical trial may receive the standard treatment or be among the first to receive a new treatment.

Patients who take part in clinical trials also help improve the way cancer will be treated in the future. Even when clinical trials do not lead to effective new treatments, they often answer important questions and help move research forward.

Patients can enter clinical trials before, during, or after starting their cancer treatment.

Some clinical trials only include patients who have not yet received treatment. Other trials test treatments for patients whose cancer has not gotten better. There are also clinical trials that test new ways to stop cancer from recurring or reduce the side effects of cancer treatment. Clinical trials are taking place in many parts of the country.

Follow-Up Tests

Some of the tests that were done to diagnose the cancer or to find out the stage of the cancer may be repeated. Some tests will be repeated in order to see how well the treatment is working. Decisions about whether to continue, change, or stop treatment may be based on the results of these tests.

Some of the tests will continue to be done from time to time after treatment has ended. The results of these tests can show if your condition has changed or if the cancer has recurred. These tests are sometimes called "follow-up tests" or "checkups."

Chapter 24

Prostate Cancer

What Is the Prostate?

The prostate is a part of the male reproductive system, which includes the penis, prostate, and testicles. The prostate is located just below the bladder and in front of the rectum. It is about the size of a walnut and surrounds the urethra (the tube that empties urine from the bladder). It produces fluid that makes up a part of semen.

As a man ages, the prostate tends to increase in size. This can cause the urethra to narrow and decrease urine flow. This is called "benign prostatic hyperplasia," and it is not the same as prostate cancer. Men may also have other prostate changes that are not cancer.

What Is Prostate Cancer?

Cancer is a disease in which cells in the body grow out of control. When cancer starts in the prostate, it is called "prostate cancer." Not including skin cancer, prostate cancer is the most common cancer in American men.

Who Is at Risk for Prostate Cancer?

All men are at risk for prostate cancer. Out of every 100 American men, about 13 will get prostate cancer during their lifetime, and about 2 to 3 men will die from prostate cancer.

This chapter includes text excerpted from "Basic Information about Prostate Cancer," Centers for Disease Control and Prevention (CDC), June 7, 2018.

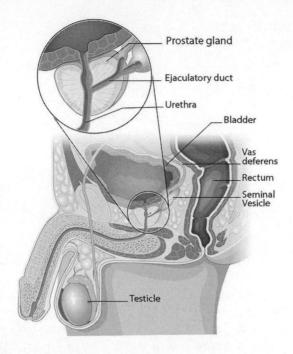

Figure 24.1. *Prostate Gland*

The most common risk factor is age. The older a man is, the greater the chance of getting prostate cancer.

Some men are at an increased risk for prostate cancer. You are at an increased risk for getting or dying from prostate cancer if you are African American or have a family history of prostate cancer.

African American Men

- Are more likely to get prostate cancer than other men

- Are more than twice as likely to die from prostate cancer than White men

- Get prostate cancer at a younger age, tend to have more advanced disease when it is found, and tend to have a more severe type of prostate cancer than other men

Family History

- Men who have a father, son, or brother who had prostate cancer are at an increased risk for getting prostate cancer.

- Men with three or more first-degree relatives (father, son, or brother), or two close relatives on the same side of the family who have had prostate cancer may have a type of prostate cancer caused by genetic changes that are inherited.

Men who are not African American and do not have a family history of prostate cancer are at average risk.

What Are the Symptoms of Prostate Cancer?

Different people have different symptoms for prostate cancer. Some men do not have symptoms at all.

Some symptoms of prostate cancer are:

- Difficulty starting urination

- Weak or interrupted flow of urine

- Frequent urination, especially at night

- Difficulty emptying the bladder completely

- Pain or burning during urination

- Blood in the urine or semen

- Pain in the back, hips, or pelvis that does not go away

- Painful ejaculation

If you have any symptoms that worry you, be sure to see your doctor right away. Keep in mind that these symptoms may be caused by conditions other than prostate cancer.

What Is Screening for Prostate Cancer?

Cancer screening means looking for cancer before it causes symptoms. The goal of screening for prostate cancer is to find cancers that may be at a high risk of spreading if they are not treated and to find them early before they spread.

Screening for prostate cancer begins with a blood test called a "prostate-specific antigen (PSA) test." This test measures the level of PSA in the blood. PSA is a substance made by the prostate. The levels of PSA in the blood can be higher in men who have prostate cancer. The PSA level may also be elevated in other conditions that affect the prostate.

As a rule, the higher the PSA level in the blood, the more likely a prostate problem is present. But many factors, such as age and race, can affect PSA levels. Some prostate glands make more PSA than others.

Prostate-specific antigen levels also can be affected by:

- Certain medical procedures

- Certain medications

- An enlarged prostate

- A prostate infection

Because many factors can affect PSA levels, your doctor is the best person to interpret your PSA test results. If the PSA test is abnormal, your doctor may recommend a biopsy to find out if you have prostate cancer.

Should I Get Screened for Prostate Cancer?

The United States Preventive Services Task Force (USPSTF) is an organization made up of doctors and disease experts who look at research on the best way to prevent diseases and make recommendations on how doctors can help patients avoid diseases or find them early.

In 2018, the USPSTF made the following recommendations about prostate cancer screening:

- Men who are between 55 and 69 years of age should make individual decisions about being screened for prostate cancer with a PSA test.

- Before making a decision, men should talk to their doctor about the benefits and harms of screening for prostate cancer, including the benefits and harms of other tests and treatment.

- Men who are 70 years of age and older should not be screened for prostate cancer routinely.

This recommendation applies to men who:

- Are at an average risk for prostate cancer

- Are at an increased risk for prostate cancer

- Do not have symptoms of prostate cancer

- Have never been diagnosed with prostate cancer

Talk to Your Doctor

If you are thinking about being screened, you and your doctor should consider:

- If you have a family history of prostate cancer

- If you are African American

- If you have other medical conditions that may make it difficult for you to be treated for prostate cancer, if it is found, or that may make you less likely to benefit from screening

- How you value the potential benefits and harms of screening, diagnosis, and treatment.

Facts about Prostate Cancer Screening

- For every 1,000 men between the ages of 55 and 69 years of age who are screened, about 1 death will be prevented, and 3 men will be prevented from getting prostate cancer that spreads to other places in the body.

- Many men with prostate cancer never experience symptoms and, without screening, would never know they had the disease.

- Half of men who die from prostate cancer are 80 years of age or older.

What Are the Benefits and Harms of Screening?
Possible Benefits of Screening

The benefits of screening for prostate cancer may include:

- Finding prostate cancers that may be at high risk of spreading, so that they can be treated before they spread. This may lower the chance of death from prostate cancer in some men.

- Some men prefer to know if they have prostate cancer.

Possible Harm from Screening

False-positive test results: This occurs when a man has an abnormal PSA test but does not have prostate cancer. False-positive test results often lead to unnecessary tests, such as a biopsy of the prostate. They may cause men to worry about their health. Older men are more likely to have false-positive test results.

Possible Harms from Diagnosis

Screening finds prostate cancer in some men who would never have had symptoms from their cancer in their lifetime. Treatment of men who would not have had symptoms or died from prostate cancer can cause them to have complications from treatment rather than benefit from the treatment. This is called "overdiagnosis."

Prostate cancer is diagnosed with a prostate biopsy. A biopsy is when a small piece of tissue is removed from the prostate and looked at under a microscope to see if there are cancer cells. Older men are more likely to have a complication after a prostate biopsy.

A prostate biopsy can cause:

- Pain
- Blood in the semen or ejaculate
- Infection

Possible Harms from Treatment

The most common treatments for prostate cancer are surgery to remove the prostate and radiation therapy.

The most common harms from prostate cancer treatment are:

- **Urinary incontinence (accidental leakage of urine).**
  About one out of every five men who have surgery to remove the prostate loses bladder control.

- **Erectile dysfunction (impotence).** About two out of every three men who have surgery to remove the prostate become impotent, and about half of men who receive radiation therapy become impotent.

Bowel problems, including fecal incontinence (accidental leakage of bowel movements) and urgency (sudden and uncontrollable urge to have a bowel movement). About one out of every six men who has radiation therapy has bowel problems.

How Is Prostate Cancer Diagnosed?

If your PSA test is abnormal, doctors may do more tests to find or diagnose prostate cancer.

A biopsy is when a small piece of tissue is removed from the prostate and looked at under a microscope to see if there are cancer cells.

A Gleason score is determined when the biopsy is looked at under the microscope. If there is cancer, the score indicates how likely it is to spread. The score ranges from 2 to 10. The lower the score, the less likely it is that the cancer will spread.

A biopsy is the main tool for diagnosing prostate cancer, but a doctor can use other tools to help make sure the biopsy is made in the right place. For example, doctors may use a transrectal ultrasound, in which a probe that is the size of a finger is inserted into the rectum and high-energy sound waves (ultrasound) bounce off the prostate to create a picture of the prostate called a "sonogram." Doctors also may use magnetic resonance imaging (MRI) to guide the biopsy.

Staging

If prostate cancer is diagnosed, other tests are done to find out if cancer cells have spread within the prostate or to other parts of the body. This process is called "staging." Whether the cancer is only in the prostate or has spread outside the prostate, determines your stage of prostate cancer. The stage of prostate cancer tells doctors what kind of treatment you need.

How Is Prostate Cancer Treated?

Different types of treatment are available for prostate cancer. You and your doctor will decide which treatment is right for you. Some common treatments are:

- **Active surveillance.** Closely monitoring the prostate cancer by performing PSA and digital rectal exam (DRE) tests and prostate biopsies regularly, and treating the cancer only if it grows or causes symptoms.

- **Surgery.** A prostatectomy is an operation where doctors remove the prostate. Radical prostatectomy removes the prostate, as well as the surrounding tissue.

- **Radiation therapy.** Using high-energy rays (similar to X-rays) to kill the cancer. There are two types of radiation therapy—

  - **External radiation therapy.** A machine outside the body directs radiation at the cancer cells.

  - **Internal radiation therapy (brachytherapy).** Radioactive seeds or pellets are surgically placed into or near the cancer to destroy the cancer cells.

347

Other therapies used in the treatment of prostate cancer that are still under investigation include:

- **Cryotherapy.** Placing a special probe inside or near the prostate cancer to freeze and kill the cancer cells.

- **Chemotherapy.** Using special drugs to shrink or kill the cancer. The drugs can be pills you take, medicines given through your veins, or, sometimes, both.

- **Biological therapy** works with your body's immune system to help it fight cancer or to control side effects from other cancer treatments. Side effects are how your body reacts to drugs or other treatments.

- **High-intensity focused ultrasound.** This therapy directs high-energy sound waves (ultrasound) at the cancer to kill cancer cells.

- **Hormone therapy.** Blocks cancer cells from getting the hormones they need to grow.

Chapter 25

Testicular Cancer

What Are Testicles?

The testicles are two egg-shaped glands located inside the scrotum (a sac of loose skin that lies directly below the penis). The testicles are held within the scrotum by the spermatic cord, which also contains the vas deferens and vessels and nerves of the testicles.

The testicles are the male sex glands and produce testosterone and sperm. Germ cells within the testicles produce immature sperm that travel through a network of tubules (tiny tubes) and larger tubes into the epididymis (a long coiled tube next to the testicles), where the sperm mature and are stored.

General Information about Testicular Cancer
What Is Testicular Cancer?

Almost all testicular cancers start in the germ cells. The two main types of testicular germ cell tumors are seminomas and nonseminomas. These two types grow and spread differently, and they are treated differently. Nonseminomas tend to grow and spread more quickly than seminomas. Seminomas are more sensitive to radiation. A testicular tumor that contains both seminoma and nonseminoma cells is treated as a nonseminoma.

This chapter includes text excerpted from "Testicular Cancer Treatment (PDQ®)—Patient Version," National Cancer Institute (NCI), April 9, 2019.

Testicular cancer is the most common cancer in men between the ages of 20 and 35.

Risks of Testicular Cancer

Anything that increases the chance of getting a disease is called a "risk factor." Having a risk factor does not mean that you will get cancer; not having risk factors does not mean that you will not get cancer. Talk with your doctor if you think you may be at risk. Risk factors for testicular cancer include:

- Having had an undescended testicle
- Having had abnormal development of the testicles
- Having a personal history of testicular cancer
- Having a family history of testicular cancer (especially in a father or brother)
- Being White

Signs and Symptoms of Testicular Cancer

These and other signs and symptoms may be caused by testicular cancer or by other conditions. Check with your doctor if you have any of the following:

- A painless lump or swelling in either testicle
- A change in how the testicle feels
- A dull ache in the lower abdomen or the groin
- A sudden buildup of fluid in the scrotum
- Pain or discomfort in a testicle or in the scrotum

Diagnosis of Testicular Cancer

The following tests and procedures may be used:

- **Physical exam and history:** An exam of the body to check general signs of health, including checking for signs of disease, such as lumps or anything else that seems unusual. The testicles will be examined to check for lumps, swelling, or pain. A history of the patient's health habits and past illnesses and treatments will also be taken.

- **Ultrasound exam of the testes:** A procedure in which high-energy sound waves (ultrasound) are bounced off internal tissues or organs and make echoes. The echoes form a picture of body tissues called a "sonogram."

- **Serum tumor marker test:** A procedure in which a sample of blood is examined to measure the amounts of certain substances released into the blood by organs, tissues, or tumor cells in the body. Certain substances are linked to specific types of cancer when found in increased levels in the blood. These are called "tumor markers." The following tumor markers are used to detect testicular cancer:

  - Alpha-fetoprotein (AFP)

  - Beta-human chorionic gonadotropin (β-hCG)

Tumor marker levels are measured before inguinal orchiectomy and biopsy to help diagnose testicular cancer.

- **Inguinal orchiectomy:** A procedure to remove the entire testicle through an incision in the groin. A tissue sample from the testicle is then viewed under a microscope to check for cancer cells. (The surgeon does not cut through the scrotum into the testicle to remove a sample of tissue for biopsy because if cancer is present, this procedure could cause it to spread into the scrotum and lymph nodes. It is important to choose a surgeon who has experience with this kind of surgery.) If cancer is found, the cell type (seminoma or nonseminoma) is determined in order to help plan treatment.

Factors Affecting Prognosis and Treatment Options

The prognosis (chance of recovery) and treatment options depend on the following:

- Stage of the cancer (whether it is in or near the testicle or has spread to other places in the body, and blood levels of AFP, β-hCG, and LDH)

- Type of cancer

- Size of the tumor

- Number and size of retroperitoneal lymph nodes

Testicular cancer can usually be cured in patients who receive adjuvant chemotherapy or radiation therapy after their primary treatment.

Testicular Cancer Treatment and Infertility

Certain treatments for testicular cancer can cause infertility that may be permanent. Patients who may wish to have children should consider sperm banking before having treatment. Sperm banking is the process of freezing sperm and storing it for later use.

Stages of Testicular Cancer

The process used to find out if cancer has spread within the testicles or to other parts of the body is called "staging." The information gathered from the staging process determines the stage of the disease. It is important to know the stage in order to plan treatment.

The following tests and procedures may be used in the staging process:

- **Chest X-ray:** An X-ray of the organs and bones inside the chest. An X-ray is a type of energy beam that can go through the body and onto film, making a picture of areas inside the body.

- **Computed tomography (CT) scan:** A procedure that makes a series of detailed pictures of areas inside the body, such as the abdomen, taken from different angles. The pictures are made by a computer linked to an X-ray machine. A dye may be injected into a vein or swallowed to help the organs or tissues show up more clearly. This procedure is also called "computed tomography," "computerized tomography," or "computerized axial tomography."

- **Magnetic resonance imaging (MRI):** A procedure that uses a magnet, radio waves, and a computer to make a series of detailed pictures of areas inside the body, such as the abdomen. This procedure is also called "nuclear magnetic resonance imaging" (NMRI).

- **Abdominal lymph node dissection:** A surgical procedure in which lymph nodes in the abdomen are removed, and a sample of tissue is checked under a microscope for signs of cancer. This procedure is also called "lymphadenectomy." For patients with nonseminoma, removing the lymph nodes may help stop the spread of disease. Cancer cells in the lymph nodes of seminoma patients can be treated with radiation therapy.

- **Serum tumor marker test:** A procedure in which a sample of blood is examined to measure the amounts of certain substances released into the blood by organs, tissues, or tumor cells in the body. Certain substances are linked to specific types of cancer when found in increased levels in the blood. These are called "tumor markers." The following three tumor markers are used in staging testicular cancer:

- Alpha-fetoprotein (AFP)
- Beta-human chorionic gonadotropin (β-hCG)
- Lactate dehydrogenase (LDH)

Tumor marker levels are measured again, after inguinal orchiectomy and biopsy, in order to determine the stage of the cancer. This helps to show if all of the cancer has been removed or if more treatment is needed. Tumor marker levels are also measured during follow-up appointments as a way of checking if the cancer has come back.

Ways Cancer Spreads in the Body

Cancer can spread through tissue, the lymph system, and the blood.

- **Tissue.** The cancer spreads from where it began by growing into nearby areas.

- **Lymph system.** The cancer spreads from where it began by getting into the lymph system. The cancer travels through the lymph vessels to other parts of the body.

- **Blood.** The cancer spreads from where it began by getting into the blood. The cancer travels through the blood vessels to other parts of the body.

When cancer spreads to another part of the body, it is called "metastasis." Cancer cells break away from where they began (the primary tumor) and travel through the lymph system or blood.

- **Lymph system.** The cancer gets into the lymph system, travels through the lymph vessels, and forms a tumor (metastatic tumor) in another part of the body.

- **Blood.** The cancer gets into the blood, travels through the blood vessels, and forms a tumor (metastatic tumor) in another part of the body.

The metastatic tumor is the same type of cancer as the primary tumor. For example, if testicular cancer spreads to the lung, the cancer cells in the lung are actually testicular cancer cells. The disease is metastatic testicular cancer, not lung cancer.

Inguinal Orchiectomy

The following stages are used for testicular cancer:

Stage 0

In stage 0, abnormal cells are found in the tiny tubules where the sperm cells begin to develop. These abnormal cells may become cancer and spread into nearby normal tissue. All tumor marker levels are normal. Stage 0 is also called "germ cell neoplasia in situ."

Stage I

In stage I, cancer has formed. Stage I is divided into stages IA, IB, and IS.

- In stage IA, cancer is found in the testicle, including the rete testis, but has not spread to the blood vessels or lymph vessels in the testicle.

All tumor marker levels are normal.

- In stage IB, cancer:
  - Is found in the testicle, including the rete testis, and has spread to the blood vessels or lymph vessels in the testicle
  - Has spread into the hilar soft tissue (tissue made of fibers and fat with blood vessels and lymph vessels), the epididymis, or the outer membranes around the testicle
  - Has spread to the spermatic cord
  - Has spread to the scrotum

All tumor marker levels are normal.

- In stage Is, cancer is found anywhere in the testicle and may have spread into the spermatic cord or scrotum.

Tumor marker levels range from slightly above normal to high.

Stage II

Stage II is divided into stages IIA, IIB, and IIC.

- In stage IIA, cancer is found anywhere in the testicle and may have spread into the spermatic cord or scrotum. Cancer has spread to one to five nearby lymph nodes, and the lymph nodes are two centimeters or smaller.

All tumor marker levels are normal or slightly above normal.

- In stage IIB, cancer is found anywhere in the testicle and may have spread into the spermatic cord or scrotum. Cancer has spread to:
  - One nearby lymph node and the lymph node is larger than two centimeters but not larger than five centimeters
  - More than five nearby lymph nodes, and the lymph nodes are not larger than five centimeters
  - A nearby lymph node and the cancer has spread outside the lymph node

All tumor marker levels are normal or slightly above normal.

- In stage IIC, cancer is found anywhere in the testicle and may have spread into the spermatic cord or scrotum. Cancer has spread to a nearby lymph node, and the lymph node is larger than five centimeters.

All tumor marker levels are normal or slightly above normal.

Stage III

Stage III is divided into stages IIIA, IIIB, and IIIC.

- In stage IIIA, cancer is found anywhere in the testicle and may have spread into the spermatic cord or scrotum. Cancer may have spread to one or more nearby lymph nodes. Cancer has spread to distant lymph nodes or to the lungs.

All tumor marker levels are normal or slightly above normal.

- In stage IIIB, cancer is found anywhere in the testicle and may have spread into the spermatic cord or scrotum. Cancer has spread:
  - To one or more nearby lymph nodes and has not spread to other parts of the body
  - To one or more nearby lymph nodes. Cancer has spread to distant lymph nodes or to the lungs.

The level of one or more tumor markers is moderately above normal.

- In stage IIIC, cancer is found anywhere in the testicle and may have spread into the spermatic cord or scrotum. Cancer has spread:

  - To one or more nearby lymph nodes and has not spread to other parts of the body

  - To one or more nearby lymph nodes. Cancer has spread to distant lymph nodes or to the lungs.

The level of one or more tumor markers is high.

Cancer is found anywhere in the testicle and may have spread into the spermatic cord or scrotum. Cancer has not spread to distant lymph nodes or the lung, but has spread to other parts of the body, such as the liver or bone.

Tumor marker levels may range from normal to high.

Recurrent Testicular Cancer

Recurrent testicular cancer is cancer that has recurred (come back) after it has been treated. The cancer may come back many years after the initial cancer, in the other testicle or in other parts of the body.

Treatment Options Overview
Types of Treatment for Patients with Testicular Cancer

Different types of treatments are available for patients with testicular cancer. Some treatments are standard (the currently used treatment), and some are being tested in clinical trials. A treatment clinical trial is a research study meant to help improve current treatments or obtain information on new treatments for patients with cancer. When clinical trials show that a new treatment is better than the standard treatment, the new treatment may become the standard treatment. Patients may want to think about taking part in a clinical trial. Some clinical trials are open only to patients who have not started treatment.

Groups of Testicular Tumors
Good Prognosis

For nonseminoma, all of the following must be true:

- The tumor is found only in the testicle or in the retroperitoneum (area outside or behind the abdominal wall).

- The tumor has not spread to organs other than the lungs.
- The levels of all the tumor markers are slightly above normal.

For seminoma, all of the following must be true:

- The tumor has not spread to organs other than the lungs.
- The level of alpha-fetoprotein (AFP) is normal. Beta-human chorionic gonadotropin (β-hCG) and lactate dehydrogenase (LDH) may be at any level.

Intermediate Prognosis

For nonseminoma, all of the following must be true:

- The tumor is found in one testicle only or in the retroperitoneum (area outside or behind the abdominal wall).
- The tumor has not spread to organs other than the lungs.
- The level of any one of the tumor markers is more than slightly above normal.

For seminoma, all of the following must be true:

- The tumor has spread to organs other than the lungs.
- The level of AFP is normal. β-hCG and LDH may be at any level.

Poor Prognosis

For nonseminoma, at least one of the following must be true:

- The tumor is in the center of the chest between the lungs.
- The tumor has spread to organs other than the lungs.
- The level of any one of the tumor markers is high.

There is no poor prognosis grouping for seminoma testicular tumors.

Types of Standard Treatment
Surgery

Surgery to remove the testicle and some of the lymph nodes may be done at diagnosis and staging.

Tumors that have spread to other places in the body may be partly or entirely removed by surgery.

357

After the doctor removes all the cancer that can be seen at the time of the surgery, some patients may be given chemotherapy or radiation therapy after surgery to kill any cancer cells that are left. Treatment given after the surgery, to lower the risk that the cancer will come back, is called "adjuvant therapy."

Radiation Therapy

Radiation therapy is a cancer treatment that uses high-energy X-rays or other types of radiation to kill cancer cells or keep them from growing. There are two types of radiation therapy:

- **External radiation therapy** uses a machine outside the body to send radiation toward the cancer.

- **Internal radiation therapy** uses a radioactive substance sealed in needles, seeds, wires, or catheters that are placed directly into or near the cancer.

The way the radiation therapy is given depends on the type and stage of the cancer being treated. External radiation therapy is used to treat testicular cancer.

Chemotherapy

Chemotherapy is a cancer treatment that uses drugs to stop the growth of cancer cells, either by killing the cells or by stopping the cells from dividing. When chemotherapy is taken by mouth or injected into a vein or muscle, the drugs enter the bloodstream and can reach cancer cells throughout the body (systemic chemotherapy). When chemotherapy is placed directly into the cerebrospinal fluid; an organ; or a body cavity, such as the abdomen, the drugs mainly affect cancer cells in those areas (regional chemotherapy). The way the chemotherapy is given depends on the type and stage of the cancer being treated.

Surveillance

Surveillance is closely following a patient's condition without giving any treatment unless there are changes in test results. It is used to find early signs that the cancer has recurred. In surveillance, patients are given certain exams and tests on a regular schedule.

High-Dose Chemotherapy with Stem Cell Transplant

High doses of chemotherapy are given to kill cancer cells. Healthy cells, including blood-forming cells, are also destroyed by the cancer treatment. Stem cell transplant is a treatment to replace the blood-forming cells. Stem cells (immature blood cells) are removed from the blood or bone marrow of the patient or a donor and are frozen and stored. After the patient completes chemotherapy, the stored stem cells are thawed and given back to the patient through an infusion. These reinfused stem cells grow into (and restore) the body's blood cells.

Clinical Trials

For some patients, taking part in a clinical trial may be the best treatment choice. Clinical trials are part of the cancer research process. Clinical trials are done to find out if new cancer treatments are safe and effective or better than the standard treatment.

Many of today's standard treatments for cancer are based on earlier clinical trials. Patients who take part in a clinical trial may receive the standard treatment or be among the first to receive a new treatment.

Patients who take part in clinical trials also help improve the way cancer will be treated in the future. Even when clinical trials do not lead to effective new treatments, they often answer important questions and help move research forward.

Some clinical trials only include patients who have not yet received treatment. Other trials test treatments for patients whose cancer has not gotten better. There are also clinical trials that test new ways to stop cancer from recurring or reduce the side effects of cancer treatment.

Follow-Up Tests

Some of the tests that were done to diagnose the cancer or to find out the stage of the cancer may be repeated. Some tests will be repeated in order to see how well the treatment is working. Decisions about whether to continue, change, or stop treatment may be based on the results of these tests.

Some of the tests will continue to be done from time to time after treatment has ended. The results of these tests can show if your condition has changed or if the cancer has recurred. These tests are sometimes called "follow-up tests" or "checkups."

Men who have had testicular cancer have an increased risk of developing cancer in the other testicle. A patient is advised to regularly check the other testicle and report any unusual symptoms to a doctor right away.

Long-term clinical exams are very important. The patient will probably have checkups frequently during the first year after surgery and less often after that.

Chapter 26

Stroke

A stroke, sometimes called a "brain attack," occurs when something blocks blood supply to part of the brain or when a blood vessel in the brain bursts. In either case, parts of the brain become damaged or die. A stroke can cause lasting brain damage, long-term disability, or even death.

Understanding Stroke

To understand stroke, it helps to understand the brain. The brain controls our movements; stores our memories; and is the source of our thoughts, emotions, and language. The brain also controls many functions of the body, such as breathing and digestion.

To work properly, your brain needs oxygen. Although your brain makes up only 2 percent of your body weight, it uses 20 percent of the oxygen you breathe. Your arteries deliver oxygen-rich blood to all parts of your brain.

What Happens during a Stroke

If something happens to block the flow of blood, brain cells start to die within minutes because they cannot get oxygen. This causes a stroke.

This chapter includes text excerpted from "About Stroke," Centers for Disease Control and Prevention (CDC), May 8, 2019.

There are two types of stroke:

- An ischemic stroke occurs when blood clots or other particles block the blood vessels to the brain. Fatty deposits called "plaque" can also cause blockages by building up in the blood vessels.

- A hemorrhagic stroke occurs when a blood vessel bursts in the brain. Blood builds up and damages surrounding brain tissue.

Both types of stroke damage brain cells. Symptoms of that damage start to show in the parts of the body controlled by those brain cells.

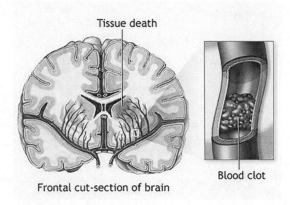

Figure 26.1. *Damaged Brain Cells*

Types of Stroke

The type of stroke you have affects your treatment and recovery. The three main types of stroke are:

Ischemic Stroke

Most strokes (87%) are ischemic strokes. An ischemic stroke happens when blood flow through the artery that supplies oxygen-rich blood to the brain becomes blocked.

Blood clots often cause the blockages that lead to ischemic strokes.

Hemorrhagic Stroke

A hemorrhagic stroke happens when an artery in the brain leaks blood or ruptures (breaks open). The leaked blood puts too much pressure on brain cells, which damages them.

High blood pressure and aneurysms—balloon-like bulges in an artery that can stretch and burst—are examples of conditions that can cause a hemorrhagic stroke.

There are two types of hemorrhagic strokes:

- **Intracerebral hemorrhage** is the most common type of hemorrhagic stroke. It occurs when an artery in the brain bursts, flooding the surrounding tissue with blood.

- **Subarachnoid hemorrhage** is a less common type of hemorrhagic stroke. It refers to bleeding in the area between the brain and the thin tissues that cover it.

Transient Ischemic Attack

A transient ischemic attack (TIA) is sometimes called a "mini-stroke." It is different from the major types of stroke because blood flow to the brain is blocked for only a short time—usually no more than five minutes.

It is important to know that:

- A TIA is a warning sign of a future stroke.

- A TIA is a medical emergency, just like a major stroke.

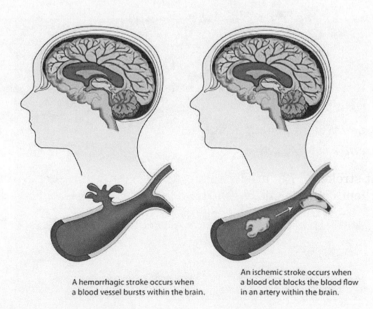

A hemorrhagic stroke occurs when a blood vessel bursts within the brain.

An ischemic stroke occurs when a blood clot blocks the blood flow in an artery within the brain.

Figure 26.2. *Stroke Types*

- Strokes and TIAs require emergency care. Call 911 right away if you feel signs of a stroke or see symptoms in someone around you.

- There is no way to know in the beginning whether symptoms are from a TIA or from a major type of stroke.

- As with ischemic strokes, blood clots often cause TIAs.

- More than a third of people who have a TIA and do not get treatment have a major stroke within 1 year. As many as 10 percent to 15 percent of people will have a major stroke within 3 months of a TIA.

Recognizing and treating TIAs can lower the risk of a major stroke. If you have a TIA, your healthcare team can find the cause and take steps to prevent a major stroke.

Signs and Symptoms of Stroke

During a stroke, every minute counts. Fast treatment can lessen the brain damage that stroke can cause.

By knowing the signs and symptoms of stroke, you can take quick action and perhaps save a life—maybe even your own.

Signs of Stroke in Men and Women

- Sudden numbness or weakness in the face, arm, or leg, especially on one side of the body

- Sudden confusion, trouble speaking, or difficulty understanding speech

- Sudden trouble seeing in one or both eyes

- Sudden trouble walking, dizziness, loss of balance, or lack of coordination

- Sudden severe headache with no known cause

Call 911 right away if you or someone else has any of these symptoms.

Acting F.A.S.T. Is Key for Stroke

Acting F.A.S.T. can help stroke patients get the treatments they desperately need. The stroke treatments that work best are available only if the stroke is recognized and diagnosed within three hours of the first symptoms. Stroke patients may not be eligible for these if they do not arrive at the hospital in time.

If you think someone may be having a stroke, act F.A.S.T. and do the following simple test:

F—Face: Ask the person to smile. Does one side of the face droop?

A—Arms: Ask the person to raise both arms. Does one arm drift downward?

S—Speech: Ask the person to repeat a simple phrase. Is the speech slurred or strange?

T—Time: If you see any of these signs, call 911 right away.

Note the time when any symptoms first appear. This information helps healthcare providers determine the best treatment for each person. Do not drive to the hospital or let someone else drive you. Call an ambulance so that medical personnel can begin lifesaving treatment on the way to the emergency room.

Treating a Transient Ischemic Attack

If your symptoms go away after a few minutes, you may have had a TIA. Although brief, a TIA is a sign of a serious condition that will not go away without medical help.

Unfortunately, because TIAs clear up, many people ignore them. But paying attention to a TIA can save your life. Tell your healthcare team about your symptoms right away.

Treatment of Stroke

Your stroke treatment begins the moment emergency medical services (EMS) arrives to take you to the hospital. Once at the hospital, you may receive emergency care, treatment to prevent another stroke, rehabilitation to treat the side effects of stroke, or all three.

On the Way to the Hospital

If someone you know shows signs of stroke, call 911 right away.

Do not drive to the hospital or let someone else drive you. The key to stroke treatment and recovery is getting to the hospital quickly. Yet, one in three stroke patients never calls 911. Calling an ambulance means that medical staff can begin lifesaving treatment on the way to the emergency room.

Stroke patients who are taken to the hospital in an ambulance may get diagnosed and treated more quickly than people who do not arrive in an ambulance. This is because emergency treatment starts on the way to the hospital. The emergency workers may take you to a specialized stroke center to ensure that you receive the quickest possible diagnosis and treatment. The emergency workers will also collect valuable information that guides treatment, and they will alert hospital medical staff before you arrive at the emergency room, giving them time to prepare.

What Happens at the Hospital

At the hospital, health professionals will ask about your medical history and about the time your symptoms started. Brain scans will show what type of stroke you had. You may also work with a neurologist who treats brain disorders, a neurosurgeon that performs surgery on the brain, or a specialist in another area of medicine.

If you get to the hospital within three hours of the first symptoms of an ischemic stroke, you may get a type of medicine called a "thrombolytic" (a "clot-busting" drug) to break up blood clots. Tissue plasminogen activator (tPA) is a thrombolytic.

tPA improves the chances of recovering from a stroke. Studies show that patients with ischemic strokes who receive tPA are more likely to recover fully or have less disability than patients who do not receive the drug. Patients treated with tPA are also less likely to need long-term care in a nursing home. Unfortunately, many stroke victims do not get to the hospital in time for tPA treatment. This is why it is so important to recognize the signs and symptoms of stroke right away and call 911.

Medicine, surgery, or other procedures may be needed to stop the bleeding and save brain tissue. For example:

Endovascular procedures. Endovascular procedures may be used to treat certain hemorrhagic strokes. The doctor inserts a long tube through a major artery in the leg or arm and then guides the tube to the site of the weak spot or break in a blood vessel. The tube is then used to install a device, such as a coil, to repair the damage or prevent bleeding.

Surgical treatment. Hemorrhagic strokes may be treated with surgery. If the bleeding is caused by a ruptured aneurysm, a metal clip may be put in place to stop the blood loss.

What Happens Next

If you have had a stroke, you are at high risk for another stroke:

- One of four stroke survivors has another stroke within five years.

- The risk of stroke within 90 days of a TIA may be as high as 17 percent, with the greatest risk during the first week.

That is why it is important to treat the underlying causes of stroke, including heart disease, high blood pressure, atrial fibrillation (fast, irregular heartbeat), high cholesterol, and diabetes. Your doctor may give you medications or tell you to change your diet, exercise, or adopt other healthy lifestyle habits. Surgery may also be helpful in some cases.

Stroke Rehabilitation

After a stroke, you may need rehabilitation (rehab) to help you recover. Before you are discharged from the hospital, social workers can help you find care services and caregiver support to continue your long-term recovery. It is important to work with your healthcare team to find out the reasons for your stroke and take steps to prevent another stroke.

Recovering from Stroke

Recovery time after a stroke is different for everyone—it can take weeks, months, or even years. Some people recover fully, but others have long-term or lifelong disabilities.

What to Expect after a Stroke

If you have had a stroke, you can make great progress in regaining your independence. However, some problems may continue:

- Paralysis (inability to move some parts of the body), weakness, or both on one side of the body

- Trouble with thinking, awareness, attention, learning, judgment, and memory

- Problems understanding or forming speech

- Trouble controlling or expressing emotions

- Numbness or strange sensations
- Pain in the hands and feet that worsens with movement and temperature changes
- Trouble with chewing and swallowing
- Problems with bladder and bowel control
- Depression

Stroke Rehabilitation

Rehab can include working with speech, physical, and occupational therapists.

- **Speech therapy** helps people who have problems producing or understanding speech.
- **Physical therapy** uses exercises to help you relearn movement and coordination skills you may have lost because of the stroke.
- **Occupational therapy** focuses on improving daily activities, such as eating, drinking, dressing, bathing, reading, and writing.

Therapy and medicine may help with depression or other mental-health conditions following a stroke. Joining a patient support group may help you adjust to life after a stroke. Talk with your healthcare team about local support groups, or check with an area medical center.

Support from family and friends can also help relieve fear and anxiety following a stroke. Let your loved ones know how you feel and what they can do to help you.

Preventing Another Stroke

If you have had a stroke, you are at high risk for another stroke:

- One in four strokes each year are recurrent.
- The chance of stroke within 90 days of a TIA may be as high as 17 percent, with the greatest risk during the first week.

That is why it is important to treat the causes of stroke, including heart disease, high blood pressure, atrial fibrillation, high cholesterol, and diabetes. Your doctor may prescribe you medicine or tell you to change your diet, exercise, or adopt other healthy lifestyle habits. Surgery may also be helpful in some cases.

Chapter 27

Suicide

What Is Suicide?

Suicide is death caused by injuring oneself with the intent to die. A suicide attempt is when someone harms themselves with the intent to end their life, but they do not die as a result of their actions.

Suicide is associated with several risk and protective factors, is connected to other forms of injury and violence, and causes serious health and economic consequences. For example, suicide risk is higher among people who have experienced violence, including child abuse, bullying, or sexual violence. Other characteristics associated with suicide include a history of suicide attempts and a lack of problem-solving skills. Protective factors, such as connectedness and easy access to healthcare, buffer individuals from suicidal thoughts and behavior.

By using a public health approach that addresses risk and protective factors for multiple types of violence, suicide and other forms of violence can be prevented.

How Big Is the Problem?

Suicide is a large and growing public-health problem. Suicide is the tenth leading cause of death in the United States. It was responsible for nearly 45,000 deaths in 2016, with approximately 1 death every 12 minutes. Many more people think about or attempt suicide

This chapter includes text excerpted from "Preventing Suicide," Centers for Disease Control and Prevention (CDC), September 29, 2018.

and survive. In 2016, 9.8 million American adults seriously thought about suicide, 2.8 million made a plan, and 1.3 million attempted suicide.

Suicide affects all ages. Suicide is a problem throughout the lifespan. It is the second leading cause of death for people between 10 and 34 years of age, the fourth leading cause among people between 35 and 54 years of age, and the eighth leading cause among people between 55 and 64 years of age.

Some groups have higher rates of suicide than others. Suicide rates vary by race/ethnicity, age, and other population characteristics, with the highest rates across the life span occurring among non-Hispanic American Indian/Alaska Native and non-Hispanic White populations. Other Americans disproportionately impacted by suicide include Veterans and other military personnel and workers in certain occupational groups. Sexual minority youth bear a large burden as well, and they experience increased suicidal ideation and behavior compared to their nonsexual minority peers.

What Are the Consequences?

Suicide, by definition, is fatal. Suicide also affects the health of others and the community. When people die by suicide, their family and friends often experience shock, anger, guilt, and depression. The economic toll of suicide on society is immense as well. Suicides and suicide attempts cost the nation approximately $70 billion per year in lifetime medical and work-loss costs alone.

People who attempt suicide and survive may experience serious injuries, such as broken bones or organ failure. These injuries can have long-term effects on their health. People who survive suicide attempts can also have depression and other mental-health problems.

In addition to the number of people who are injured or die, many other people are impacted by knowing someone who dies or by personally experiencing suicidal thoughts. Additionally, being a survivor or someone with lived experience increases one's risk of suicide.

How Can We Prevent Suicide?

The Centers for Disease Control and Prevention (CDC) has developed a technical package, Preventing Suicide: A Technical Package of Policy, Programs, and Practices. The technical package can be used to inform a comprehensive, multi-level, and multi-sectoral approach within communities and states. It includes strategies to prevent suicide in the first place, by decreasing suicide risk factors and increasing protective factors. Strategies range from a focus on the whole population, regardless of risk, to strategies designed to support people at the highest risk. Importantly, this technical package extends typical prevention strategies to approaches that go beyond individual behavior change to better address factors impacting communities and populations more broadly.

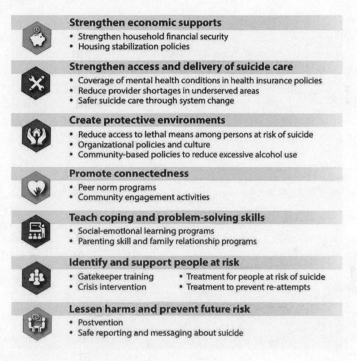

Figure 27.1. *Suicide Prevention Tips*

Part Three

Sexual and Reproductive Concerns

Chapter 28

Kidney and Urological Disorders

Chapter Contents

Section 28.1—Kidney Stones 376

Section 28.2—Urinary Incontinence in Men 388

Section 28.1

Kidney Stones

This section includes text excerpted from "Kidney Stones,"
National Institute of Diabetes and Digestive and
Kidney Diseases (NIDDK), September 2016.

What Are Kidney Stones?

Kidney stones are hard, pebble-like pieces of material that form in one or both of your kidneys when high levels of certain minerals are in your urine. Kidney stones rarely cause permanent damage if treated by a healthcare professional.

Kidney stones vary in size and shape. They may be as small as a grain of sand or as large as a pea. Rarely, some kidney stones are as big as golf balls. Kidney stones may be smooth or jagged and are usually yellow or brown.

A small kidney stone may pass through your urinary tract on its own, causing little or no pain. A larger kidney stone may get stuck along the way. A kidney stone that gets stuck can block your flow of urine, causing severe pain or bleeding.

If you have symptoms of kidney stones, including severe pain or bleeding, seek care right away. A doctor, such as a urologist, can treat any pain and prevent further problems, such as a urinary tract infection (UTI).

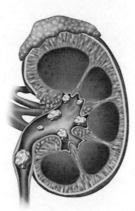

Figure 28.1. *Kidney Stone*

A small kidney stone may pass through your urinary tract on its own, causing little or no pain. A larger kidney stone may get stuck along the way.

How Common Are Kidney Stones?

Kidney stones are common and are on the rise. About 11 percent of men and 6 percent of women in the United States have kidney stones at least once during their lifetime.

Who Is More Likely to Develop Kidney Stones?

Men are more likely to develop kidney stones than women. If you have a family history of kidney stones, you are more likely to develop them. You are also more likely to develop kidney stones again if you have had them once.

You may also be more likely to develop a kidney stone if you do not drink enough liquids.

People with Certain Conditions

You are more likely to develop kidney stones if you have certain conditions, including:

- A blockage of the urinary tract

- Chronic, or long-lasting, inflammation of the bowel

- Cystic kidney diseases, which are disorders that cause fluid-filled sacs to form on the kidneys

- Cystinuria

- Digestive problems or a history of gastrointestinal (GI) tract surgery

- Gout, a disorder that causes painful swelling of the joints

- Hypercalciuria, a condition that runs in families in which urine contains unusually large amounts of calcium; this is the most common condition found in people who form calcium stones.

- Hyperoxaluria, a condition in which urine contains unusually large amounts of oxalate

- Hyperparathyroidism, a condition in which the parathyroid glands release too much parathyroid hormone (PTH), causing extra calcium in the blood

- Hyperuricosuria, a disorder in which too much uric acid is in the urine

377

- Obesity

- Repeated, or recurrent, UTIs

- Renal tubular acidosis (RTA), a disease that occurs when the kidneys fail to remove acids into the urine, which causes a person's blood to remain too acidic

People Who Take Certain Medicines

You are more likely to develop kidney stones if you are taking one or more of the following medicines over a long period of time:

- Diuretics, often called "water pills," which help rid your body of water

- Calcium-based antacids

- Indinavir, a protease inhibitor (PI) used to treat human immunodeficiency virus (HIV) infection

- Topiramate, an anti-seizure medication

What Are the Complications of Kidney Stones?

Complications of kidney stones are rare if you seek treatment from a healthcare professional before problems occur.
If kidney stones are not treated, they can cause:

- Hematuria, or blood in the urine

- Severe pain

- UTIs, including kidney infections

- Loss of kidney function

What Are the Symptoms of Kidney Stones?

Symptoms of kidney stones include:

- Sharp pains in your back, side, lower abdomen, or groin

- Hematuria

- A constant need to urinate

- Pain while urinating

- Inability to urinate or can only urinate a small amount

- Cloudy or bad-smelling urine

See a healthcare professional right away if you have any of these symptoms. These symptoms may mean you have a kidney stone or a more serious condition.

Your pain may last for a short or long time, or it may come and go in waves. Along with pain, you may have:

- Nausea

- Vomiting

Other symptoms include:

- Fever

- Chills

What Causes Kidney Stones

Kidney stones are caused by high levels of calcium, oxalate, and phosphorus in the urine. These minerals are normally found in urine and do not cause problems at low levels.

Certain foods may increase the chances of having a kidney stone in people who are more likely to develop them.

How Do Healthcare Professionals Diagnose Kidney Stones?

Healthcare professionals use your medical history, a physical exam, and lab and imaging tests to diagnose kidney stones.

A healthcare professional will ask if you have a history of health conditions that make you more likely to develop kidney stones. The healthcare professional also may ask if you have a family history of kidney stones and about what you typically eat. During a physical exam, the healthcare professional usually examines your body. The healthcare professional will ask you about your symptoms.

What Tests Do Healthcare Professionals Use to Diagnose Kidney Stones?

Healthcare professionals may use lab or imaging tests to diagnose kidney stones.

Lab Tests

Urine tests can show whether your urine contains high levels of minerals that form kidney stones. Urine and blood tests can also help a healthcare professional find out what type of kidney stones you have.

Urinalysis. Urinalysis involves a healthcare professional testing your urine sample. You will collect a urine sample at a doctor's office or at a lab, and a healthcare professional will test the sample. Urinalysis can show whether your urine has blood in it and minerals that can form kidney stones. White blood cells (WBCs) and bacteria in the urine mean you may have a UTI.

Blood tests. A healthcare professional may take a blood sample from you and send the sample to a lab to test. The blood test can show if you have high levels of certain minerals in your blood that can lead to kidney stones.

Imaging Tests

Healthcare professionals use imaging tests to find kidney stones. The tests may also show problems that caused a kidney stone to form, such as a blockage in the urinary tract or a birth defect. You do not need anesthesia for these imaging tests.

Abdominal X-ray. An abdominal X-ray is a picture of the abdomen that uses low levels of radiation and is recorded on film or on a computer. An X-ray technician takes an abdominal X-ray at a hospital or outpatient center, and a radiologist reads the images. During an abdominal X-ray, you will lie on a table or stand up. The X-ray technician will position the X-ray machine over or in front of your abdomen and ask you to hold your breath so the picture will not be blurry. The X-ray technician then may ask you to change position for additional pictures. Abdominal X-rays can show the location of kidney stones in the urinary tract. Not all stones are visible on abdominal X-ray.

Computed tomography (CT) scans. CT scans use a combination of X-rays and computer technology to create images of your urinary tract. Although a CT scan without contrast medium is most commonly used to view your urinary tract, a healthcare professional may give you an injection of contrast medium. Contrast medium is a dye or other substance that makes structures inside your body easier to see during imaging tests. You will lie on a table that slides into a tunnel-shaped device that takes the X-rays. CT scans can show the size and location of a kidney stone, if the stone is blocking the urinary tract, and conditions that may have caused the kidney stone to form.

How Do Healthcare Professionals Treat Kidney Stones?

Healthcare professionals usually treat kidney stones based on their size, location, and what type they are.

Small kidney stones may pass through your urinary tract without treatment. If you are able to pass a kidney stone, a healthcare professional may ask you to catch the kidney stone in a special container. A healthcare professional will send the kidney stone to a lab to find out what type it is. A healthcare professional may advise you to drink plenty of liquids if you are able to help move a kidney stone along. The healthcare professional also may prescribe pain medicine.

Larger kidney stones or kidney stones that block your urinary tract or cause great pain may need urgent treatment. If you are vomiting and dehydrated, you may need to go to the hospital and get fluids through an IV.

Kidney Stone Removal

A urologist can remove the kidney stone or break it into small pieces with the following treatments:

Shock wave lithotripsy. The doctor can use shock wave lithotripsy to blast the kidney stone into small pieces. The smaller pieces of the kidney stone then pass through your urinary tract. A doctor can give you anesthesia during this outpatient procedure.

Cystoscopy and ureteroscopy. During cystoscopy, the doctor uses a cystoscope to look inside the urethra and bladder to find a stone in your urethra or bladder. During ureteroscopy, the doctor uses a ureteroscope, which is longer and thinner than a cystoscope, to see detailed images of the lining of the ureters and kidneys. The doctor inserts the cystoscope or ureteroscope through the urethra to see the rest of the urinary tract. Once the stone is found, the doctor can remove it or break it into smaller pieces. The doctor performs these procedures in the hospital with anesthesia. You can typically go home the same day.

Percutaneous nephrolithotomy (PNL). The doctor uses a thin viewing tool, called a "nephroscope," to locate and remove the kidney stone. The doctor inserts the tool directly into your kidney through a small cut made in your back. For larger kidney stones, the doctor also may use a laser to break the kidney stones into smaller pieces. The doctor performs percutaneous nephrolithotomy in a hospital with anesthesia. You may have to stay in the hospital for several days after the procedure.

After these procedures, sometimes the urologist may leave a thin flexible tube, called a "ureteral stent," in your urinary tract to help urine flow or a stone to pass. Once the kidney stone is removed, your doctor sends the kidney stone or its pieces to a lab to find out what type it is.

The healthcare professional also may ask you to collect your urine for 24 hours after the kidney stone has passed or been removed. The healthcare professional can then measure how much urine you produce in a day, along with mineral levels in your urine. You are more likely to form stones if you do not make enough urine each day or have a problem with high mineral levels.

How Can I Prevent Kidney Stones?

To help prevent future kidney stones, you also need to know what caused your previous kidney stones. Once you know what type of kidney stone you had, a healthcare professional can help you make changes to your eating, diet, and nutrition to prevent future kidney stones.

Drinking Liquids

In most cases, drinking enough liquids each day is the best way to help prevent most types of kidney stones. Drinking enough liquids keeps your urine diluted and helps flush away minerals that might form stones.

Though water is best, other liquids, such as citrus drinks, may also help prevent kidney stones. Some studies show that citrus drinks, such as lemonade and orange juice, protect against kidney stones because they contain citrate, which stops crystals from turning into stones.

Unless you have kidney failure, you should drink six to eight 8-ounce glasses a day. If you previously had cystine stones, you may need to drink even more. Talk with a healthcare professional if you cannot drink the recommended amount due to other health problems, such as urinary incontinence, urinary frequency, or kidney failure.

The amount of liquid you need to drink depends on the weather and your activity level. If you live, work, or exercise in hot weather, you may need more liquid to replace the fluid you lose through sweat. A healthcare professional may ask you to collect your urine for 24 hours to determine the amount of urine you produce a day. If the amount of urine is too low, the healthcare professional may advise you to increase your liquid intake.

Medicines

If you have had a kidney stone, a healthcare professional also may prescribe medicines to prevent future kidney stones. Depending on the type of kidney stone you had and what type of medicine the healthcare professional prescribes, you may have to take the medicine for a few weeks, several months, or longer.

For example, if you had struvite stones, you may have to take an oral antibiotic for one to six weeks, or possibly longer.

If you had another type of stone, you may have to take a potassium citrate tablet one to three times daily. You may have to take potassium citrate for months or even longer until a healthcare professional says you are no longer at risk for kidney stones.

Table 28.1. Types of Stones and Prescribed Medicines

Type of Kidney Stone	Possible Medicines Prescribed by Your Doctor
Calcium Stones	• Potassium citrate, which is used to raise the citrate and pH levels in urine • Diuretics, often called water pills, help rid your body of water
Uric Acid Stones	• Allopurinol, which is used to treat high levels of uric acid in the body • Potassium citrate
Struvite Stones	• Antibiotics, which are bacteria-fighting medications • Acetohydroxamic acid, a strong antibiotic, used with another long-term antibiotic medication to prevent infection
Cystine Stones	• Mercaptopropionyl glycine, an antioxidant used for heart problems • Potassium citrate

Talk with a healthcare professional about your health history prior to taking kidney stone medicines. Some kidney stone medicines have minor to serious side effects. Side effects are more likely to occur the longer you take the medicine and the higher the dose. Tell the healthcare professional about any side effects that occur when you take kidney stone medicine.

Hyperparathyroidism Surgery

People with hyperparathyroidism, a condition that results in too much calcium in the blood, sometimes develop calcium stones. Treatment for hyperparathyroidism may include surgery to remove the abnormal parathyroid gland. Removing the parathyroid gland cures hyperparathyroidism and can prevent kidney stones. Surgery sometimes causes complications, including infection.

Eating, Diet, and Nutrition

Can I Help Prevent Kidney Stones by Changing What I Eat or Drink?

Drinking enough liquid, mainly water, is the most important thing you can do to prevent kidney stones. Unless you have kidney failure, many healthcare professionals recommend that you drink six to eight, 8-ounce glasses a day. Talk with a healthcare professional about how much liquid you should drink.

Studies have shown that the Dietary Approaches to Stop Hypertension (DASH) diet can reduce the risk of kidney stones.

Studies have shown that being overweight increases your risk of kidney stones. A dietitian can help you plan meals to help you lose weight.

Does the Type of Kidney Stone I Had Affect Food Choices I Should Make?

Yes. If you have already had kidney stones, ask your healthcare professional which type of kidney stone you had. Based on the type of kidney stone you had, you may be able to prevent kidney stones by making changes in how much sodium, animal protein, calcium, or oxalate is in the food you eat.

You may need to change what you eat and drink for these types of kidney stones:

- Calcium oxalate stones

- Calcium phosphate stones

- Uric acid stones

- Cystine stones

A dietitian who specializes in kidney stone prevention can help you plan meals to prevent kidney stones. Find a dietitian who can help you.

Calcium Oxalate Stones

Reduce oxalate. If you have had calcium oxalate stones, you may want to avoid these foods to help reduce the amount of oxalate in your urine:

- Nuts and nut products

- Peanuts—which are legumes, not nuts, and are high in oxalate

- Rhubarb

- Spinach

- Wheat bran

Talk with a healthcare professional about other food sources of oxalate and how much oxalate should be in what you eat.

Reduce sodium. Your chance of developing kidney stones increases when you eat more sodium. Sodium is a part of salt. Sodium is in many canned, packaged, and fast foods. It is also in many condiments, seasonings, and meats.

Talk with a healthcare professional about how much sodium should be in what you eat.

Limit animal protein. Eating animal protein may increase your chances of developing kidney stones.

A healthcare professional may tell you to limit eating animal protein, including:

- Beef, chicken, and pork, especially organ meats

- Eggs

- Fish and shellfish

- Milk, cheese, and other dairy products

Although you may need to limit how much animal protein you eat each day, you still need to make sure you get enough protein. Consider replacing some of the meat and animal protein you would typically eat with beans, dried peas, and lentils, which are plant-based foods that are high in protein and low in oxalate.

Talk with a healthcare professional about how much total protein you should eat and how much should come from animal or plant-based foods.

Get enough calcium from foods. Even though calcium sounds like it would be the cause of calcium stones, it is not. In the right amounts, calcium can block other substances in the digestive tract that may cause stones. Talk with a healthcare professional about how much calcium you should eat to help prevent getting more calcium oxalate stones and to support strong bones. It may be best to get calcium from low-oxalate, plant-based foods, such as calcium-fortified juices, cereals, bread, some kinds of vegetables, and some types of beans. Ask a dietitian or other healthcare professional which foods are the best sources of calcium for you.

Calcium Phosphate Stones

Reduce sodium. Your chance of developing kidney stones increases when you eat more sodium. Sodium is a part of salt. Sodium is in many canned, packaged, and fast foods. It is also in many condiments, seasonings, and meats.

Talk with a healthcare professional about how much sodium should be in what you eat.

Limit animal protein. Eating animal protein may increase your chances of developing kidney stones.

A healthcare professional may tell you to limit eating animal protein, including:

- Beef, chicken, and pork, especially organ meats
- Eggs
- Fish and shellfish
- Milk, cheese, and other dairy products

Although you may need to limit how much animal protein you have each day, you still need to make sure you get enough protein. Consider replacing some of the meat and animal protein you would typically eat with some of these plant-based foods that are high in protein:

- Legumes, such as beans, dried peas, lentils, and peanuts
- Soy foods, such as soy milk, soy nut butter, and tofu
- Nuts and nut products, such as almonds and almond butter, cashews and cashew butter, walnuts, and pistachios
- Sunflower seeds

Talk with a healthcare professional about how much total protein you should eat and how much should come from animal or plant-based foods.

Get enough calcium from foods. Even though calcium sounds like it would be the cause of calcium stones, it is not. In the right amounts, calcium can block other substances in the digestive tract that may lead to stones. Talk with a healthcare professional about how much calcium you should eat to help prevent getting more calcium phosphate stones and to support strong bones. It may be best to get calcium from plant-based foods, such as calcium-fortified juices, cereals, bread, some kinds of vegetables, and some types of beans. Ask a dietitian or other healthcare professional which foods are the best sources of calcium for you.

Uric Acid Stones

Limit animal protein. Eating animal protein may increase your chances of developing kidney stones.

A healthcare professional may tell you to limit eating animal protein, including:

- Beef, chicken, and pork, especially organ meats

- Eggs

- Fish and shellfish

- Milk, cheese, and other dairy products

Although you may need to limit how much animal protein you have each day, you still need to make sure you get enough protein. Consider replacing some of the meat and animal protein you would typically eat with some of these plant-based foods that are high in protein:

- Legumes, such as beans, dried peas, lentils, and peanuts

- Soy foods, such as soy milk, soy nut butter, and tofu

- Nuts and nut products, such as almonds and almond butter, cashews and cashew butter, walnuts, and pistachios

- Sunflower seeds

Talk with a healthcare professional about how much total protein you should eat and how much should come from animal or plant-based foods.

Losing weight if you are overweight is especially important for people who have had uric acid stones.

Cystine Stones

Drinking enough liquid, mainly water, is the most important lifestyle change you can make to prevent cystine stones. Talk with a healthcare professional about how much liquid you should drink.

Section 28.2

Urinary Incontinence in Men

This section includes text excerpted from "Urinary Incontinence in Older Adults," National Institute on Aging (NIA), National Institutes of Health (NIH), May 16, 2017.

Urinary incontinence means a person leaks urine by accident. While it may happen to anyone, urinary incontinence is more common in older people. Incontinence can often be cured or controlled. Talk to your healthcare provider about what you can do.

What happens in the body to cause bladder control problems? The body stores urine in the bladder. During urination, muscles in the bladder tighten to move urine into a tube called the "urethra." At the same time, the muscles around the urethra relax and let the urine pass out of the body. When the muscles in and around the bladder do not work the way they should, urine can leak. Incontinence typically occurs if the muscles relax without warning.

Causes of Urinary Incontinence

Incontinence can happen for many reasons. For example, urinary tract infections (UTIs) or constipation. Some medicines can cause bladder control problems that last a short time. When incontinence lasts longer, it may be due to:

- Weak bladder muscles
- Overactive bladder muscles

- Weak pelvic floor muscles

- Damage to nerves that control the bladder from diseases, such as multiple sclerosis (MS), diabetes, or Parkinson disease (PD)

- Blockage from an enlarged prostate in men

- Diseases, such as arthritis that may make it difficult to get to the bathroom in time

- Pelvic organ prolapse, which is when pelvic organs (such as the bladder, or rectum) shift out of their normal place into the vagina. When pelvic organs are out of place, the bladder and urethra are not able to work normally, which may cause urine to leak.

Most incontinence in men is related to the prostate gland. Male incontinence may be caused by:

- Prostatitis—a painful inflammation of the prostate gland

- Injury, or damage to nerves or muscles from surgery

- An enlarged prostate gland, which can lead to Benign prostate hyperplasia (BPH), a condition where the prostate grows as men age

Diagnosis of Urinary Incontinence

The first step in treating incontinence is to see a doctor. She or he will give you a physical exam and take your medical history. The doctor will ask about your symptoms and the medicines you use. She or he will want to know if you have been sick recently or had surgery. Your doctor also may do a number of tests. These might include:

- Urine and blood tests

- Tests that measure how well you empty your bladder

In addition, your doctor may ask you to keep a daily diary of when you urinate and when you leak urine. Your family doctor may also send you to a urologist, a doctor who specializes in urinary tract problems.

Types of Urinary Incontinence

There are different types of incontinence:

- **Stress incontinence** occurs when urine leaks as pressure is put on the bladder, for example, during exercise, coughing, sneezing, laughing, or lifting heavy objects.

- **Urge incontinence** happens when people have a sudden need to urinate and cannot hold their urine long enough to get to the toilet. It may be a problem for people who have diabetes, Alzheimer disease (AD), Parkinson disease, multiple sclerosis, or stroke.

- **Overflow incontinence** happens when small amounts of urine leak from a bladder that is always full. A man can have trouble emptying his bladder if an enlarged prostate is blocking the urethra. Diabetes and spinal cord injuries (SCIs) can also cause this type of incontinence.

- **Functional incontinence** occurs in many older people who have normal bladder control. They just have a problem getting to the toilet because of arthritis or other disorders that make it hard to move quickly.

Treatment for Urinary Incontinence

Nowadays, there are more treatments for urinary incontinence than ever before. The choice of treatment depends on the type of bladder control problem you have, how serious it is, and what best fits your lifestyle. As a general rule, the simplest and safest treatments should be tried first.

Bladder control training may help you get better control of your bladder. Your doctor may suggest you try the following:

- **Pelvic muscle exercises** (also known as "Kegel exercises") work the muscles that you use to stop urinating. Making these muscles stronger helps you hold urine in your bladder longer.

- **Biofeedback** uses sensors to make you aware of signals from your body. This may help you regain control over the muscles in your bladder and urethra. Biofeedback can be helpful when learning pelvic muscle exercises.

- **Timed voiding** may help you control your bladder. In timed voiding, you urinate on a set schedule, for example, every hour. You can slowly extend the time between bathroom trips. When timed voiding is combined with biofeedback and pelvic muscle exercises, you may find it easier to control urge and overflow incontinence.

- **Lifestyle changes** may help with incontinence. Losing weight, quitting smoking, saying "no" to alcohol, drinking less caffeine (found in coffee, tea, and many sodas), preventing constipation, and avoiding lifting heavy objects may help with incontinence.

Choosing water instead of other drinks and limiting drinks before bedtime may also help.

Incontinence and Alzheimer Disease

People in the later stages of Alzheimer disease often have problems with urinary incontinence. This can be a result of not realizing they need to urinate, forgetting to go to the bathroom, or not being able to find the toilet. To minimize the chance of accidents, the caregiver can:

- Avoid giving drinks, such as caffeinated coffee, tea, and sodas, which may increase urination. But do not limit water.

- Keep pathways clear and the bathroom clutter-free, with a light on at all times.

- Make sure you provide regular bathroom breaks.

- Supply underwear that is easy to get on and off.

- Use absorbent underclothes for trips away from home.

Managing Urinary Incontinence

Besides bladder control training, you may want to talk with your doctor about other ways to help manage incontinence:

- Medicines can help the bladder empty more fully during urination. Other drugs tighten muscles and can lessen leakage.

- A doctor may inject a substance that thickens the area around the urethra to help close the bladder opening. This treatment may need to be repeated.

- Nerve stimulation, which sends mild electric current to the nerves around the bladder that help control urination, may be another option.

- Surgery can sometimes improve or cure incontinence if it is caused by a change in the position of the bladder or blockage due to an enlarged prostate.

- Even after treatment, some people still leak urine from time to time. There are bladder control products and other solutions, including adult diapers, furniture pads, urine deodorizing pills, and special skin cleansers, that may make leaking urine bother you a little less.

Chapter 29

Penile Concerns

Chapter Contents

Section 29.1—Circumcision.. 394

Section 29.2—Balanitis 395

Section 29.3—Penile Intraepithelial Neoplasia 398

Section 29.4—Penile Trauma.. 400

Section 29.5—Peyronie Disease 402

Section 29.6—Phimosis and Paraphimosis 409

Section 29.1

Circumcision

This section includes text excerpted from "Circumcision,"
MedlinePlus, National Institutes of Health (NIH), March 22, 2016.

What Is Circumcision?

Circumcision is a surgical procedure to remove the foreskin, the skin that covers the tip of the penis. In the United States, it is often done before a new baby leaves the hospital. According to the American Academy of Pediatrics (AAP), there are medical benefits and risks to circumcision.

What Are the Medical Benefits of Circumcision?

The possible medical benefits of circumcision include:

- A lower risk of human immunodeficiency virus (HIV)
- A slightly lower risk of other sexually transmitted diseases (STDs)
- A slightly lower risk of urinary tract infections (UTIs) and penile cancer. However, these are both rare in all males.

What Are the Risks of Circumcision?

The risks of circumcision include:

- A low risk of bleeding or infection
- Pain. The AAP suggests that providers use pain medicines to reduce pain from circumcision.

What Are the American Academy of Pediatrics Recommendations on Circumcision?

The AAP does not recommend routine circumcision. However, they said that because of the possible benefits, parents should have the option to circumcise their sons if they want to. They recommend that parents discuss circumcision with their baby's healthcare provider. Parents should make their decision based on the benefits and risks, as well as their own religious, cultural, and personal preferences.

Section 29.2

Balanitis

Balanitis is a condition in which the head of the penis (glans) becomes inflamed. Although it rarely occurs among circumcised adult males, it affects approximately 3.3 percent of uncircumcised males at some point in their lives, as well as 4 percent of all boys under the age of 4. A related condition, posthitis, involves inflammation of the foreskin that covers the head of the penis in uncircumcised males. When both the glans and foreskin are affected, the condition is known as "balanoposthitis."

Symptoms of Balanitis

The primary symptoms of balanitis include:

- Swelling, redness, and tenderness of the glans
- Skin irritation or rash on the end of the penis
- Itching and discomfort
- Thick, lumpy discharge under the foreskin
- Unpleasant smell
- Painful urination
- Difficulty retracting the foreskin (phimosis)

Causes and Risk Factors of Balanitis

Balanitis has many possible causes, ranging from skin conditions and allergic reactions that affect the penis to sexually transmitted infections (STIs) and poor hygiene. Men with phimosis are particularly susceptible to balanitis. Diabetes also increases the risk of developing balanitis because glucose in the urine can remain on the penis, creating a favorable environment for bacteria to grow. Some of the main causes of balanitis include the following:

- Skin conditions, such as eczema, psoriasis, or lichen planus
- Dermatitis (inflammation of the skin) due to contact with an irritant or allergen, such as latex condoms, lubricants,

spermicides, medicated ointments, detergents, fabric softeners, or perfumed bath products

- Irritation or minor trauma to the skin of the penis from friction, sexual intercourse, excessive washing with harsh soap, or vigorous drying with an abrasive towel

- Candida (also known as "yeast infection" or "thrush")

- Sexually transmitted infections, such as genital herpes, chlamydia, or syphilis

- Bacterial infection from poor hygiene practices, such as infrequent washing of the glans or failure to dry the tissue beneath the foreskin after washing

Diagnosis and Treatment of Balanitis

To make a diagnosis of balanitis, a doctor merely needs to observe inflammation of the glans. In order to treat the condition effectively, however, the doctor must also determine the underlying cause. This process may involve examining the skin for evidence of eczema, psoriasis, or other skin conditions that may affect the penis. The doctor may also advise the patient to avoid potential skin irritants or allergens, such as lubricants or perfumed bath products, to see whether the balanitis resolves itself. Finally, the doctor may order diagnostic tests—such as blood tests, urine tests, or a swab of the glans—to see whether the patient has diabetes, a yeast infection, or an STI.

If the balanitis appears to be related to a skin condition, the patient will likely be referred to a dermatologist for treatment. For balanitis caused by an allergic reaction, the patient may be prescribed a mild topical steroid cream, such as 1% hydrocortisone, to help relieve the swelling and other symptoms. If the cause is candida, the recommended treatment will include an antifungal cream—such as clotrimazole or miconazole—for both the patient and his sex partner. For balanitis caused by a bacterial infection, the patient will likely be prescribed an oral antibiotic, such as penicillin or erythromycin. If no infection or irritant can be identified, treatment may include astringent compresses with diluted vinegar or potassium permanganate. In rare cases, if the patient has phimosis and the balanitis recurs frequently, the doctor may recommend circumcision.

Prevention of Balanitis

Left untreated, chronic balanitis can lead to health complications, including:

- Phimosis (may require surgery to correct)

- Balanitis xerotica obliterans (chronic dermatitis affecting the glans and foreskin)

- Scarring and narrowing of the opening of the penis

- Reduction in blood supply to the tip of the penis

- Increased risk of penile cancer

Good hygiene is key to preventing the occurrence or recurrence of balanitis. Doctors recommend washing the penis daily with warm water, making sure to pull back the foreskin to expose the glans. Although regular soap may cause irritation, an aqueous cream or other nonsoap cleanser may be used as long as it is completely rinsed off. It is important to dry the head of the penis thoroughly before replacing the foreskin because moisture promotes the growth of bacteria. Men who tend to develop balanitis following sexual intercourse should wash the penis after sex. Finally, men who are prone to balanitis should avoid contact with potential irritants, such as lubricants, detergents, or other chemicals.

References

1. Ngan, Vanessa. "Balanitis," DermNet NZ, 2016.

2. Nordqvist, Christian. "Balanitis: Causes, Symptoms, and Treatments," Medical News Today, September 28, 2015.

3. Sobol, Jennifer. "Balanitis," MedlinePlus, August 31, 2015.

Section 29.3

Penile Intraepithelial Neoplasia

Penile intraepithelial neoplasia (PEIN) is a precancerous condition in which abnormal cell growth occurs in the outer layer of skin on the penis. Intraepithelial refers to the layer of cells that forms the surface or lining of an organ, while neoplasia refers to cystic lesions or tumors. Penile intraepithelial neoplasia is also known as "erythroplasia of Queyrat," "Bowen disease of the penis," "squamous intraepithelial lesion," or "squamous cell carcinoma in-situ of the penis." Although PEIN is not a form of cancer, up to 30 percent of cases may develop into penile cancer (invasive squamous cell carcinoma of the penis) if left untreated.

Risk Factors of Penile Intraepithelial Neoplasia

Penile cancer is rare in the United States, with only about 2,000 new cases diagnosed each year. Some studies suggest that human papillomavirus (HPV) infection in the genital area, which also causes genital warts, is a significant risk factor in the development of penile intraepithelial cancer. As a result, many developed nations have instituted immunization programs aimed at vaccinating both boys and girls against HPV.

Studies have also shown that PEIN is most likely to affect uncircumcised males over the age of 50. Other risk factors include chronic skin diseases, such as lichen planus or lichen sclerosus; chronic irritation of the penis by friction, urine, allergens, or injury; suppression of the immune system by medications or disease; and smoking.

Symptoms and Diagnosis of Penile Intraepithelial Neoplasia

The main symptom of PEIN is the presence of one or more lesions, growths, or tumors on the glans or foreskin of the penis. The surface of these lesions may appear smooth, velvety, crusty, scaly, or bumpy. Men with PEIN may also experience inflammation, redness, itching, or pain in the area. In advanced stages, PEIN may cause bleeding, discharge, difficulty retracting the foreskin, or difficulty with urination.

Some of the symptoms of penile intraepithelial neoplasia may resemble other conditions, such as balanitis or dermatitis, so a skin biopsy should be performed to confirm the diagnosis and rule out invasive squamous cell carcinoma.

Treatment of Penile Intraepithelial Neoplasia

Penile intraepithelial neoplasia can be treated with medications, surgery, or both. In addition to practicing good genital hygiene, men with PEIN may benefit from the use of topical medications, such as 5-fluorouracil cream, which destroys abnormal skin cells, or imiquimod cream, which stimulates the immune system's response to abnormal cells. The lesions may also be removed using a variety of techniques, such as cryotherapy, curettage and cautery, excision, laser vaporization, Mohs micrographic surgery, photodynamic therapy, and radiotherapy. Since up to 10 percent of patients may experience a recurrence of PEIN following successful treatment, it is important to maintain a regular schedule of follow-up examinations.

Patients diagnosed with PEIN should undergo treatment promptly to prevent the precancerous lesions from becoming cancerous. Although penile cancer is highly curable in its early stages, the prognosis declines sharply for more advanced stages. Finally, sexual partners of patients with penile intraepithelial neoplasia should be screened for related conditions—such as cervical, vulvar, and anal cancer—which can also be caused by HPV.

References

1. Ngan, Vanessa. "Penile Intraepithelial Neoplasia," DermNet NZ, April 25, 2016.

2. "Penile Cancer Treatment," National Cancer Institute (NCI), February 18, 2016.

Section 29.4

Penile Trauma

Penile trauma can describe any sort of injury or wound that affects the penis. Since the penis contains no bone and is very flexible in its regular, flaccid state, penile injuries are rare when compared to injuries affecting most other parts of the body. Trauma usually occurs when the penis is in its erect state, with between 30 percent and 50 percent of penile injuries resulting from sexual intercourse. Although most types of penile trauma will heal with appropriate treatment, many men resist seeking medical attention for penis injuries. Left untreated, however, penile trauma may result in pain, swelling, infection, sexual dysfunction, or permanent curvature of the penis (Peyronie disease).

Causes of Penile Trauma

Although most cases of penile trauma are related to sexual inter-course, injuries to the penis may result from a variety of other causes. Some of the most common types of injuries and associated causes include:

Blunt Force Trauma

Sports-related injuries—such as being hit in the groin by a ball, stick, foot, or knee—are a leading cause of blunt force trauma to the penis, which can result in pain, swelling, and bruising. Other common sources of blunt force trauma to the penis include automobile accidents and industrial accidents.

Cuts, Abrasions, and Burns

Penis abrasion can result from vigorous, repetitive exercise, chafing from coarse fabrics, or rug burns. Minor cuts and bruises to the penis may occur from being caught in a zipper or from using a penile pump or other stretching device in an effort to enlarge the penis. Burns to the penis can result from hot liquids being spilled or clothing catching on fire.

Punctures

Inserting objects into the tip of the penis can damage the urethra (the tube that carries urine and semen out of the penis). Bleeding from the penis or blood in the urine are indications of a serious injury to the urethra.

Severe Trauma or Amputation

Part or all of the penis may be damaged or severed as a result of gunshot wounds, automobile accidents, or industrial accidents. In addition, placing a rubber tube, metal ring, or other constricting device around the base of the penis can block blood flow and cause lasting damage to the organ.

Penis "Fracture"

The most common form of penile trauma occurs when an erect penis is bent sharply, resulting in a tear or rupture in the tube-like structures (tunica albuginea) that carry blood to the penis. It usually occurs during sexual intercourse as a result of vigorous thrusting. Men who experience this type of injury typically feel a sharp pain and hear a popping or cracking sound. Discoloration and swelling usually occur as blood collects under the skin of the penis. Although urologists often refer to this particular injury as a "penile fracture," the term is somewhat misleading since there is no bone in the penis.

Diagnosis and Treatment of Penile Trauma

To diagnose an injury to the penis, a urologist will discuss the patient's medical history and conduct a physical examination, checking the organ carefully for bruises, cuts, abrasions, dents, sensitive areas, or bleeding. The urologist may also order blood and urine tests, as well as diagnostic tests, such as an ultrasound or magnetic resonance imaging (MRI) exam, to determine the extent of damage to the penis. Another diagnostic tool involves inserting a tiny fiber-optic camera into the urethra. Finally, the urologist may perform a retrograde urethrogram—an X-ray study that is performed by injecting a special dye into the urethra and checking to see whether it leaks out.

Treatment of penile trauma varies depending on the type and extent of injury. Many minor injuries can be treated with rest and anti-inflammatory medications. The usual treatment for penile fracture is surgery to repair tears or ruptures in the tunica albuginea and to remove any blood clots. Studies have shown that surgery offers the lowest rates of penile scarring, curvature, and sexual dysfunction. The typical procedure is performed under general anesthesia. It involves making an incision around the shaft near the head of the penis and retracting the skin to locate and repair tissue damage. Afterward, the area is bandaged, and a catheter is placed in the urethra to drain urine from the bladder and allow the penis to heal. Most patients remain in the hospital under observation for one to two days and take antibiotics and pain relievers for one to two weeks after returning home.

Surgery is also the preferred option for patients with severe penile trauma or amputation. In cases where part or all of the penis has been severed, surgical reattachment may be possible for up to 16 hours if the organ is wrapped in gauze, placed in a plastic bag containing a sterile salt solution, and stored in a cooler of ice-cold water. Surgical reconstruction of the penis may also be possible following massive injuries, although the extent of the damage will determine how much function the organ retains afterward.

References

1. "What Is Penile Trauma?" Urology Care Foundation, 2016.

2. "Your Guide to Penis Pain and Injury," Herbal Love, 2016.

Section 29.5

Peyronie Disease

This section includes text excerpted from "Penile Curvature (Peyronie Disease)," National Institute of Diabetes and Digestive and Kidney Diseases (NIDDK), July 2014. Reviewed June 2019.

What Is Peyronie Disease?

Peyronie disease is a disorder in which scar tissue, called a "plaque," forms in the penis—the male organ used for urination and sex. The plaque builds up inside the tissues of a thick, elastic membrane called the "tunica albuginea." The most common area for the plaque is on the top or bottom of the penis. As the plaque builds up, the penis will curve or bend, which can cause painful erections. Curves in the penis can make sexual intercourse painful, difficult, or impossible. Peyronie disease begins with inflammation, or swelling, which can become a hard scar.

The plaque that develops in Peyronie disease is not the same plaque that can develop in a person's arteries. The plaque seen in Peyronie disease is benign, or noncancerous, and is not a tumor. Peyronie disease is not contagious or caused by any known transmittable disease.

Early researchers thought Peyronie disease was a form of impotence, now called "erectile dysfunction" (ED). ED happens when a man is unable to achieve or keep an erection firm enough for sexual intercourse. Some men with Peyronie disease may have ED. Usually, men with Peyronie disease are referred to a urologist—a doctor who specializes in sexual and urinary problems.

How Does an Erection Occur?

An erection occurs when blood flow increases into the penis, making it expand and become firm. Two long chambers inside the penis, called the "corpora cavernosa," contain a spongy tissue that draws blood into the chambers. The spongy tissue contains smooth muscles, fibrous tissues, spaces, veins, and arteries. The tunica albuginea encases the corpora cavernosa. The urethra, which is the tube that carries urine and semen outside of the body, runs along the underside of the corpora cavernosa in the middle of a third chamber called the "corpus spongiosum." An erection requires a precise sequence of events:

- An erection begins with sensory or mental stimulation, or both. The stimulus may be physical contact or a sexual image or thought.

- When the brain senses a sexual urge, it sends impulses to local nerves in the penis that cause the muscles of the corpora cavernosa to relax. As a result, blood flows in through the arteries and fills the spaces in the corpora cavernosa like water filling a sponge.

- The blood creates pressure in the corpora cavernosa, making the penis expand.

- The tunica albuginea helps trap the blood in the corpora cavernosa, thereby sustaining the erection.

- The erection ends after climax or after the sexual urge has passed. The muscles in the penis contract to stop the inflow of blood. The veins open, and the extra blood flows out of the penis and back into the body.

What Causes Peyronie Disease

Medical experts do not know the exact cause of Peyronie disease. Many believe that Peyronie disease may be the result of:

- Acute injury to the penis

- Chronic, or repeated, injury to the penis

- Autoimmune disease—a disorder in which the body's immune system attacks the body's own cells and organs

Injury to the Penis

Medical experts believe that hitting or bending the penis may injure the tissues inside. A man may injure the penis during sex, athletic activity, or an accident. Injury ruptures blood vessels, which leads to bleeding and swelling inside the layers of the tunica albuginea. Swelling inside the penis will block blood flow through the layers of tissue inside the penis. When the blood cannot flow normally, clots can form and trap immune system cells. As the injury heals, the immune system cells may release substances that lead to the formation of too much scar tissue. The scar tissue builds up and forms a plaque inside the penis. The plaque reduces the elasticity of tissues and flexibility of the penis during erection, leading to curvature. The plaque may further harden because of calcification—the process in which calcium builds up in body tissue.

Autoimmune Disease

Some medical experts believe that Peyronie disease may be part of an autoimmune disease. Normally, the immune system is the body's way of protecting itself from infection by identifying and destroying bacteria, viruses, and other potentially harmful foreign substances. Men who have autoimmune diseases may develop Peyronie disease when the immune system attacks cells in the penis. This can lead to inflammation in the penis and can cause scarring. Medical experts do not know what causes autoimmune diseases. Some of the autoimmune diseases associated with Peyronie disease affect connective tissues. Connective tissue is specialized tissue that supports, joins, or separates different types of tissues and organs of the body.

How Common Is Peyronie Disease?

Researchers estimate that Peyronie disease may affect 1 to 23 percent of men between 40 and 70 years of age. However, the actual occurrence of Peyronie disease may be higher due to men's embarrassment and healthcare providers' limited reporting. The disease is rare in young men, although it has been reported in men in their thirties. The chance of developing Peyronie disease increases with age.

Who Is Most Likely to Develop Peyronie Disease?

The following factors may increase a man's chance of developing Peyronie disease:

Vigorous Sexual and Nonsexual Activities

Men whose sexual or nonsexual activities cause microscopic injury to the penis are more likely to develop Peyronie disease.

Connective Tissue and Autoimmune Disorders

Men who have certain connective tissue and autoimmune disorders may have a higher chance of developing Peyronie disease. A common example is a condition known as "Dupuytren disease," an abnormal cordlike thickening across the palm of the hand. Dupuytren disease is also known as "Dupuytren contracture." Although Dupuytren disease is fairly common in older men, only about 15 percent of men with Peyronie disease will also have Dupuytren disease. Other connective tissue disorders associated with Peyronie disease include:

- Plantar fasciitis—inflammation of the plantar fascia, thick tissue on the bottom of the foot that connects the heel bone to the toes and creates the arch of the foot

- Scleroderma—abnormal growth of connective tissue, causing it to get thick and hard; scleroderma can cause swelling or pain in muscles and joints.

Autoimmune disorders associated with Peyronie disease include:

- Systemic lupus erythematosus (SLE)—inflammation and damage to various body tissues, including the joints, skin, kidneys, heart, lungs, blood vessels, and brain

- Sjögren syndrome—inflammation and damage to the glands that make tears and saliva

- Behcet syndrome—inflammation of the blood vessels

405

Family History of Peyronie Disease

Medical experts believe that Peyronie disease may run in some families. For example, a man whose father or brother has Peyronie disease may have an increased chance of getting the disease.

Aging

The chance of getting Peyronie disease increases with age. Age-related changes in the elasticity of tissues in the penis may cause it to be more easily injured and less likely to heal well.

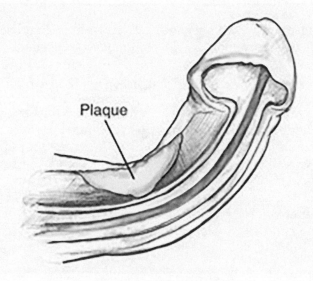

Plaque

Figure 29.1. *Cross Section of a Curved Penis during Erection*

What Are the Signs and Symptoms of Peyronie Disease?

The signs and symptoms of Peyronie disease may include:

- Hard lumps on one or more sides of the penis
- Pain during sexual intercourse or during an erection
- A curve in the penis either with or without an erection
- Narrowing or shortening of the penis
- Erectile dysfunction

Symptoms of Peyronie disease range from mild to severe. Symptoms may develop slowly or appear quickly. In many cases, the pain decreases over time, although the curve in the penis may remain. In milder cases, symptoms may go away without causing a permanent curve.

What Are the Complications of Peyronie Disease?

Complications of Peyronie disease may include:

- The inability to have sexual intercourse
- Erectile dysfunction
- Anxiety, or stress, about sexual abilities or the appearance of the penis
- Stress on a relationship with a sexual partner
- Problems fathering a child because intercourse is difficult

How Is Peyronie Disease Diagnosed?

A urologist diagnoses Peyronie disease based on a number of factors.

Medical and Family History

Taking a medical and family history is one of the first things a urologist may do to help diagnose Peyronie disease. She or he will ask the man to provide a medical and family history, which may include the following questions:

- What is the man's ability to have an erection?
- What are the problems with sexual intercourse?
- When did the symptoms begin?
- What is the family medical history?
- What medications is the man taking?
- What other symptoms is the man experiencing?
- What other medical conditions does the man have?

Physical Exam

A physical exam may help diagnose Peyronie disease. During a physical exam, a urologist usually examines the man's body, including the penis.

407

A urologist can usually feel the plaque in the penis with or without an erection. Sometimes the urologist will need to examine the penis during an erection. The urologist will give the man an injectable medication to cause an erection.

Imaging Tests

To help pinpoint the location of the plaque buildup inside the penis, a urologist may perform:

• Ultrasound of the penis

• An X-ray of the penis

For both tests, a specially trained technician performs the procedure in a healthcare provider's office, an outpatient center, or a hospital, and a radiologist—a doctor who specializes in medical imaging—interprets the images. The patient does not need anesthesia.

Ultrasound. Ultrasound uses a device, called a "transducer," that bounces safe, painless sound waves off organs to create an image of their structure.

X-ray. An X-ray is a picture created by using radiation and recorded on film or on a computer. The amount of radiation used is small. The man will lie on a table or stand during the X-ray, and the technician may ask the man to change positions for additional pictures.

Section 29.6

Phimosis and Paraphimosis

What Is Phimosis?

Phimosis is a condition in which the foreskin (prepuce) of an uncircumcised male cannot be retracted over the head (glans) of the penis. It often appears to be a tight ring around the tip of the penis.

Causes of Phimosis

Phimosis can either be physiologic or pathologic.

- Physiologic phimosis occurs when a child is born with a tight foreskin. The condition generally corrects itself without intervention sometime between late childhood and early adolescence. In the United States, about 10 percent of boys are born with phimosis.

- Pathologic phimosis occurs in older boys and adult men, often due to poor hygiene, infection, inflammation, or other medical conditions. Forceful retraction of the foreskin can lead to scarring and repeated swelling of the foreskin and glans.

Symptoms of Phimosis

Symptoms of phimosis include:

- Ballooning of the foreskin during urination
- Difficulty or pain during urination
- Urinary tract infections (UTIs)
- Painful erection
- Paraphimosis

Diagnosis of Phimosis

Phimosis is diagnosed by a physical examination, in which the doctor can observe the symptoms, and does not usually require additional tests.

Treatment of Phimosis

Treatment depends on such factors as the age of the individual, type of symptoms, and the severity of the condition. Phimosis may be treated by gently retracting the foreskin manually and applying topical corticosteroid ointment. Steroid ointment softens the foreskin, and full retraction may be possible in four to six weeks, following which this treatment is discontinued. In rare cases—such as unsuccessful steroid treatment, recurrent or severe inflammation, paraphimosis, or recurrent UTIs—circumcision might be required.

What Is Paraphimosis?

Paraphimosis is a condition in which the retracted foreskin cannot be returned to its normal position. This leads to decreased blood flow to the glans penis, which then becomes a urologic emergency.

Causes of Paraphimosis

Paraphimosis is most often observed in children and the elderly. It can be caused by an injury to the area, failure to return the foreskin to its original position after retraction, or infection that may occur when the area is not washed properly. It commonly occurs in hospitals and nursing homes when the foreskin is retracted by a healthcare professional to prepare a patient for a medical procedure, such as the insertion of a Foley catheter.

Symptoms of Paraphimosis

When a retracted foreskin stays behind the glans penis for too long, it causes the glans and the foreskin to become swollen. This swelling often aggravates the restriction, forming a tight tissue ring around the head of the penis. This in turn worsens the swelling and causes considerable pain.

Diagnosis of Paraphimosis

Paraphimosis is diagnosed by a physical examination, in which a "doughnut" is usually observed close to the head of the penis.

Treatment of Paraphimosis

The first option is to reduce the swelling manually by pushing the foreskin forward while simultaneously pressing on the glans penis. The

410

application of ice to the swollen area can also help. To reduce discomfort, the person may be given pain medication or a local anesthetic or anesthetic cream, applied to the penis. Another effective option, used to decrease swelling, is a local injection of hyaluronidase.

In circumstances in which none of these options are successful, or if a faster reduction is required, the doctor may make a small surgical incision on the back (dorsal) side of the constricting ring. If this procedure is followed, circumcision must be done at a later time to prevent recurrence.

References

1. Balentine, Jerry R. "Phimosis and Paraphimosis (Penis Disorders)," MedicineNet, Inc., March 23, 2016.

2. "Phimosis," Department of Urology, University of California, San Francisco, n.d.

3. Zieve, David. "Paraphimosis," A.D.A.M., Inc., January 21, 2015.

Chapter 30

Disorders of the Scrotum and Testicles

Chapter Contents

Section 30.1—Epididymitis 414

Section 30.2—Hydrocele 418

Section 30.3—Inguinal Hernia.. 421

Section 30.4—Spermatocele 428

Section 30.5—Perineal Injury 430

Section 30.1

Epididymitis

This section includes text excerpted from "Epididymitis,"
Centers for Disease Control and Prevention (CDC),
June 4, 2015. Reviewed June 2019.

Acute epididymitis is a clinical syndrome consisting of pain, swelling, and inflammation of the epididymis that lasts less than six weeks. Sometimes, the testis is also involved—a condition referred to as "epididymo-orchitis." A high index of suspicion for spermatic cord (testicular) torsion must be maintained in men who present with a sudden onset of symptoms associated with epididymitis, as this condition is a surgical emergency.

Among sexually active men 35 years of age and younger, acute epididymitis is most frequently caused by *C. trachomatis* or *N. gonorrhoeae*. Acute epididymitis caused by sexually transmitted enteric organisms (e.g., *Escherichia coli*) also occurs among men who are the insertive partner during anal intercourse. Sexually transmitted acute epididymitis usually is accompanied by urethritis, which frequently is asymptomatic. Other nonsexually transmitted infectious causes of acute epididymitis (e.g., Fournier gangrene) are uncommon and should be managed in consultation with a urologist.

In men 35 years of age and younger who do not report insertive anal intercourse, sexually transmitted acute epididymitis is less common. In this group, the epididymis usually becomes infected in the setting of bacteriuria secondary to bladder outlet obstruction (e.g., benign prostatic hyperplasia). In older men, nonsexually transmitted acute epididymitis is also associated with prostate biopsy, urinary tract instrumentation or surgery, systemic disease, and/or immunosuppression.

Chronic epididymitis is characterized by a less than six-week history of symptoms of discomfort and/or pain in the scrotum, testicle, or epididymis. Chronic infectious epididymitis is most frequently seen in conditions associated with a granulomatous reaction; Mycobacterium tuberculosis (TB) is the most common granulomatous disease affecting the epididymis and should be suspected, especially in men with a known history of or recent exposure to TB. The differential diagnosis of chronic noninfectious epididymitis, sometimes termed "orchialgia/epididymalgia" is broad (i.e., trauma, cancer, autoimmune, and idiopathic conditions); men with this diagnosis should be referred to a urologist for clinical management.

Diagnostic Considerations

Men who have acute epididymitis typically have unilateral testicular pain and tenderness, hydrocele, and palpable swelling of the epididymis. Although inflammation and swelling usually begins in the tail of the epididymis, it can spread to involve the rest of the epididymis and testicle. The spermatic cord is usually tender and swollen. Spermatic cord (testicular) torsion, a surgical emergency, should be considered in all cases, but it occurs more frequently among adolescents and in men without evidence of inflammation or infection. In men with severe, unilateral pain with sudden onset, those whose test results do not support a diagnosis of urethritis or urinary tract infection (UTI), or men in whom diagnosis of acute epididymitis is questionable, immediate referral to a urologist for evaluation of testicular torsion is important because testicular viability might be compromised.

Bilateral symptoms should raise suspicion of other causes of testicular pain. Radionuclide scanning of the scrotum is the most accurate method to diagnose epididymitis, but it is not routinely available. Ultrasound should be primarily used for ruling out torsion of the spermatic cord in cases of acute, unilateral, painful scrotum swelling. However, because partial spermatic cord torsion can mimic epididymitis on scrotal ultrasound, when torsion is not ruled out by ultrasound, differentiation between spermatic cord torsion and epididymitis must be made on the basis of clinical evaluation. Although ultrasound can demonstrate epididymal hyperemia and swelling associated with epididymitis, it provides minimal utility for men with a clinical presentation consistent with epididymitis, because a negative ultrasound does not alter clinical management. Ultrasound should be reserved for men with scrotal pain who cannot receive an accurate diagnosis by history, physical examination, and objective laboratory findings or if torsion of the spermatic cord is suspected.

All suspected cases of acute epididymitis should be evaluated for objective evidence of inflammation by one of the following point-of-care tests.

- Gram or methylene blue or gentian violet (MB/GV) stain of urethral secretions demonstrating more than two white blood cell (WBC) per oil immersion field. These stains are preferred point-of-care diagnostic tests for evaluating urethritis because they are highly sensitive and specific for documenting both urethral inflammation and the presence or absence of gonococcal infection. Gonococcal infection is established by documenting the presence of WBC-containing intracellular Gram-negative or purple diplococci on an urethral Gram stain or MB/GV smear, respectively.

- Positive leukocyte esterase test on first-void urine

- Microscopic examination of sediment from a spun first-void urine demonstrating more than 10 WBC per high power field

All suspected cases of acute epididymitis should be tested for *C. trachomatis* and for *N. gonorrhoeae* by nucleic acid amplification tests (NAAT). Urine is the preferred specimen for NAAT testing in men. Urine cultures for chlamydia and gonococcal epididymitis are insensitive and not recommended. Urine bacterial culture might have a higher yield in men with sexually transmitted enteric infections and in older men with acute epididymitis caused by genitourinary bacteriuria.

Treatment

To prevent complications and transmission of STIs, presumptive therapy is indicated at the time of the visit before all laboratory test results are available. Selection of presumptive therapy is based on the risk for chlamydia and gonorrhea and/or enteric organisms. The goals of treatment of acute epididymitis are microbiologic cure of infection, improvement of signs and symptoms, prevention of transmission of chlamydia and gonorrhea to others, and a decrease in potential chlamydia/gonorrhea epididymitis complications (e.g., infertility and chronic pain). Although most men with acute epididymitis can be treated on an outpatient basis, referral to a specialist and hospitalization should be considered when severe pain or fever suggests other diagnoses (e.g., torsion, testicular infarction, abscess, and necrotizing fasciitis) or when men are unable to comply with an antimicrobial regimen. Because high fever is uncommon and indicates a complicated infection, hospitalization for further evaluation is recommended.

Therapy including levofloxacin or ofloxacin should be considered if the infection is most likely caused by enteric organisms and gonorrhea has been ruled out by gram, MB, or GV stain. This includes men who have undergone prostate biopsy, vasectomy, and other urinary-tract instrumentation procedures. As an adjunct to therapy, bed rest, scrotal elevation, and nonsteroidal anti-inflammatory drugs (NSAIDs) are recommended until fever and local inflammation have subsided. Complete resolution of discomfort might not occur until a few weeks after completion of the antibiotic regimen.

Other Management Considerations

Men who have acute epididymitis confirmed or suspected to be caused by *N. gonorrhoeae* or *C. trachomatis* should be advised to abstain from sexual intercourse until they and their partners have been adequately treated and symptoms have resolved. All men with acute epididymitis should be tested for other sexually transmitted diseases (STDs), including human immunodeficiency virus (HIV).

Follow-Up

Men should be instructed to return to their healthcare providers if their symptoms fail to improve within 72 hours of the initiation of treatment. Signs and symptoms of epididymitis that do not subside within 3 days require reevaluation of the diagnosis and therapy. Men who experience swelling and tenderness that persist after completion of antimicrobial therapy should be evaluated for alternative diagnoses, including tumor, abscess, infarction, testicular cancer, tuberculosis, and fungal epididymitis.

Management of Sex Partners

Men who have acute sexually transmitted epididymitis confirmed or suspected to be caused by *N. gonorrhoeae* or *C. trachomatis* should be instructed to refer for evaluation, testing, and presumptive treatment all sex partners with whom they have had sexual contact within the 60 days preceding onset of symptoms. If the last sexual intercourse was greater than 60 days before onset of symptoms or diagnosis, the most recent sex partner should be treated. Arrangements should be made to link female partners to care. EPT and enhanced referral are effective strategies for treating female sex partners of men who have chlamydia or gonorrhea for whom linkage to care is anticipated to be delayed. Partners should be instructed to abstain from sexual intercourse until they and their sex partners are adequately treated and symptoms have resolved.

Special Considerations
Allergy, Intolerance, and Adverse Reactions

The cross-reactivity between penicillins and cephalosporins is less than 2.5 percent in persons with a history of penicillin allergy. The risk for penicillin cross-reactivity is highest with first-generation cephalosporins but is negligible between most second-generation (cefoxitin) and all third-generation (ceftriaxone) cephalosporins. Alternative regimens have not been studied; therefore, clinicians should consult infectious-disease specialists if such regimens are required.

Human Immunodeficiency Virus Infection

Men with HIV infection who have uncomplicated acute epididymitis should receive the same treatment regimen as those who are HIV negative. Other etiologic agents have been implicated in acute epididymitis in men with HIV infection, including CMV, salmonella, toxoplasmosis, Ureaplasma urealyticum, Corynebacterium sp., Mycoplasma sp., and Mima polymorpha. Fungi and mycobacteria also are more likely to cause acute epididymitis in men with HIV infection than in those who are immunocompetent.

Section 30.2

Hydrocele

"Hydrocele," © 2017 Omnigraphics.
Reviewed June 2019.

A hydrocele is a generally harmless, painless buildup of fluid around one or both testicles that causes swelling in the scrotum. Hydroceles can be described as primary or secondary. A primary hydrocele, also called an "idiopathic hydrocele," often occurs as a result of an imbalance between the secretion and absorption of fluids in the membranes covering the testes. A secondary hydrocele may follow trauma, infection, or neoplasms.

Common in newborns, congenital hydroceles may form a few weeks prior to birth when the testes descend from the abdomen into the scrotum, surrounded by a fluid-filled sac. Normally, this sac closes, and the fluid is absorbed. In some newborns, however, the sac fails to close, which causes a route to the abdominal cavity to remain open. This is called a "communicating hydrocele" since it allows the passage of fluid between the abdomen and scrotum. A noncommunicating hydrocele, on the other hand, develops when the sac closes but traps some fluid in the scrotum. Congenital hydroceles are found in about 10 percent of newborns and may regress spontaneously within the first 2 years of life.

Hydroceles may also affect adolescents and adults, most often men older than 40 years of age. In these cases, the hydrocele may be caused by a condition in which the passage from abdomen to scrotum either has not closed all the way or has reopened. Other causes of hydroceles in adults include injury to the scrotum or inflammation resulting from an infection.

Symptoms of Hydrocele

A hydrocele commonly presents as an enlargement of the scrotum, just below the testes, and is usually painless unless there is infection or some other underlying cause of discomfort. In the case of communicating hydroceles, the size of the swelling may vacillate during the day, typically growing larger with coughing, straining, crying, or any activity that raises intra-abdominal pressure.

Diagnosis of Hydrocele

A simple physical examination involving palpation (feeling with the hand) is the first step in diagnosing a hydrocele. The doctor may also use a technique called "transillumination," in which a bright light is focused on the scrotum. The presence of clear fluid allows transmission of light, and the scrotum "lights up," revealing the presence of a hydrocele or other testicular abnormalities. The doctor may also recommend blood and urine tests or a scrotal ultrasound to confirm the initial diagnosis.

Treatment of Hydrocele

Hydroceles generally do not require treatment unless they attain a critical size, and the patient experiences discomfort or difficulty moving. However, it is prudent to check with your healthcare provider to rule out other complications, such as infection, a testicular tumor, or an inguinal hernia. An inguinal hernia, one of the most common risks associated with hydrocele, develops when a loop of the intestine protrudes into the scrotum and may require surgical intervention.

When medical intervention is required, some possible treatments for hydrocele include:

Needle Aspiration

The safest, cheapest, and most noninvasive treatment option involves drainage of fluid from the hydrocele using a syringe. While this procedure is often successful in providing symptomatic relief in large hydroceles, it carries a high likelihood of recurrence and is most often recommended when surgery is not an option.

Sclerotherapy

This form of treatment is often used in conjunction with aspiration to prevent or delay the recurrence of a hydrocele. Sclerotherapy involves the injection of medication after the fluid has been drained.

Hydrocelectomy

A hydrocelectomy is a surgical repair that is used to correct large, painful, recurring hydroceles. If the hydrocele is uncomplicated, the surgery generally takes less than an hour and is typically performed on an outpatient basis under either general or local anesthesia. An incision is made in the scrotum or lower abdomen. The hydrocele sac is drained of its fluid and is partially or totally removed. Related conditions, such as an inguinal hernia, may also be corrected during hydrocelectomy. Some surgeons use laparoscopy—a minimally invasive procedure using a camera-tipped instrument called a "laparoscope"—to repair hydroceles. Hydrocelectomy is generally considered safe, and most patients experience minimal complications and have a successful long-term outcome.

References

1. "Hydrocele: Topic Overview," WebMD, November 14, 2014.

2. Parks, Kelly and Leung, Lawrence. "Recurrent Hydrocoele," National Center for Biotechnology Information (NCBI), 2013.

3. "Hydrocele," Mayo Clinic, October 9, 2014.

Section 30.3

Inguinal Hernia

This section includes text excerpted from "Inguinal Hernia,"
National Institute of Diabetes and Digestive and Kidney
Diseases (NIDDK), June 2014. Reviewed June 2019.

What Is an Inguinal Hernia?

An inguinal hernia happens when contents of the abdomen—usually fat or part of the small intestine—bulge through a weak area in the lower abdominal wall. The abdomen is the area between the chest and the hips. The area of the lower abdominal wall is also called the "inguinal" or "groin region."
Two types of inguinal hernias:

- Indirect inguinal hernias, which are caused by a defect in the abdominal wall that is congenital, or present at birth

- Direct inguinal hernias, which usually occur only in male adults and are caused by a weakness in the muscles of the abdominal wall that develops over time

Inguinal hernias occur at the inguinal canal in the groin region.

What Is the Inguinal Canal?

The inguinal canal is a passage through the lower abdominal wall. People have two inguinal canals—one on each side of the lower abdomen. In males, the spermatic cords pass through the inguinal canals and connect to the testicles in the scrotum—the sac around the testicles. The spermatic cords contain blood vessels, nerves, and a duct, called the "spermatic duct," that carries sperm from the testicles to the penis.

What Causes Inguinal Hernias

The cause of inguinal hernias depends on the type of inguinal hernia.

Indirect inguinal hernias. A defect in the abdominal wall that is present at birth causes an indirect inguinal hernia.
During the development of the fetus in the womb, the lining of the abdominal cavity forms and extends into the inguinal canal. In

males, the spermatic cord and testicles descend out from inside the abdomen and through the abdominal lining to the scrotum through the inguinal canal.

Sometimes the lining of the abdomen does not close as it should, leaving an opening in the abdominal wall at the upper part of the inguinal canal. Fat or part of the small intestine may slide into the inguinal canal through this opening, causing a hernia.

Indirect hernias are the most common type of inguinal hernia. Indirect inguinal hernias may appear in two to three percent of male children; however, they are much less common in female children, occurring in less than one percent.

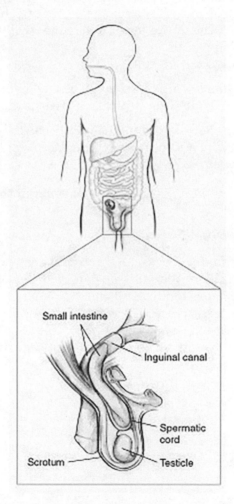

Figure 30.1. *Indirect Inguinal Hernia in a Male*

Direct inguinal hernias. Direct inguinal hernias usually occur only in male adults as aging and stress or strain weaken the abdominal muscles around the inguinal canal. Previous surgery in the lower abdomen can also weaken the abdominal muscles.

Who Is More Likely to Develop an Inguinal Hernia?

Males are much more likely to develop inguinal hernias than females. About 25 percent of males and about 2 percent of females will develop an inguinal hernia in their lifetimes. Some people who have an inguinal hernia on one side will have or will develop a hernia on the other side.

People of any age can develop inguinal hernias. Indirect hernias can appear before 1 year of age and often appear before 30 years of age; however, they may appear later in life. Premature infants have a higher chance of developing an indirect inguinal hernia. Direct hernias, which usually only occur in male adults, are much more common in men older than the age of 40 because the muscles of the abdominal wall weaken with age.

People with a family history of inguinal hernias are more likely to develop inguinal hernias. Studies also suggest that people who smoke have an increased risk of inguinal hernias.

What Are the Signs and Symptoms of an Inguinal Hernia?

The first sign of an inguinal hernia is a small bulge on one or, rarely, on both sides of the groin—the area just above the groin crease between the lower abdomen and the thigh. The bulge may increase in size over time and usually disappears when lying down.

Other signs and symptoms can include:

- Discomfort or pain in the groin—especially when straining, lifting, coughing, or exercising—that improves when resting

- Feelings, such as weakness, heaviness, burning, or aching in the groin

- A swollen or an enlarged scrotum in men or boys

Indirect and direct inguinal hernias may slide in and out of the abdomen into the inguinal canal. A healthcare provider can often move them back into the abdomen with a gentle massage.

What Are the Complications of Inguinal Hernias?

Inguinal hernias can cause the following complications:

- **Incarceration.** An incarcerated hernia happens when part of the fat or small intestine from inside the abdomen becomes stuck in the groin or scrotum and cannot go back into the abdomen. A healthcare provider is unable to massage the hernia back into the abdomen.

- **Strangulation.** When an incarcerated hernia is not treated, the blood supply to the small intestine may become obstructed, causing a "strangulation" of the small intestine. This lack of blood supply is an emergency situation and can cause the section of the intestine to die.

Seek Immediate Care

People who have symptoms of an incarcerated or a strangulated hernia should seek emergency medical help immediately. A strangulated hernia is a life-threatening condition. Symptoms of an incarcerated or a strangulated hernia include:

- Extreme tenderness or painful redness in the area of the bulge in the groin

- Sudden pain that worsens quickly and does not go away

- The inability to have a bowel movement and pass gas

- Nausea and vomiting

- Fever

How Are Inguinal Hernias Diagnosed?

A healthcare provider diagnoses an inguinal hernia with:

- A medical and family history

- A physical exam

- Imaging tests, including X-rays

Medical and family history. Taking a medical and family history may help a healthcare provider diagnose an inguinal hernia. Often, the symptoms that the patient describes will be signs of an inguinal hernia.

Physical exam. A physical exam may help diagnose an inguinal hernia. During a physical exam, a healthcare provider usually examines the patient's body. The healthcare provider may ask the patient to stand and cough or strain so the healthcare provider can feel for a bulge caused by the hernia as it moves into the groin or scrotum. The healthcare provider may gently try to massage the hernia back into its proper position in the abdomen.

Imaging tests. A healthcare provider does not usually use imaging tests, including X-rays, to diagnose an inguinal hernia unless he:

- Is trying to diagnose a strangulation or an incarceration

- Cannot feel the inguinal hernia during a physical exam, especially in patients who are overweight

- Is uncertain if the hernia or another condition is causing the swelling in the groin or other symptoms

Specially trained technicians perform imaging tests at a healthcare provider's office, an outpatient center, or a hospital.

A radiologist—a doctor who specializes in medical imaging—interprets the images. A patient does not usually need anesthesia.

Tests may include the following:

- **Abdominal X-ray.** An X-ray is a picture recorded on film or on a computer using a small amount of radiation. The patient will lie on a table or stand during the X-ray. The technician positions the X-ray machine over the abdominal area. The patient will hold his or her breath as the technician takes the picture so that the picture will not be blurry. The technician may ask the patient to change position for additional pictures.

- **Computerized tomography (CT) scan.** CT scans use a combination of X-rays and computer technology to create images. For a CT scan, the technician may give the patient a solution to drink and an injection of a special dye, called "contrast medium." A healthcare provider injects the contrast medium into a vein, and the injection will make the patient feel warm all over for a minute or two. The contrast medium allows the healthcare provider to see the blood vessels and blood flow on the X-rays. CT scans require the patient to lie on a table that slides into a tunnel-shaped device where the technician takes the X-rays. A healthcare provider may give children a sedative to help them fall asleep for the test.

- **Abdominal ultrasound.** Ultrasound uses a device, called a "transducer," that bounces safe, painless sound waves off organs to create an image of their structure.

How Are Inguinal Hernias Treated?

Repair of an inguinal hernia via surgery is the only treatment for inguinal hernias and can prevent incarceration and strangulation. Healthcare providers recommend surgery for most people with inguinal hernias and especially for people with hernias that cause symptoms. Research suggests that men with hernias that cause few or no symptoms may be able to safely delay surgery until their symptoms increase. Men who delay surgery should watch for symptoms and see a healthcare provider regularly. Healthcare providers usually recommend surgery for infants and children to prevent incarceration. Emergent, or immediate, surgery is necessary for incarcerated or strangulated hernias.

A general surgeon—a doctor who specializes in abdominal surgery—performs hernia surgery at a hospital or surgery center, usually on an outpatient basis. Recovery time varies depending on the size of the hernia, the technique used, and the age and health of the person.

Hernia surgery is also called "herniorrhaphy." The two main types of surgery for hernias are:

- Open hernia repair. During an open hernia repair, a healthcare provider usually gives a patient local anesthesia in the abdomen with sedation; however, some patients may have:

  - Sedation with a spinal block, in which a healthcare provider injects anesthetics around the nerves in the spine, making the body numb from the waist down

  - General anesthesia

- The surgeon makes an incision in the groin, moves the hernia back into the abdomen, and reinforces the abdominal wall with stitches. Usually, the surgeon also reinforces the weak area with a synthetic mesh or "screen" to provide additional support.

- Laparoscopic hernia repair. A surgeon performs laparoscopic hernia repair with the patient under general anesthesia. The surgeon makes several small, half-inch incisions in the lower abdomen and inserts a laparoscope—a thin tube with a tiny video camera attached. The camera sends a magnified image from inside the body to a video monitor, giving the surgeon a close-up view of the hernia and surrounding tissue. While watching the monitor, the surgeon repairs the hernia using synthetic mesh or "screen."

People who undergo laparoscopic hernia repair generally experience a shorter recovery time than those who have an open hernia repair. However, the surgeon may determine that laparoscopy is not the best option if the hernia is large or if the person has had previous pelvic surgery.

Most adults experience discomfort and require pain medication after either an open hernia repair or a laparoscopic hernia repair. Intense activity and heavy lifting are restricted for several weeks. The surgeon will discuss when a person may safely return to work. Infants and children also experience some discomfort; however, they usually resume normal activities after several days.

Surgery to repair an inguinal hernia is quite safe, and complications are uncommon. People should contact their healthcare provider if any of the following symptoms appear:

• Redness around or drainage from the incision

• Fever

• Bleeding from the incision

• Pain that is not relieved by medication or pain that suddenly worsens

Possible long-term complications include:

• Long-lasting pain in the groin

• Recurrence of the hernia, requiring a second surgery

• Damage to nerves near the hernia

How Can Inguinal Hernias Be Prevented?

People cannot prevent the weakness in the abdominal wall that causes indirect inguinal hernias. However, people may be able to prevent direct inguinal hernias by maintaining a healthy weight and not smoking.

People can keep inguinal hernias from getting worse or keep inguinal hernias from recurring after surgery by:

• Avoiding heavy lifting

• Using the legs, not the back, when lifting objects

- Preventing constipation and straining during bowel movements
- Maintaining a healthy weight
- Not smoking

Eating, Diet, and Nutrition

Researchers have not found that eating, diet, and nutrition play a role in causing inguinal hernias. A person with an inguinal hernia may be able to prevent symptoms by eating high-fiber foods. Fresh fruits, vegetables, and whole grains are high in fiber and may help prevent the constipation and straining that cause some of the painful symptoms of a hernia.

The surgeon will provide instructions on eating, diet, and nutrition after inguinal hernia surgery. Most people drink liquids and eat a light diet the day of the operation and then resume their usual diet the next day.

Section 30.4

Spermatocele

What Is Spermatocele?

A spermatocele—often called a "spermatic cyst"—is a benign fluid-filled mass within the scrotum. The cyst is an accumulation of fluid and sperm cells that typically arises from the caput (head) of the epididymis, a tightly coiled tube located above each testicle that collects and transports sperm. Spermatoceles are common and generally do not require treatment. However, discomfort, pain, or a bothersome enlargement may require surgical intervention.

Spermatoceles are found in an estimated 30 percent of adult men. They are usually asymptomatic, do not affect fertility, and are most often discovered during self-examination or in an imaging test carried out for other conditions.

Causes of Spermatocele

The exact cause of spermatoceles is unknown, although a number of possible etiologies have been proposed:

- They could be caused by an obstruction in the epididymal ducts.
- Sperm may accumulate in the head of the epididymis and lead to the formation of a cyst.
- Although they usually form spontaneously without any preceding injury, infection, or inflammation, they could result from a previous medical condition.

Symptoms of Spermatocele

Symptoms of spermatoceles include the following:

- A lump or mass in the scrotum
- Enlarged scrotum
- Pain, swelling, or redness of the scrotum
- Pressure felt at the base of the penis

Diagnosis of Spermatocele

A spermatocele can be felt as a firm, smooth lump by palpating (feeling) the scrotum during a medical examination or self-exam.

Diagnosis can be confirmed by a transillumination exam, in which a doctor shines a light behind each testicle. An ultrasound may be used for further confirmation, and a sonogram can help determine if the lump is a spermatocele or a benign or cancerous tumor. If the lump is painful, a blood count and urinalysis may be required to detect infection or inflammation.

Treatment of Spermatocele

Spermatoceles are not dangerous, and if the cyst is small and does not change in size, treatment may not be needed. However, treatment might be required for pain alleviation or, in rare cases, if there is decreased blood supply to the penis.

Oral analgesics are often prescribed for symptomatic pain relief. If the pain and discomfort are caused by underlying epididymitis—inflammation of the epididymis—antibiotics may be prescribed.

If the spermatocele becomes larger and causes considerable discomfort, a procedure to remove it surgically, known as a "spermatocelectomy," may be carried out. Needle aspiration, often used to treat other types of cysts, is contraindicated in spermatoceles because it could result in infection due to spillage of sperm within the scrotum.

Spermatocelectomy is generally an outpatient surgical procedure, performed under anesthesia. A postoperative evaluation is done after 2–6 weeks to ensure that the incision is healing properly and that there are no complications. Spermatocelectomy has an excellent outcome and prognosis, with a 94 percent recovery rate.

References

1. Mayo Clinic Staff. "Diseases and Conditions: Spermatocele," Mayo Clinic, December 16, 2014.

2. "Spermatoceles," Urology Care Foundation, n.d.

3. Paris, Vernon M. "Spermatocele Treatment and Management," Medscape, October 15, 2015.

Section 30.5

Perineal Injury

This section includes text excerpted from "Perineal Injury in Males," National Institute of Diabetes and Digestive and Kidney Diseases (NIDDK), March 2014. Reviewed June 2019.

What Is Perineal Injury in Males?

Perineal injury is an injury to the perineum, the part of the body between the anus and the genitals, or sex organs. In males, the perineum is the area between the anus and the scrotum, the external pouch of skin that holds the testicles. Injuries to the perineum can happen suddenly, such as in an accident, or gradually, such as the result of an activity that persistently puts pressure on the perineum. Sudden damage to the perineum is called an "acute injury," while gradual damage is called a "chronic injury."

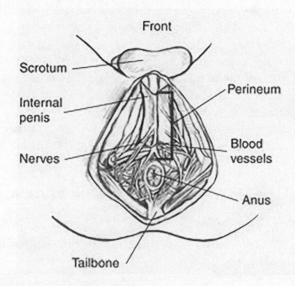

Figure 30.2. *Male Perineum*

In males, the perineum is the area between the anus and the scrotum.

Why Is the Perineum Important?

The perineum is important because it contains blood vessels and nerves that supply the urinary tract and genitals with blood and nerve signals. The perineum lies just below a sheet of muscles called the "pelvic floor muscles." Pelvic floor muscles support the bladder and bowel.

What Are the Complications of Perineal Injury?

Injury to the blood vessels, nerves, and muscles in the perineum can lead to complications, such as:

Bladder control problems. The nerves in the perineum carry signals from the bladder to the spinal cord and brain, telling the brain when the bladder is full. Those same nerves carry signals from the brain to the bladder and pelvic floor muscles, directing those muscles to hold or release urine. Injury to those nerves can block or interfere with the signals, causing the bladder to squeeze at the wrong time or not to squeeze at all. Damage to the pelvic floor muscles can cause bladder and bowel control problems.

Sexual problems. The perineal nerves also carry signals between the genitals and the brain. Injury to those nerves can interfere with the sensations of sexual contact.

Signals from the brain direct the smooth muscles in the genitals to relax, causing greater blood flow into the penis. In men, damaged blood vessels can cause erectile dysfunction (ED), the inability to achieve or maintain an erection firm enough for sexual intercourse. An internal portion of the penis runs through the perineum and contains a section of the urethra. As a result, damage to the perineum may also injure the penis and urethra.

What Are the Most Common Causes of Acute Perineal Injury?

Common causes of acute perineal injury in males include:

Perineal Surgery

Acute perineal injury may result from surgical procedures that require an incision in the perineum:

- A prostatectomy is the surgical removal of the prostate to treat prostate cancer and other prostate problems. The prostate, a walnut-shaped gland in men, surrounds the urethra at the neck of the bladder and supplies fluid that goes into semen. The surgeon chooses the location for the incision based on the patient's physical characteristics, such as size and weight, and the surgeon's experience and preferences. In one approach, called the "radical perineal prostatectomy," the surgeon makes an incision between the scrotum and the anus. In a retropubic prostatectomy, the surgeon makes the incision in the lower abdomen, just above the penis. Both approaches can damage blood vessels and nerves affecting sexual function and bladder control.

- Perineal urethroplasty is surgery to repair stricture, or narrowing, of the portion of the urethra that runs through the perineum. Without this procedure, some men would not be able to pass urine. However, the procedure does require an incision in the perineum, which can damage blood vessels or nerves.

- Colorectal or anal cancer surgery can injure the perineum by cutting through some of the muscle around the anus to remove a tumor. One approach to anal cancer surgery involves making incisions in the abdomen and the perineum.

Surgeons try to avoid procedures that damage a person's blood vessels, perineal nerves, and muscles. However, sometimes a perineal incision may achieve the best angle to remove a life-threatening cancer.

People should discuss the risks of any planned surgery with their healthcare provider so they can make an informed decision and understand what to expect after the operation.

Straddle Injuries

Straddle injuries result from falls onto objects, such as metal bars, pipes, or wooden rails, where the person's legs are on either side of the object and the perineum strikes the object forcefully. These injuries include motorcycle and bike riding accidents; saddle horn injuries during horseback riding; falls on playground equipment, such as monkey bars; and gymnastic accidents on an apparatus, such as the parallel bars or pommel horse.

In rare situations, a blunt injury to the perineum may burst a blood vessel inside the erectile tissue of the penis, causing a persistent partial erection that can last for days to years. This condition is called "high-flow priapism." If not treated, ED may result.

Sexual Abuse

Forceful and inappropriate sexual contact can result in perineal injury. When healthcare providers evaluate injuries in the genital area, they should consider the possibility of sexual abuse, even if the person or family members say the injury is the result of an accident, such as a straddle injury. The law requires that healthcare providers report cases of sexual abuse that come to their attention. The person and family members should understand that the healthcare provider may ask some uncomfortable questions about the circumstances of the injury.

Impalement

Impalement injuries may involve metal fence posts, rods, or weapons that pierce the perineum. Impalement is rare, although it may occur where moving equipment and pointed tools are in use, such as on farms or construction sites. Impalement can also occur as the result of a fall, such as from a tree or playground equipment, onto something sharp. Impalement injuries are most common in combat situations. If an impalement injury pierces the skin and muscles, the injured person needs immediate medical attention to minimize blood loss and repair the injury.

What Are the Most Common Causes of Chronic Perineal Injury?

Chronic perineal injury most often results from a job-or sport-related practice—such as bike, motorcycle, or horseback riding—or a long-term condition, such as chronic constipation.

Bike Riding

Sitting on a narrow, saddle-style bike seat—which has a protruding "nose" in the front—places far more pressure on the perineum than sitting in a regular chair. In a regular chair, the flesh and bone of the buttocks partially absorb the pressure of sitting, and the pressure occurs farther toward the back than on a bike seat. The straddling position on a narrow seat pinches the perineal blood vessels and nerves, possibly causing blood vessel and nerve damage over time. Research shows wider, noseless seats reduce perineal pressure.

Occasional bike riding for short periods of time may pose no risk. However, men who ride bikes several hours a week—such as competitive bicyclists, bicycle couriers, and bicycle patrol officers—have a significantly higher risk of developing mild to severe ED. The ED may be caused by repetitive pressure on blood vessels, which constricts them and results in plaque buildup in the vessels.

Other activities that involve riding saddle-style include motorcycle and horseback riding. Researchers have studied bike riding more extensively than these other activities; however, the few studies published regarding motorcycle and horseback riding suggest motorcycle riding increases the risk of ED and urinary symptoms. Horseback riding appears relatively safe in terms of chronic injury, although the action of bouncing up and down, repeatedly striking the perineum, has the potential for causing damage.

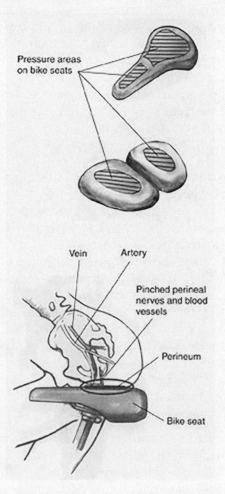

Figure 30.3. *Pinched Perineal Nerves and Blood Vessels*

Constipation

Constipation is defined as having a bowel movement fewer than three times per week. People with constipation usually have hard, dry stools that are small in size and difficult to pass. Some people with constipation need to strain to pass stools. This straining creates internal pressure that squeezes the perineum and can damage the perineal blood vessels and nerves.

Who Is Most at Risk for Perineal Injury?

Men who have perineal surgery are most likely to have an acute perineal injury. Straddle injuries are most common among people who ride motorcycles, bikes, or horses and children who use playground equipment. Impalement injuries are most common in military personnel engaged in combat. Impalement injuries can also occur in construction or farm workers.

Chronic perineal injuries are most common in people who ride bikes as part of a job or sport, or in people with constipation.

How Is Perineal Injury Evaluated?

Healthcare providers evaluate perineal injury based on the circumstances and severity of the injury. In general, the evaluation process includes a physical examination and one or more imaging tests.

During a physical examination, the patient lies face up with legs spread and feet in stirrups. The healthcare provider looks for cuts, bruises, or bleeding from the anus. The healthcare provider may insert a gloved, lubricated finger into the rectum to feel for internal injuries.

To look for internal injuries, the healthcare provider may order one or more imaging tests. Imaging is the general term for any technique used to provide pictures of bones and organs inside the body. An X-ray technician performs these procedures in an outpatient center or a hospital, and a radiologist—a doctor who specializes in medical imaging—interprets the images. The person does not need anesthesia. However, people with a fear of confined spaces may receive light sedation before a magnetic resonance imaging (MRI) test.

- **Computerized tomography (CT)** scans use a combination of X-rays and computer technology to create images. For a CT scan, a healthcare provider may give the patient a solution to drink and an injection of a special dye, called "contrast medium." CT scans require the patient to lie on a table that slides into a tunnel-shaped device where an X-ray technician takes the X-rays. CT scans can show traumatic injury to the perineum.

- **Magnetic resonance imaging** is a test that takes pictures of the body's internal organs and soft tissues without using X-rays. An MRI may include the injection of contrast medium. With most MRI machines, the patient will lie on a table that slides into a tunnel-shaped device that may be open ended or closed at one end. During an MRI, the patient, although usually awake, remains perfectly still while the technician takes the images, which usually only takes a few minutes. The technician will take a sequence of images from different angles to create a detailed picture of the perineum. The patient will hear loud mechanical knocking and humming noises. MRI results can show damage to blood vessels and muscles.

- **Ultrasound** uses a device, called a "transducer," that bounces safe, painless sound waves off organs to create an image of their structure. Color Doppler is enhanced ultrasound technology that shows blood flowing through arteries and veins. Blood flowing through arteries appears red, and while blood flowing through veins appears blue. The color Doppler is useful in showing damage to blood vessels in the perineum.

Chapter 31

Noncancerous
Prostate Disorders

Chapter Contents

Section 31.1—Benign Prostatic Hyperplasia 440

Section 31.2—Prostatitis 459

Section 31.1

Benign Prostatic Hyperplasia

This section includes text excerpted from "Prostate Enlargement
(Benign Prostatic Hyperplasia)," National Institute of
Diabetes and Digestive and Kidney Diseases (NIDDK),
September 2014. Reviewed June 2019.

What Is Benign Prostatic Hyperplasia?

Benign prostatic hyperplasia is a condition in men in which the
prostate gland is enlarged and not cancerous. Benign prostatic hyperplasia is also called "benign prostatic hypertrophy" or "benign prostatic
obstruction."

The prostate goes through two main growth periods as a man ages.
The first occurs early in puberty, when the prostate doubles in size.
The second phase of growth begins around the age of 25 and continues
during most of a man's life. Benign prostatic hyperplasia often occurs
with the second growth phase.

As the prostate enlarges, the gland presses against and pinches
the urethra. The bladder wall becomes thicker. Eventually, the
bladder may weaken and lose the ability to empty completely,
leaving some urine in the bladder. The narrowing of the urethra
and urinary retention—the inability to empty the bladder completely—causes many of the problems associated with benign prostatic hyperplasia.

What Is the Prostate?

The prostate is a walnut-shaped gland that is part of the male
reproductive system. The main function of the prostate is to make
a fluid that goes into semen. Prostate fluid is essential for a man's
fertility. The gland surrounds the urethra at the neck of the bladder.
The bladder neck is the area where the urethra joins the bladder.
The bladder and urethra are parts of the lower urinary tract. The
prostate has two or more lobes, or sections, enclosed by an outer
layer of tissue, and it is in front of the rectum, just below the bladder. The urethra is the tube that carries urine from the bladder to
the outside of the body. In men, the urethra also carries semen out
through the penis.

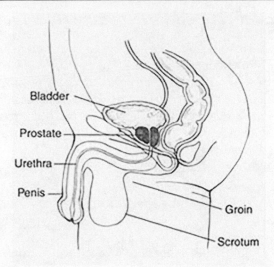

Figure 31.1. *Prostate*

The prostate is a walnut-shaped gland that is part of the male reproductive system.

What Causes Benign Prostatic Hyperplasia

The cause of benign prostatic hyperplasia is not well understood; however, it occurs mainly in older men. Benign prostatic hyperplasia does not develop in men whose testicles were removed before puberty. For this reason, some researchers believe that factors related to aging and the testicles may cause benign prostatic hyperplasia.

Throughout their lives, men produce testosterone, a male hormone, and small amounts of estrogen, a female hormone. As men age, the amount of active testosterone in their blood decreases, which leaves a higher proportion of estrogen. Scientific studies have suggested that benign prostatic hyperplasia may occur because the higher proportion of estrogen within the prostate increases the activity of substances that promote prostate cell growth.

Another theory focuses on dihydrotestosterone (DHT), a male hormone that plays a role in prostate development and growth. Some research has indicated that even with a drop in blood testosterone levels, older men continue to produce and accumulate high levels of DHT in the prostate. This accumulation of DHT may encourage prostate cells to continue to grow. Scientists have noted that men who do not produce DHT do not develop benign prostatic hyperplasia.

How Common Is Benign Prostatic Hyperplasia?

Benign prostatic hyperplasia is the most common prostate problem for men older than the age of 50. In 2010, as many as 14 million men in the United States had lower urinary tract symptoms suggestive of benign prostatic hyperplasia. Although benign prostatic hyperplasia rarely causes symptoms before the age of 40, the occurrence and symptoms increase with age. Benign prostatic hyperplasia affects about 50 percent of men between the ages of 51 and 60 and up to 90 percent of men older than 80 years of age.

Who Is More Likely to Develop Benign Prostatic Hyperplasia?

Men with the following factors are more likely to develop benign prostatic hyperplasia:

- 40 years of age and older
- Family history of benign prostatic hyperplasia
- Medical conditions, such as obesity, heart and circulatory disease, and type 2 diabetes
- Lack of physical exercise
- Erectile dysfunction

What Are the Symptoms of Benign Prostatic Hyperplasia?

Lower urinary tract symptoms suggestive of benign prostatic hyperplasia may include:

- Urinary frequency—urination eight or more times a day
- Urinary urgency—the inability to delay urination
- Trouble starting a urine stream
- A weak or an interrupted urine stream
- Dribbling at the end of urination
- Nocturia—frequent urination during periods of sleep
- Urinary retention
- Urinary incontinence—the accidental loss of urine

- Pain after ejaculation or during urination
- Urine that has an unusual color or smell

Symptoms of benign prostatic hyperplasia most often come from:

- A blocked urethra
- A bladder that is overworked from trying to pass urine through the blockage

The size of the prostate does not always determine the severity of the blockage or symptoms. Some men with greatly enlarged prostates have little blockage and few symptoms, while other men who have minimally enlarged prostates have greater blockage and more symptoms. Less than half of all men with benign prostatic hyperplasia have lower urinary tract symptoms.

Sometimes, men may not know they have a blockage until they cannot urinate. This condition, called "acute urinary retention" (AUR), can result from taking over-the-counter (OTC) cold or allergy medications that contain decongestants, such as pseudoephedrine and oxymetazoline. A potential side effect of these medications may prevent the bladder neck from relaxing and releasing urine. Medications that contain antihistamines, such as diphenhydramine, can weaken the contraction of bladder muscles and cause urinary retention, difficulty urinating, and painful urination. When men have partial urethra blockage, urinary retention also can occur as a result of alcohol consumption, cold temperatures, or a long period of inactivity.

What Are the Complications of Benign Prostatic Hyperplasia?

The complications of benign prostatic hyperplasia may include:

- Acute urinary retention
- Chronic, or long lasting, urinary retention
- Blood in the urine
- Urinary tract infections (UTIs)
- Bladder damage
- Kidney damage
- Bladder stones

Most men with benign prostatic hyperplasia do not develop these complications. However, kidney damage in particular can be a serious health threat when it occurs.

When to Seek Medical Care

A person may have urinary symptoms unrelated to benign prostatic hyperplasia that are caused by bladder problems, UTIs, or prostatitis—inflammation of the prostate. Symptoms of benign prostatic hyperplasia also can signal more serious conditions, including prostate cancer. Men with symptoms of benign prostatic hyperplasia should see a healthcare provider.

Men with the following symptoms should seek immediate medical care:

- Complete inability to urinate

- Painful, frequent, and urgent need to urinate, with fever and chills

- Blood in the urine

- Great discomfort or pain in the lower abdomen and urinary tract

How Is Benign Prostatic Hyperplasia Diagnosed?

A healthcare provider diagnoses benign prostatic hyperplasia based on:

Personal and Family Medical History

Taking a personal and family medical history is one of the first things a healthcare provider may do to help diagnose benign prostatic hyperplasia. A healthcare provider may ask a man:

- What symptoms are present

- When the symptoms began and how often they occur

- Whether he has a history of recurrent UTIs

- What medications he takes, both prescription and over-the-counter

- How much liquid he typically drinks each day

- Whether he consumes caffeine and alcohol

- About his general medical history, including any significant illnesses or surgeries

Physical Exam

A physical exam may help diagnose benign prostatic hyperplasia. During a physical exam, a healthcare provider most often:

- Examines a patient's body, which can include checking for:
  - Discharge from the urethra
  - Enlarged or tender lymph nodes in the groin
  - A swollen or tender scrotum
- Taps on specific areas of the patient's body
- Performs a digital rectal exam

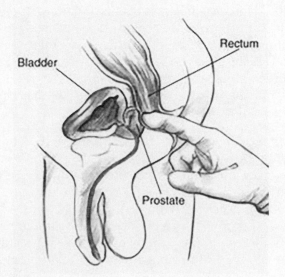

Figure 31.2. *Rectal Exam*

A digital rectal exam, or rectal exam, is a physical exam of the prostate. To perform the exam, the healthcare provider asks the man to bend over a table or lie on his side while holding his knees close to his chest. The healthcare provider slides a gloved, lubricated finger into the rectum and feels the part of the prostate that lies next to the rectum. The man may feel slight, brief discomfort during the rectal exam. A healthcare provider most often performs a rectal exam during an office visit, and men do not require anesthesia. The exam helps the healthcare provider see if the prostate is enlarged or tender or has any abnormalities that require more testing.

Many healthcare providers perform a rectal exam as part of a routine physical exam for men age 40 years of age or older, whether or not they have urinary problems.

Medical Tests

A healthcare provider may refer men to a urologist—a doctor who specializes in urinary problems and the male reproductive system—though the healthcare provider most often diagnoses benign prostatic hyperplasia on the basis of symptoms and a digital rectal exam. A urologist uses medical tests to help diagnose lower urinary tract problems related to benign prostatic hyperplasia and recommend treatment. Medical tests may include:

Urinalysis. Urinalysis involves testing a urine sample. The patient collects a urine sample in a special container in a healthcare provider's office or a commercial facility. A healthcare provider tests the sample during an office visit or sends it to a lab for analysis. For the test, a nurse or technician places a strip of chemically treated paper, called a "dipstick," into the urine. Patches on the dipstick change color to indicate signs of infection in urine.

Prostate-specific antigen (PSA) blood test. A healthcare provider may draw blood for a PSA test during an office visit or in a commercial facility and send the sample to a lab for analysis. Prostate cells create a protein called "prostate-specific antigen" (PSA). Men who have prostate cancer may have a higher amount of PSA in their blood. However, a high PSA level does not necessarily indicate prostate cancer. In fact, benign prostatic hyperplasia, prostate infections, inflammation, aging, and normal fluctuations often cause high PSA levels. Much remains unknown about how to interpret a PSA blood test, the test's ability to discriminate between cancer and prostate conditions, such as benign prostatic hyperplasia, and the best course of action to take if the PSA level is high.

Urodynamic tests. Urodynamic tests include a variety of procedures that look at how well the bladder and urethra store and release urine. A healthcare provider performs urodynamic tests during an office visit or in an outpatient center or a hospital. Some urodynamic tests do not require anesthesia; others may require local anesthesia. Most urodynamic tests focus on the bladder's ability to hold urine and empty steadily and completely and may include the following:

- Uroflowmetry, which measures how rapidly the bladder releases urine

- Postvoid residual measurement, which evaluates how much urine remains in the bladder after urination

- Reduced urine flow or residual urine in the bladder, which often suggests urine blockage due to benign prostatic hyperplasia

Cystoscopy. Cystoscopy is a procedure that uses a tube-like instrument, called a "cystoscope," to look inside the urethra and bladder. A urologist inserts the cystoscope through the opening at the tip of the penis and into the lower urinary tract. A urologist performs cystoscopy during an office visit or in an outpatient center or a hospital. The urologist will give the patient local anesthesia; however, in some cases, the patient may require sedation and regional or general anesthesia. A urologist may use cystoscopy to look for blockage or stones in the urinary tract.

Transrectal ultrasound. Transrectal ultrasound uses a device, called a "transducer," that bounces safe, painless sound waves off organs to create an image of their structure. The healthcare provider can move the transducer to different angles to make it possible to examine different organs. A specially trained technician performs the procedure in a healthcare provider's office, an outpatient center, or a hospital, and a radiologist—a doctor who specializes in medical imaging—interprets the images; the patient does not require anesthesia. Urologists most often use transrectal ultrasound to examine the prostate. In a transrectal ultrasound, the technician inserts a transducer slightly larger than a pen into the man's rectum, next to the prostate. The ultrasound image shows the size of the prostate and any abnormalities, such as tumors. Transrectal ultrasound cannot reliably diagnose prostate cancer.

Biopsy. Biopsy is a procedure that involves taking a small piece of prostate tissue for examination with a microscope. A urologist performs the biopsy in an outpatient center or a hospital. The urologist will give the patient light sedation and local anesthetic; however, in some cases, the patient will require general anesthesia. The urologist uses imaging techniques, such as ultrasound, a computerized tomography (CT) scan, or magnetic resonance imaging (MRI) to guide the biopsy needle into the prostate. A pathologist—a doctor who specializes in examining tissues to diagnose diseases—examines the prostate tissue in a lab. The test can show whether prostate cancer is present.

How Is Benign Prostatic Hyperplasia Treated?

Treatment options for benign prostatic hyperplasia may include:

- Lifestyle changes
- Medications
- Minimally invasive procedures
- Surgery

A healthcare provider treats benign prostatic hyperplasia based on the severity of symptoms, how much the symptoms affect a man's daily life, and a man's preferences.

Men may not need treatment for a mildly enlarged prostate unless their symptoms are bothersome and affecting their quality of life. In these cases, instead of treatment, a urologist may recommend regular checkups. If benign prostatic hyperplasia symptoms become bothersome or present a health risk, a urologist most often recommends treatment.

Lifestyle Changes

A healthcare provider may recommend lifestyle changes for men whose symptoms are mild or slightly bothersome. Lifestyle changes can include:

- Reducing intake of liquids, particularly before going out in public or before periods of sleep
- Avoiding or reducing intake of caffeinated beverages and alcohol
- Avoiding or monitoring the use of medications, such as decongestants, antihistamines, antidepressants, and diuretics
- Training the bladder to hold more urine for longer periods
- Exercising pelvic floor muscles
- Preventing or treating constipation

Medications

A healthcare provider or urologist may prescribe medications that stop the growth of or shrink the prostate or reduce symptoms associated with benign prostatic hyperplasia:

- Alpha-blockers

- Phosphodiesterase-5 inhibitors
- 5-alpha reductase inhibitors
- Combination medications

Alpha-blockers. These medications relax the smooth muscles of the prostate and bladder neck to improve urine flow and reduce bladder blockage:

- Terazosin (Hytrin)
- Doxazosin (Cardura)
- Tamsulosin (Flomax)
- Alfuzosin (Uroxatral)
- Silodosin (Rapaflo)

Phosphodiesterase-5 inhibitors. Urologists prescribe these medications mainly for erectile dysfunction. Tadalafil (Cialis) belongs to this class of medications and can reduce lower urinary tract symptoms by relaxing smooth muscles in the lower urinary tract. Researchers are working to determine the role of erectile dysfunction drugs in the long-term treatment of benign prostatic hyperplasia.

5-alpha reductase inhibitors. These medications block the production of DHT, which accumulates in the prostate and may cause prostate growth:

- Finasteride (Proscar)
- Dutasteride (Avodart)

These medications can prevent the progression of prostate growth or actually shrink the prostate in some men. Finasteride and dutasteride act more slowly than alpha-blockers and are useful for only moderately enlarged prostates.

Combination medications. Several studies, such as the Medical Therapy of Prostatic Symptoms (MTOPS) study, have shown that combining two classes of medications, instead of using just one, can more effectively improve symptoms, urinary flow, and quality of life. The combinations include:

- Finasteride and doxazosin
- Dutasteride and tamsulosin (Jalyn), a combination of both medications that is available in a single tablet

- Alpha-blockers and antimuscarinics

A urologist may prescribe a combination of alpha-blockers and anti-muscarinics for patients with overactive bladder symptoms. Overactive bladder is a condition in which the bladder muscles contract uncontrollably and cause urinary frequency, urinary urgency, and urinary incontinence. Antimuscarinics are a class of medications that relax the bladder muscles.

Minimally Invasive Procedures

Researchers have developed a number of minimally invasive procedures that relieve benign prostatic hyperplasia symptoms when medications prove ineffective. These procedures include:

- Transurethral needle ablation

- Transurethral microwave thermotherapy

- High-intensity focused ultrasound

- Transurethral electrovaporization

- Water-induced thermotherapy

- Prostatic stent insertion

Minimally invasive procedures can destroy enlarged prostate tissue or widen the urethra, which can help relieve blockage and urinary retention caused by benign prostatic hyperplasia.

Urologists perform minimally invasive procedures using the transurethral method, which involves inserting a catheter—a thin, flexible tube—or cystoscope through the urethra to reach the prostate. These procedures may require local, regional, or general anesthesia. Although destroying troublesome prostate tissue relieves many benign prostatic hyperplasia symptoms, tissue destruction does not cure benign prostatic hyperplasia. A urologist will decide which procedure to perform based on the man's symptoms and overall health.

Transurethral needle ablation. This procedure uses heat generated by radiofrequency energy to destroy prostate tissue. A urologist inserts a cystoscope through the urethra to the prostate. A urologist then inserts small needles through the end of the cystoscope and into the prostate. The needles send radiofrequency energy that heats and destroys selected portions of prostate tissue. Shields protect the urethra from heat damage.

Transurethral microwave thermotherapy. This procedure uses microwaves to destroy prostate tissue. A urologist inserts a catheter through the urethra to the prostate, and a device called an "antenna" sends microwaves through the catheter to heat selected portions of the prostate. The temperature becomes high enough inside the prostate to destroy enlarged tissue. A cooling system protects the urinary tract from heat damage during the procedure.

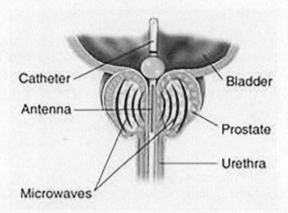

Figure 31.3. *Transurethral Microwave Thermotherapy*

High-intensity focused ultrasound. For this procedure, a urologist inserts a special ultrasound probe into the rectum, near the prostate. Ultrasound waves from the probe heat and destroy enlarged prostate tissue.

Transurethral electrovaporization. For this procedure, a urologist inserts a tube-like instrument called a "resectoscope" through the urethra to reach the prostate. An electrode attached to the resectoscope moves across the surface of the prostate and transmits an electric current that vaporizes prostate tissue. The vaporizing effect penetrates below the surface area being treated and seals blood vessels, which reduces the risk of bleeding.

Water-induced thermotherapy. This procedure uses heated water to destroy prostate tissue. A urologist inserts a catheter into the urethra so that a treatment balloon rests in the middle of the prostate. Heated water flows through the catheter into the treatment balloon, which heats and destroys the surrounding prostate tissue. The treatment balloon can target a specific region of the prostate, while surrounding tissues in the urethra and bladder remain protected.

Prostatic stent insertion. This procedure involves a urologist inserting a small device called a "prostatic stent" through the urethra to the area narrowed by the enlarged prostate. Once in place, the stent expands like a spring, and it pushes back the prostate tissue, widening the urethra. Prostatic stents may be temporary or permanent. Urologists generally use prostatic stents in men who may not tolerate or be suitable for other procedures.

Surgery

For long-term treatment of benign prostatic hyperplasia, a urologist may recommend removing enlarged prostate tissue or making cuts in the prostate to widen the urethra. Urologists recommend surgery when:

- Medications and minimally invasive procedures are ineffective
- Symptoms are particularly bothersome or severe
- Complications arise

Although removing troublesome prostate tissue relieves many benign prostatic hyperplasia symptoms, tissue removal does not cure benign prostatic hyperplasia.

Surgery to remove enlarged prostate tissue includes:

- Transurethral resection of the prostate (TURP)
- Laser surgery
- Open prostatectomy
- Transurethral incision of the prostate (TUIP)

A urologist performs these surgeries, except for open prostatectomy, using the transurethral method. Men who have these surgical procedures require local, regional, or general anesthesia and may need to stay in the hospital.

The urologist may prescribe antibiotics before or soon after surgery to prevent infection. Some urologists prescribe antibiotics only when an infection occurs.

Immediately after benign prostatic hyperplasia surgery, a urologist may insert a special catheter, called a "Foley catheter," through the opening of the penis to drain urine from the bladder into a drainage pouch.

Transurethral resection of the prostate. With TURP, a urologist inserts a resectoscope through the urethra to reach the prostate and cuts pieces of enlarged prostate tissue with a wire loop. Special fluid carries the tissue pieces into the bladder, and the urologist flushes them out at the end of the procedure. TURP is the most common surgery for benign prostatic hyperplasia and is considered the gold standard for treating blockage of the urethra due to benign prostatic hyperplasia.

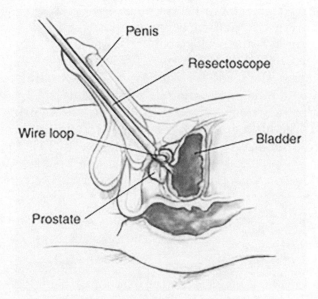

Figure 31.4. *Transurethral Resection of the Prostate*

Laser surgery. With this surgery, a urologist uses a high-energy laser to destroy prostate tissue. The urologist uses a cystoscope to pass a laser fiber through the urethra into the prostate. The laser destroys the enlarged tissue. The risk of bleeding is lower than in TURP and TUIP because the laser seals blood vessels as it cuts through the prostate tissue. However, laser surgery may not effectively treat greatly enlarged prostates.

Open prostatectomy. In an open prostatectomy, a urologist makes an incision, or cut, through the skin to reach the prostate. The urologist can remove all or part of the prostate through the incision. This surgery is used most often when the prostate is greatly enlarged, complications occur, or the bladder is damaged and needs repair. Open prostatectomy requires general anesthesia, a longer hospital stay than other surgical procedures for benign prostatic hyperplasia, and a longer rehabilitation period. The three open prostatectomy procedures are retropubic prostatectomy, suprapubic prostatectomy, and perineal prostatectomy. The recovery period for open prostatectomy is different for each man who undergoes the procedure.

Transurethral incision of the prostate. A TUIP is a surgical procedure to widen the urethra. During a TUIP, the urologist inserts a cystoscope and an instrument that uses an electric current or a laser beam through the urethra to reach the prostate. The urologist widens the urethra by making a few small cuts in the prostate and in the bladder neck. Some urologists believe that TUIP gives the same relief as TURP except with less risk of side effects.

After surgery, the prostate, urethra, and surrounding tissues may be irritated and swollen, causing urinary retention. To prevent urinary retention, a urologist inserts a Foley catheter so urine can drain freely out of the bladder. A Foley catheter has a balloon on the end that the urologist inserts into the bladder. Once the balloon is inside the bladder, the urologist fills it with sterile water to keep the catheter in place. Men who undergo minimally invasive procedures may not need a Foley catheter.

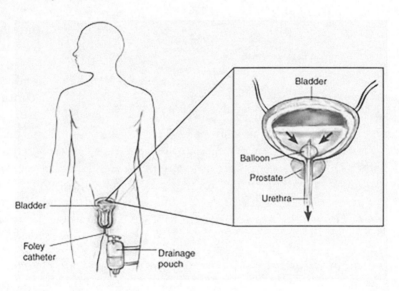

Figure 31.5. *Foley Catheter*

The Foley catheter most often remains in place for several days. Sometimes, the Foley catheter causes recurring, painful, difficult-to-control bladder spasms the day after surgery. However, these spasms will eventually stop. A urologist may prescribe medications to relax bladder muscles and prevent bladder spasms.

These medications include:

- Oxybutynin chloride (Ditropan)
- Solifenacin (VESIcare)
- Darifenacin (Enablex)
- Tolterodine (Detrol)
- Hyoscyamine (Levsin)
- Propantheline bromide (Pro-Banthine)

What Are the Complications of Benign Prostatic Hyperplasia Treatment?

The complications of benign prostatic hyperplasia treatment depend on the type of treatment.

Medications

Medications used to treat benign prostatic hyperplasia may have side effects that sometimes can be serious. Men who are prescribed medications to treat benign prostatic hyperplasia should discuss possible side effects with a healthcare provider before taking the medications. Men who experience the following side effects should contact a healthcare provider right away or get emergency medical care:

- Hives
- Rash
- Itching
- Shortness of breath
- Rapid, pounding, or irregular heartbeat
- Painful erection of the penis that lasts for hours
- Swelling of the eyes, face, tongue, lips, throat, arms, hands, feet, ankles, or lower legs
- Difficulty breathing or swallowing
- Chest pain
- Dizziness or fainting when standing up suddenly
- Sudden decrease or loss of vision

- Blurred vision

- Sudden decrease or loss of hearing

- Chest pain, dizziness, or nausea during sexual activity

These side effects are mostly related to phosphodiesterase-5 inhibitors. Side effects related to alpha-blockers include:

- Dizziness or fainting when standing up suddenly

- Decreased sexual drive

- Problems with ejaculation

Minimally Invasive Procedures

Complications after minimally invasive procedures may include:

- UTIs

- Painful urination

- Difficulty urinating

- An urgent or a frequent need to urinate

- Urinary incontinence

- Blood in the urine for several days after the procedure

- Sexual dysfunction

- Chronic prostatitis—long-lasting inflammation of the prostate

- Recurring problems, such as urinary retention and UTIs

Most of the complications of minimally invasive procedures go away within a few days or weeks. Minimally invasive procedures are less likely to have complications than surgery.

Surgery

Complications after surgery may include:

- Problems urinating

- Urinary incontinence

- Bleeding and blood clots

- Infection

- Scar tissue

- Sexual dysfunction

- Recurring problems, such as urinary retention and UTIs

Problems urinating. Men may initially have painful urination or difficulty urinating. They may experience urinary frequency, urgency, or retention. These problems will gradually lessen, and after a couple of months, urination will be easier and less frequent.

Urinary incontinence. As the bladder returns to normal, men may have some temporary problems controlling urination. However, long-term urinary incontinence rarely occurs. The longer urinary problems existed before surgery, the longer it takes for the bladder to regain its full function after surgery.

Bleeding and blood clots. After benign prostatic hyperplasia surgery, the prostate or tissues around it may bleed. Blood or blood clots may appear in urine. Some bleeding is normal and should clear up within several days. However, men should contact a healthcare provider right away if:

- They experience pain or discomfort.

- Their urine contains large clots.

- Their urine is so red it is difficult to see through.

Blood clots from benign prostatic hyperplasia surgery can pass into the bloodstream and lodge in other parts of the body—most often in the legs. Men should contact a healthcare provider right away if they experience swelling or discomfort in their legs.

Infection. Use of a Foley catheter after benign prostatic hyperplasia surgery may increase the risk of a UTI. Anesthesia during surgery may cause urinary retention and also increase the risk of a UTI. In addition, the incision site of an open prostatectomy may become infected. A healthcare provider will prescribe antibiotics to treat infections.

Scar tissue. In the year after the original surgery, scar tissue sometimes forms and requires surgical treatment. Scar tissue may form in the urethra and cause it to narrow. A urologist can solve this problem during an office visit by stretching the urethra. Rarely, the opening of the bladder becomes scarred and shrinks, causing blockage. This problem may require a surgical procedure similar to TUIP.

Sexual dysfunction. Some men may experience temporary problems with sexual function after benign prostatic hyperplasia surgery. The length of time for restored sexual function depends on the type of benign prostatic hyperplasia surgery performed and how long symptoms were present before surgery. Many men have found that concerns about sexual function can interfere with sex as much as the benign prostatic hyperplasia surgery itself. Understanding the surgical procedure and talking about concerns with a healthcare provider before surgery often help men regain sexual function earlier. Many men find it helpful to talk with a counselor during the adjustment period after surgery. Even though it can take a while for sexual function to fully return, with time, most men can enjoy sex again.

Most healthcare providers agree that if men with benign prostatic hyperplasia were able to maintain an erection before surgery, they will probably be able to have erections afterward. Surgery rarely causes a loss of erectile function. However, benign prostatic hyperplasia surgery most often cannot restore function that was lost before the procedure. Some men find a slight difference in the quality of orgasm after surgery. However, most report no difference.

Prostate surgery may make men sterile, or unable to father children, by causing retrograde ejaculation—the backward flow of semen into the bladder. Men flush the semen out of the bladder when they urinate. In some cases, medications, such as pseudoephedrine, found in many cold medications, or imipramine can treat retrograde ejaculation. These medications improve muscle tone at the bladder neck and keep semen from entering the bladder.

Recurring problems. Men may require further treatment if prostate problems, including benign prostatic hyperplasia, return. Problems may arise when treatments for benign prostatic hyperplasia leave a good part of the prostate intact. About 10 percent of men treated with TURP or TUIP require additional surgery within 5 years. About 2 percent of men who have an open prostatectomy require additional surgery within 5 years.

In the years after benign prostatic hyperplasia surgery or treatment, men should continue having a digital rectal exam once a year and have any symptoms checked by a healthcare provider. In some cases, the healthcare provider may recommend a digital rectal exam and checkup more than once a year.

How Can Benign Prostatic Hyperplasia Be Prevented?

Researchers have not found a way to prevent benign prostatic hyperplasia. Men with risk factors for benign prostatic hyperplasia should talk with a healthcare provider about any lower urinary tract symptoms and the need for regular prostate exams. Men can get early treatment and minimize benign prostatic hyperplasia effects by recognizing lower urinary tract symptoms and identifying an enlarged prostate.

Eating, Diet, and Nutrition

Researchers have not found that eating, diet, and nutrition play a role in causing or preventing benign prostatic hyperplasia. However, a healthcare provider can give information about how changes in eating, diet, or nutrition could help with treatment. Men should talk with a healthcare provider or dietitian about what diet is right for them.

Section 31.2

Prostatitis

This section includes text excerpted from "Prostatitis: Inflammation of the Prostate," National Institute of Diabetes and Digestive and Kidney Diseases (NIDDK), July 2014. Reviewed June 2019.

What Is Prostatitis?

Prostatitis is a frequently painful condition that involves inflammation of the prostate and sometimes the areas around the prostate. Scientists have identified four types of prostatitis:

- Chronic prostatitis or chronic pelvic pain syndrome
- Acute bacterial prostatitis
- Chronic bacterial prostatitis
- Asymptomatic inflammatory prostatitis

Men with asymptomatic inflammatory prostatitis do not have symptoms. A healthcare provider may diagnose asymptomatic inflammatory prostatitis when testing for other urinary tract or reproductive tract disorders. This type of prostatitis does not cause complications and does not need treatment.

What Causes Prostatitis

The causes of prostatitis differ depending on the type.

Chronic prostatitis or chronic pelvic pain syndrome. The exact cause of chronic prostatitis/chronic pelvic pain syndrome is unknown. Researchers believe a microorganism, though not a bacterial infection, may cause the condition. This type of prostatitis may relate to chemicals in the urine, the immune system's response to a previous urinary tract infection (UTI), or nerve damage in the pelvic area.

Acute and chronic bacterial prostatitis. A bacterial infection of the prostate causes bacterial prostatitis. The acute type happens suddenly and lasts a short time, while the chronic type develops slowly and lasts a long time, often years. The infection may occur when bacteria travel from the urethra into the prostate.

How Common Is Prostatitis?

Prostatitis is the most common urinary tract problem for men younger than the age of 50 and the third most common urinary tract problem for men older than the age of 50. Prostatitis accounts for about two million visits to healthcare providers in the United States each year.

Chronic prostatitis or chronic pelvic pain syndrome is:

- The most common and least understood form of prostatitis
- Can occur in men of any age group
- Affects 10 to 15 percent of the U.S. male population

Who Is More Likely to Develop Prostatitis?

The factors that affect a man's chances of developing prostatitis differ depending on the type.

Chronic prostatitis/chronic pelvic pain syndrome. Men with nerve damage in the lower urinary tract due to surgery or trauma may be more likely to develop chronic prostatitis/chronic pelvic pain syndrome. Psychological stress may also increase a man's chances of developing the condition.

Acute and chronic bacterial prostatitis. Men with lower UTIs may be more likely to develop bacterial prostatitis. UTIs that recur or are difficult to treat may lead to chronic bacterial prostatitis.

What Are the Symptoms of Prostatitis?

Each type of prostatitis has a range of symptoms that vary depending on the cause and may not be the same for every man. Many symptoms are similar to those of other conditions.

Chronic prostatitis/chronic pelvic pain syndrome. The main symptoms of chronic prostatitis/chronic pelvic pain syndrome can include pain or discomfort lasting three or more months in one or more of the following areas:

• Between the scrotum and anus

• The central lower abdomen

• The penis

• The scrotum

• The lower back

Pain during or after ejaculation is another common symptom. A man with chronic prostatitis/chronic pelvic pain syndrome may have pain spread out around the pelvic area or may have pain in one or more areas at the same time. The pain may come and go and appear suddenly or gradually.

Other symptoms may include:

• Pain in the urethra during or after urination

• Pain in the penis during or after urination

• Urinary frequency—urination eight or more times a day. The bladder begins to contract even when it contains small amounts of urine, causing more frequent urination.

• Urinary urgency—the inability to delay urination

• A weak or an interrupted urine stream

Acute bacterial prostatitis. The symptoms of acute bacterial prostatitis come on suddenly and are severe. Men should seek immediate medical care. Symptoms of acute bacterial prostatitis may include:

- Urinary frequency
- Urinary urgency
- Fever
- Chills
- A burning feeling or pain during urination
- Pain in the genital area, groin, lower abdomen, or lower back
- Nocturia—frequent urination during periods of sleep
- Nausea and vomiting
- Body aches
- Urinary retention—the inability to empty the bladder completely
- Trouble starting a urine stream
- A weak or an interrupted urine stream
- Urinary blockage—the complete inability to urinate
- A UTI—as shown by bacteria and infection-fighting cells in the urine

Chronic bacterial prostatitis. The symptoms of chronic bacterial prostatitis are similar to those of acute bacterial prostatitis, though not as severe. This type of prostatitis often develops slowly and can last three months or more. The symptoms may come and go, or they may be mild all the time. Chronic bacterial prostatitis may occur after previous treatment of acute bacterial prostatitis or a UTI. The symptoms of chronic bacterial prostatitis may include:

- Urinary frequency
- Urinary urgency
- A burning feeling or pain during urination
- Pain in the genital area, groin, lower abdomen, or lower back
- Nocturia
- Painful ejaculation
- Urinary retention

- Trouble starting a urine stream
- A weak or an interrupted urine stream
- Urinary blockage
- A UTI

What Are the Complications of Prostatitis?

The complications of prostatitis may include:

- Bacterial infection in the bloodstream
- Prostatic abscess—a pus-filled cavity in the prostate
- Sexual dysfunction
- Inflammation of reproductive organs near the prostate

When to Seek Medical Care

A person may have urinary symptoms unrelated to prostatitis that are caused by bladder problems, UTIs, or benign prostatic hyperplasia. Symptoms of prostatitis also can signal more serious conditions, including prostate cancer. Men with symptoms of prostatitis should see a healthcare provider.

Men with the following symptoms should seek immediate medical care:

- Complete inability to urinate
- Painful, frequent, and urgent need to urinate, with fever and chills
- Blood in the urine
- Great discomfort or pain in the lower abdomen and urinary tract

How Is Prostatitis Treated?

Treatment depends on the type of prostatitis.

Chronic prostatitis/chronic pelvic pain syndrome. Treatment for chronic prostatitis/chronic pelvic pain syndrome aims to decrease pain, discomfort, and inflammation. A wide range of symptoms exists and no single treatment works for every man. Although antibiotics will not help treat nonbacterial prostatitis, a urologist may prescribe them, at least initially, until the urologist can rule out a bacterial infection. A urologist may prescribe other medications:

- Silodo

- Sin (Rapaflo)

- 5-alpha reductase inhibitors, such as finasteride (Proscar) and dutasteride (Avodart)

- Nonsteroidal anti-inflammatory drugs—also called "nonsteroidal anti-inflammatory drugs" (NSAIDs)—such as aspirin, ibuprofen, and Naproxen sodium

- Glycosaminogly

- Cans, such as chondroitin sulfate

- Muscle relaxants, such as cyclobenzaprine (Amrix, Flexeril) and clonazepam (Klonopin)

- Neuromodulators, such as amitriptyline, nortriptyline (Aventyl, Pamelor), and pregabalin (Lyrica)

Alternative treatments may include:

- Warm baths, called "sitz baths"

- Local heat therapy with hot water bottles or heating pads

- Physical therapy, such as:

- Kegel exercises—tightening and relaxing the muscles that hold urine in the bladder and hold the bladder in its proper position. Also called "pelvic muscle exercises."

- Myofascial release—pressing and stretching, sometimes with cooling and warming, of the muscles and soft tissues in the lower back, pelvic region, and upper legs. Also known as "myofascial trigger point release."

- Relaxation exercises

- Biofeedback

- Phytotherapy with plant extracts, such as quercetin, bee pollen, and saw palmetto

- Acupuncture

To help ensure coordinated and safe care, people should discuss their use of complementary and alternative medical practices, including their use of dietary supplements, with their healthcare provider.

For men whose chronic prostatitis/chronic pelvic pain syndrome symptoms are affected by psychological stress, appropriate psychiatric treatment and stress reduction may reduce the recurrence of symptoms.

Acute bacterial prostatitis. A urologist treats acute bacterial prostatitis with antibiotics. The antibiotic prescribed may depend on the type of bacteria causing the infection. Urologists usually prescribe oral antibiotics for at least two weeks. The infection may come back; therefore, some urologists recommend taking oral antibiotics for six to eight weeks. Severe cases of acute prostatitis may require a short hospital stay so men can receive fluids and antibiotics through an intravenous (IV) tube. After the IV treatment, the man will need to take oral antibiotics for two to four weeks. Most cases of acute bacterial prostatitis clear up completely with medication and slight changes to diet. The urologist may recommend:

- Avoiding or reducing intake of substances that irritate the bladder, such as alcohol, caffeinated beverages, and acidic and spicy foods

- Increasing intake of liquids—64 to 128 ounces per day—to urinate often and help flush bacteria from the bladder

Chronic bacterial prostatitis. A urologist treats chronic bacterial prostatitis with antibiotics; however, treatment requires a longer course of therapy. The urologist may prescribe a low dose of antibiotics for up to six months to prevent recurrent infection. The urologist may also prescribe a different antibiotic or use a combination of antibiotics if the infection keeps coming back. The urologist may recommend increasing intake of liquids and avoiding or reducing intake of substances that irritate the bladder.

A urologist may use alpha-blockers that treat chronic prostatitis/chronic pelvic pain syndrome to treat urinary retention caused by chronic bacterial prostatitis. These medications help relax the bladder muscles near the prostate and lessen symptoms, such as painful urination. Men may require surgery to treat urinary retention caused by chronic bacterial prostatitis. Surgically removing scar tissue in the urethra often improves urine flow and reduces urinary retention.

How Can Prostatitis Be Prevented?

Men cannot prevent prostatitis. Researchers are currently seeking to better understand what causes prostatitis and develop prevention strategies.

Chapter 32

Sexual Dysfunction

Sexual dysfunction can refer to any physical or psychological problem that disrupts the sexual response cycle and prevents an individual or couple from achieving satisfaction. More than 30 percent of men report experiencing some sort of sexual dysfunction during their lives. The most common types of male sexual dysfunction include erectile dysfunction (ED) and premature ejaculation (PE). Less common conditions that may result in male sexual dysfunction include priapism and retrograde ejaculation. A variety of treatment options are available to help men overcome sexual dysfunction and enjoy satisfying intimate relations.

Erectile Dysfunction

Erectile dysfunction (formerly known as "impotence") is a condition in which a man has trouble achieving an erection or sustaining it long enough for sexual intercourse. Researchers believe that ED affects 30 million men in the United States, including about 30 percent of men over the age of 70. ED can be caused by a variety of diseases and conditions that affect the nerves and arteries, as well as by some medications commonly prescribed to treat such conditions. Lifestyle choices can also contribute to ED, as can psychological or emotional issues. Some of the conditions that are often related to ED include:

- High blood pressure

"Sexual Dysfunction," © 2017 Omnigraphics. Reviewed June 2019.

- Diabetes

- Cardiovascular disease

- Atherosclerosis (formation of plaque in the arteries)

- Kidney disease

- Multiple sclerosis

- Peyronie disease (formation of scar tissue in the penis)

- Injury to the penis, prostate, pelvis, or spinal cord

- Prostate cancer and related treatments

- Lifestyle choices, such as smoking, excessive alcohol consumption, illegal-drug use, poor diet, lack of exercise, and being overweight

- Psychological issues, such as anxiety, depression, stress, guilt, low self-esteem, or fear of sexual failure

- Medications, such as antihistamines, antidepressants, appetite suppressants, blood pressure medications, and ulcer medications

Although some men may feel reluctant to acknowledge or discuss erectile dysfunction, it is important to seek medical attention if the problem persists for more than a few weeks or months. ED can be a sign of other health conditions, such as diabetes or heart disease, that may be developing or worsening. In addition, ED can cause both health and relationship complications if left untreated.

Diagnosis of Erectile Dysfunction

To diagnose erectile dysfunction, a urologist or other healthcare provider will typically begin by discussing the patient's medical and sexual history. The doctor will ask about health conditions, medications, and lifestyle decisions that may contribute to ED. They will also inquire about the patient's ability to get an erection, maintain an erection hard enough for penetration and intercourse, and reach climax and ejaculate. The doctor may also use a questionnaire or other tools to assess psychological or emotional factors that may contribute to ED.

The next step in diagnosing ED typically involves a physical examination. The doctor may check for high blood pressure, circulatory problems, or hormonal changes that may contribute to ED. Blood tests may be ordered to check for signs of underlying health conditions, such as diabetes, cardiovascular disease, or kidney disease.

The doctor may also examine the penis for unusual characteristics or lack of sensitivity.

There are three main diagnostic tests that are used to help determine the underlying cause of ED:

- Injection test

  This test involves injecting medication into the urethra or into the base of the penis to cause an erection. It allows the doctor to evaluate the hardness of the penis and the duration of the erection.

- Doppler ultrasound

  This imaging exam, which is often conducted in combination with an injection test, enables the doctor to measure the speed and direction of blood flow through the penis.

- Nocturnal erection test

  Most men have between three and five erections each night while asleep. This test is used to determine whether a patient is physically capable of having an erection, which may indicate that the cause of ED is psychological in nature. It may be performed in a sleep laboratory using electronic monitoring equipment to record the number of erections, their firmness, and how long they last. A simpler version may be done at home by placing a plastic ring around the penis that will break if the patient has a nocturnal erection.

Treatment of Erectile Dysfunction

Erectile dysfunction can be treated in a variety of ways, depending on the extent of the problem and the underlying cause. Some of the treatment options include:

- Lifestyle changes, such as eating a healthy diet, exercising regularly, losing weight, and not smoking or consuming excessive alcohol

- Treatment of underlying health conditions, such as diabetes or cardiovascular disease

- Psychological counseling to address self-esteem issues or performance anxiety

- Oral medications designed to increase blood flow to the penis, such as sildenafil (Viagra), vardenafil (Levitra), or tadalafil (Cialis)

- Medications, such as alprostadil (Caverject, Edex) that are administered directly to the penis, either via injection or a suppository that is inserted into the urethra

- Use of a vacuum device to pump blood into the penis manually, coupled with an elastic ring at the base of the penis to help maintain the erection

- Surgery to reconstruct arteries that supply blood to the penis

- Surgery to implant an inflatable or malleable prosthetic device in the penis

Some forms of treatment involve risks or side effects, so men with ED should research their options carefully and choose the one that works best for them and their partners.

Premature Ejaculation

Premature ejaculation (PE) is a common form of sexual dysfunction in which a man consistently reaches orgasm and ejaculates sooner than he or his partner would like during sexual activity. Ejaculation occurs when muscles at the base of the penis contract, forcing semen from the prostate gland to be released from the erect penis. It usually takes place at the same time as orgasm or sexual climax, and the erection typically dissipates afterward. Premature ejaculation usually occurs with very little stimulation, or within one to two minutes of penetration.

Surveys suggest that one-third of men experience PE at least occasionally, although doctors believe that only about two percent suffer from primary or lifelong PE, meaning that they climax too early during nearly every sexual encounter. PE can lead to negative personal consequences for men, including frustration, embarrassment, worry, anxiety, and avoidance of sexual intimacy. In many cases, however, the man who experiences PE is much more concerned about it than is his sexual partner.

Causes of Premature Ejaculation

Some cases of PE are related to underlying medical conditions, such as diabetes, high blood pressure, multiple sclerosis, prostate disease, thyroid problems, or nerve damage due to injury or surgery. Lifestyle choices, such as illegal drug use or alcohol abuse, can also increase the likelihood of PE. In addition, some studies suggest that low levels of serotonin in the brain may act to shorten the time to ejaculation.

In most cases, however, the primary causes of PE are not biological but psychological in nature. Some of the common factors that can lead to PE include:

- Sexual inexperience

- Overexcitement or overstimulation

- Unrealistic expectations about sexual performance

- Lack of confidence or self-esteem

- Relationship problems

- Intimacy issues

- Guilt, anxiety, stress, or depression

- Early sexual trauma or history of sexual repression

- Conditioning oneself to ejaculate quickly while masturbating

Diagnosis and Treatment of Premature Ejaculation

To diagnose PE, a urologist or other healthcare provider will usually take a medical and sexual history and conduct a physical examination. They will typically ask a series of questions to assess the patient's symptoms and help determine the cause of the problem, such as how often PE occurs, whether it happens in every sexual encounter or only under certain circumstances, how long the patient is able to delay ejaculation, and the extent to which PE has affected the patient's sexual activity and quality of life.

Most treatments for PE involve therapy to address the psychological issues that contribute to the problem, as well as exercises and medications to help the patient delay ejaculation. Up to 95 percent of patients with PE show improvement through some combination of the following treatments:

- Psychological therapy to help patients uncover the source of negative feelings that may interfere with sexual performance

- Couples counseling or sex therapy to improve communication, intimacy, and sexual satisfaction

- Relaxation techniques to reduce performance anxiety and increase confidence

- Exercises to help the patient learn to control and delay ejaculation, such as the squeeze method (squeezing the penis firmly just before the point of climax) or the start-stop method (stimulating the penis to the point of climax and then stopping until the patient regains control)

- Condom use to reduce sensation in the penis

- Topical anesthetic creams or sprays, such as lidocaine or prilocaine, applied 30 minutes before intercourse to numb the penis

- Antidepressant medications, such as fluoxetine, paroxetine, sertraline, and clomipramine that affect serotonin levels in the brain and delay orgasm in some patients

Priapism

Priapism is a rare but serious medical condition in which an erection lasts more than four hours. This persistent erection is not caused by sexual stimulation, and it does not dissipate after ejaculation. Instead, it occurs when blood becomes trapped in the penis due to problems with nerves or blood vessels. Left untreated, priapism can cause permanent damage to the penis and result in sexual dysfunction. There are three main types of priapism:

- Low blood flow or ischemic priapism

  The most common form of priapism, it occurs due to blockage of a blood vessel that prevents blood from flowing normally through the penis. The blockage prevents oxygen- and nutrient-rich blood from reaching the penile tissue, which can cause permanent damage if not treated promptly.

- High blood flow priapism

  This rare condition occurs when a blood vessel ruptures, causing excessive blood to flow into the penile tissue. It usually results from an injury to the genital area.

- Stuttering or episodic priapism

  This condition involves recurring, painful erections that last between two and three hours. They may occur during sleep or before or after sexual stimulation, and their frequency may increase over time. The causes and risk factors are usually similar to low blood flow priapism.

Causes of Priapism

Priapism can have a number of underlying causes, including the following:

- Prescription medications that are commonly used to treat high blood pressure, attention deficit hyperactivity disorder (ADHD), depression, schizophrenia, and hormone imbalances

- Injectable medications that are used to treat ED

- Illegal drugs, such as marijuana, ecstasy, cocaine, or methamphetamine (crystal meth)

- Sickle cell disease (an inherited condition in which the body produces abnormally shaped red blood cells that can interfere with the function of blood vessels)

- Blood cancers, such as leukemia and multiple myeloma

- Injuries or medical conditions that affect the nervous system, brain, or spinal cord

- Tumors of the prostate, bladder, or kidney

- Infections in the genital area

Diagnosis and Treatment of Priapism

In addition to taking a medical history and performing a physical examination, a urologist or other practitioner will likely order blood tests and diagnostic tests to determine the type of priapism. These tests may include blood-gas analysis of blood taken from the penile tissue, color duplex ultrasound to measure blood flow in the penis, or magnetic resonance imaging (MRI) to detect possible tumors or blood clots.

To relieve the immediate symptoms of priapism and restore normal blood flow, applying ice packs to the penis and perineum or exercising vigorously may be helpful. In other cases, a doctor may need to drain the trapped blood manually by inserting a needle into the penis. A vasoconstrictor medication may also be injected to help reduce the size of blood vessels and improve blood flow.

The recommended treatment for priapism depends on the underlying cause. If priapism occurs as a side effect of medication, the doctor may recommend stopping the medication and trying an alternative prescription. For stuttering priapism, a medication called "phenylephrine" may be prescribed to help control blood flow to the penis and prevent further episodes. For priapism resulting from a blood clot, surgery may be needed to remove the clot. High blood flow priapism resolves itself without treatment in about two-thirds of men, while the remaining cases require surgery to repair the ruptured blood vessels. If priapism causes tissue damage, resulting in sexual dysfunction, the patient may require surgery to implant a penile prosthesis.

Retrograde Ejaculation

Retrograde ejaculation (also known as "dry climax") is a rare condition in which semen flows backward and enters the bladder during ejaculation, rather than flowing out of the body through the penis. Under normal circumstances, the bladder sphincter muscle contracts just before ejaculation, which prevents semen from entering the bladder and forces it out through the urethra. In retrograde ejaculation, the sphincter malfunctions and remains open. The condition is not harmful—and the semen is soon eliminated in the form of urine—but it can decrease fertility.

Symptoms and Causes of Retrograde Ejaculation

Men with retrograde ejaculation will notice that little to no fluid is released from the penis when they ejaculate. In addition, their urine may appear cloudy following orgasms, and urinalysis results will show the presence of sperm.

The most common causes of retrograde ejaculation include uncontrolled diabetes and side effects of medications used to treat high blood pressure, depression, and anxiety. Surgery for prostate or urethra disorders can also cause retrograde ejaculation. Nerve damage from multiple sclerosis or a spinal cord injury can also affect the function of the bladder sphincter muscle.

Treatment of Retrograde Ejaculation

Since retrograde ejaculation is not harmful, no treatment is needed unless the condition interferes with fertility. In that case, a urologist or other healthcare provider may recommend that the patient reduce the dosage or stop taking any medications that may contribute to the condition. For retrograde ejaculation caused by diabetes, the condition may improve if the patient maintains good control over blood sugar. Medications, such as pseudoephedrine or imipramine have also shown positive results in improving muscle tone in the bladder sphincter so that it closes during ejaculation. Collagen injections into the bladder neck or surgical reconstruction of the sphincter muscles are other possible treatments to improve contraction.

If retrograde ejaculation persists following treatment, assisted reproductive technologies can be used to improve the chances of conception. One approach involves harvesting sperm from the bladder or gathering them from a urine sample for use in artificial insemination procedures. Of course, the success of such infertility procedures depends not only on the viability of the man's sperm but also on his partner's fertility.

References

1. "Erectile Dysfunction," National Institute of Diabetes and Digestive and Kidney Diseases (NIDDK), November 2015.

2. MacGill, Markus. "Premature Ejaculation: Causes and Treatments," Medical News Today, July 5, 2016.

3. "Priapism," MyDr, June 25, 2016.

4. "Retrograde Ejaculation," Norman Regional Health Center, 2012.

5. "Retrograde Ejaculation Treatments," Urologists.org, n.d.

6. "What Is Premature Ejaculation?" Urology Care Foundation, 2016.

Chapter 33

Male Infertility

What Is Infertility?

In general, "infertility" is defined as not being able to get pregnant (conceive) after 1 year (or longer) of unprotected sex.

Pregnancy is the result of a process that has many steps.

To get pregnant:

- A woman's body must release an egg from one of her ovaries, (ovulation)

- A man's sperm must join with the egg along the way (fertilize)

- The fertilized egg must go through a fallopian tube toward the uterus (womb)

- The fertilized egg must attach to the inside of the uterus (implantation)

Infertility may result from a problem with any or several of these steps.

Impaired fecundity is a condition related to infertility and refers to women who have difficulty getting pregnant or carrying a pregnancy to term.

This chapter includes text excerpted from "Infertility FAQs," Centers for Disease Control and Prevention (CDC), January 16, 2019.

Is Infertility Just a Woman's Problem?

No, infertility is not always a woman's problem. Both men and women can contribute to infertility.

Many couples struggle with infertility and seek help to become pregnant, but it is often thought of as only a woman's condition. However, in about 35 percent of couples with infertility, a male factor is identified along with a female factor. In about 8 percent of couples with infertility, a male factor is the only identifiable cause.

Almost 9 percent of men between 25 and 44 years of age in the United States reported that they or their partner saw a doctor for advice, testing, or treatment for infertility during their lifetime.

What Causes Infertility in Men

Infertility in men can be caused by different factors and is typically evaluated by a semen analysis. When a semen analysis is performed, the number of sperm (concentration), motility (movement), and morphology (shape) are assessed by a specialist. A slightly abnormal semen analysis does not mean that a man is necessarily infertile. Instead, a semen analysis helps determine if and how malefactors are contributing to infertility.

Disruption of Testicular or Ejaculatory Function

- Varicoceles, a condition in which the veins on a man's testicles are large and cause them to overheat. The heat may affect the number or shape of the sperm.

- Trauma to the testes may affect sperm production and result in lower number of sperm.

- Unhealthy habits, such as heavy alcohol use, smoking, anabolic steroid use, and illicit drug use

- Use of certain medications and supplements

- Cancer treatment involving the use of certain types of chemotherapy, radiation, or surgery to remove one or both testicles

- Medical conditions, such as diabetes, cystic fibrosis, certain types of autoimmune disorders, and certain types of infections, may cause testicular failure.

Hormonal Disorders

- Improper function of the hypothalamus or pituitary glands. The hypothalamus and pituitary glands in the brain produce hormones that maintain normal testicular function. Production of too much prolactin, a hormone made by the pituitary gland (often due to the presence of a benign pituitary gland tumor), or other conditions that damage or impair the function of the hypothalamus or the pituitary gland may result in low or no sperm production.

- These conditions may include benign and malignant (cancerous) pituitary tumors, congenital adrenal hyperplasia, exposure to too much estrogen, exposure to too much testosterone, Cushing syndrome, and chronic use of medications called "glucocorticoids."

Genetic Disorders

- Genetic conditions, such as a Klinefelter syndrome; Y-chromosome microdeletion; myotonic dystrophy; and other, less common genetic disorders, may cause no sperm to be produced, or low numbers of sperm to be produced.

What Increases a Man's Risk of Infertility

- Age. Although advanced age plays a much more important role in predicting female infertility, couples in which the male partner is 40 years of age or older are more likely to report difficulty conceiving.

- Being overweight or obese

- Smoking

- Excessive alcohol use

- Use of marijuana

- Exposure to testosterone. This may occur when a doctor prescribes testosterone injections, implants, or topical gel for low testosterone, or when a man takes testosterone or similar medications illicitly for the purposes of increasing their muscle mass.

- Exposure to radiation

- Frequent exposure of the testes to high temperatures, such as that which may occur in men confined to a wheelchair, or through frequent sauna or hot tub use

- Exposure to certain medications, such as flutamide, cyproterone, bicalutamide, spironolactone, ketoconazole, or cimetidine

- Exposure to environmental toxins including exposure to pesticides, lead, cadmium, or mercury

What Are Some of the Specific Treatments for Male Infertility?

Male infertility may be treated with medical, surgical, or assisted reproductive therapies depending on the underlying cause. Medical and surgical therapies are usually managed by an urologist who specializes in infertility. A reproductive endocrinologist may offer intrauterine inseminations (IUIs) or in vitro fertilization (IVF) to help overcome male factor infertility.

Chapter 34

Vasectomy and Vasectomy Reversal

A vasectomy is a surgical procedure performed as a method of birth control. It involves cutting the vas deferens in order to close off the tubes that carry sperm from the testicles (there is one vas deferens per testicle). If a man has a successful vasectomy, he can no longer get a woman pregnant.

Sperm are made in the two testicles, which are inside the scrotum. Sperm is stored in a tube attached to each testicle called the "epididymis." When a man ejaculates, the sperm travel from the epididymis, through the vas deferens, and then mix with seminal fluid to form semen. The semen then travels through the urethra and out the penis.

Before a vasectomy, semen contains sperm and seminal fluid. After a vasectomy, sperm are no longer in the semen. The man's testicles will make less sperm over time, and his body will harmlessly absorb any sperm that are made.

How Is a Vasectomy Done?

A vasectomy is usually performed in the office of urologist, a doctor who specializes in the male urinary tract and reproductive

This chapter includes text excerpted from "Vasectomy: Condition Information," *Eunice Kennedy Shriver* National Institute of Child Health and Human Development (NICHD), December 1, 2016.

system. In some cases, the urologist may decide to do a vasectomy in an outpatient surgery center or a hospital. This could be because of patient anxiety or because other procedures will be done at the same time.

There are two ways to perform a vasectomy. In either case, the patient is awake during the procedure, but the urologist uses a local anesthetic to numb the scrotum.

With the conventional method, the doctor makes one or two small cuts in the scrotum to access the vas deferens. A small section of the vas deferens is cut out and then removed. The urologist may cauterize (seal with heat) the ends and then tie the ends with stitches. The doctor will then perform the same procedure on the other testicle, either through the same opening or through a second scrotal incision. For both testicles, when the vas deferens has been tied off, the doctor will use a few stitches or skin "glue" to close the opening(s) in the scrotum.

With the "no-scalpel" method, a small puncture hole is made on one side of the scrotum. The healthcare provider will find the vas deferens under the skin and pull it through the hole. The vas deferens is then cut and a small section is removed. The ends are either cauterized or tied off and then put back in place. The procedure is then performed on the other testicle. No stitches are needed with this method because the puncture holes are so small.

After a vasectomy, most men go home the same day and fully recover in less than a week.

How Effective Is Vasectomy?

Vasectomy is one of the most effective forms of birth control. In the first year after a man has a vasectomy, a few couples will still get pregnant. But, the number is far lower than the rates of pregnancy among couples using condoms or oral contraceptive pills.

However, a vasectomy is not effective right away. Men still need to use other birth control until the remaining sperm are cleared out of the semen. This takes 15 to 20 ejaculations, or about 3 months. Even then, 1 of every 5 men will still have sperm in his semen and will need to wait longer for the sperm to clear.

A healthcare provider will check a man's semen for sperm at least once after the surgery. Once the sperm count has dropped to zero, it is safe to assume that a vasectomy is now an effective form of birth control. Until that time, men need to use another form of birth control to make sure their partner does not become pregnant.

What Are the Risks of Vasectomy?

Although vasectomy is safe and highly effective, men should be aware of problems that could occur after surgery and over time.

Surgical Risks

After surgery, most men have discomfort, bruising, and some swelling, all of which usually go away within two weeks. Problems that can occur after surgery and need to be checked by a healthcare provider include:

- Hematoma, which is bleeding under the skin that can lead to painful swelling

- Infection. Fever and scrotal redness and tenderness are signs of infection.

Other Risks

The risk of other problems is small, but they do occur. These include:

- A lump in the scrotum, called a "granuloma." This is formed from sperm that leak out of the vas deferens into the tissue.

- This is called "postvasectomy pain syndrome" (PVPS) and occurs in some men.

- Vasectomy failure. There is a small risk that the vasectomy will fail. This can lead to unintended pregnancy. Among 1,000 vasectomies, 11 will likely fail over 2 years; and half of these failures will occur within the first 3 months after surgery. The risk of failure depends on a number of factors. For example, some surgical techniques are more likely to fail than others. Additionally, there is a very small risk that the 2 ends of the vas deferens will grow back together. If this happens, sperm may be able to enter the semen and make pregnancy possible.

- Risk of regret. Vasectomy may be a good choice for men and/ or couples who are certain that they do not want more or any children. Most men who have vasectomy, as well as spouses of men who have vasectomy, do not regret the decision. Men who have vasectomy before the age of 30 are the group most likely to want a vasectomy reversal in the future.

Will Vasectomy Affect Sex Life?

Vasectomy will not affect your sex life. It does not decrease your sex drive because it does not affect the production of the male hormone testosterone. It also does not affect your ability to get an erection or ejaculate semen. Because the sperm make up a very small amount of the semen, you will not notice a difference in the amount of semen you ejaculate.

Is Vasectomy Linked to Cancer?

Research shows that vasectomy does not increase a man's risk of cancer. Some studies in the 1990s found that men who had undergone vasectomy had higher rates of prostate cancer. But findings from more recent studies have conclusively shown no link between vasectomy and prostate cancer. Indeed, men who have vasectomy are no more likely to get prostate cancer than men who do not have vasectomy. Vasectomy also does not increase a man's risk of testicular cancer.

Does Having a Vasectomy Change My Risk for Sexually Transmitted Diseases?

A vasectomy does not protect you from getting or passing on any sexually transmitted disease (STD), including human immunodeficiency virus (HIV). You must still use condoms or another barrier method to protect yourself from STDs.

Vasectomy Reversal

Almost all vasectomies can be reversed. In a reversal, the cut ends of the vas deferens are surgically reattached. Or, one end of the vas deferens is surgically connected to the part of the testicle where mature sperm are stored.

Vasectomy reversal is usually done in an outpatient surgery center or the outpatient area of a hospital. The surgeon may use general anesthesia.

To reverse a vasectomy, the surgeon makes a small cut in the side of the scrotum and finds the closed ends of the vas deferens. Then, a fluid sample is taken from the end closest to the testicle to test for the presence of sperm. If sperm is found in the fluid, the two closed ends of the vas deferens can be reattached.

Many doctors perform the reversal using a microsurgical approach. Here, a high-powered microscope is used to magnify the ends of the vas deferens. It allows the surgeon to use smaller stitches—as small as an eyelash—which reduces scarring. Microsurgery returns sperm to the semen in the majority of reversals.

If no sperm is found in the fluid, there is a blockage in the epididymis or vas deferens. The surgeon gets around this by attaching the upper part of the vas deferens to the epididymis in a place that bypasses the blockage. This procedure is more involved but has nearly as high a success rate as a standard reversal.

Recovery from a reversal usually takes one to three weeks. As with vasectomy, complications from surgery are possible. Most men who undergo vasectomy reversal report the same or less discomfort during recovery than they had after vasectomy.

Sperm start appearing in the semen about 3 months after the surgery. However, if the surgeon has to work around a blockage, it can take as long as 15 months for sperm to reappear.

On average, it takes 1 year to achieve a pregnancy after a vasectomy reversal. However, a successful reversal (sperm is returned to the semen) does not guarantee pregnancy. The chance of restored fertility and pregnancy is highest when the reversal is performed not long after the vasectomy. The likelihood of restored fertility and pregnancy decreases as more time elapses between the vasectomy and the vasectomy reversal.

Chapter 35

Nonsurgical Contraception

Chapter Contents

Section 35.1—Condoms 488
Section 35.2—Withdrawal 490

Section 35.1

Condoms

This section includes text excerpted from "Male Condom,"
U.S. Department of Health and Human Services (HHS), May 5, 2019.

What Is the Male Condom?

A male condom is a thin film cover that is placed over the penis.
Condoms prevent pregnancy by keeping sperm from entering a woman's body.

Condoms made from latex rubber are the most common type. For
people who get skin irritation from latex, polyurethane condoms are
a good choice.

Condoms are either lubricated or nonlubricated. You can also add a
water-based lubricant to a condom to make sex more comfortable and,
more important, to help prevent breakage. At your local pharmacy, ask
which brands of lubricant are water based. Avoid oil-based lubricants
(for example, petroleum jelly, massage oil, body lotion) as they weaken
condoms and may cause them to break.

Used correctly each time you have sex, latex and polyurethane
condoms are a good option to prevent pregnancy and many sexually
transmitted diseases (STDs). Condoms made from natural or lambskin
materials also protect against pregnancy, but they will not protect
against some STDs.

How to Use It

Condoms can be damaged by heat, so store them somewhere cool
and dry. Do not store them in a wallet or in a car. Condoms have a
limited shelf-life, and they will expire. Check the expiration date on
the packaging to make sure the condom is still good.

- Place on the erect penis before any sexual contact occurs.

- Use water- or silicone-based lubricants to decrease risk of
  condom breakage.

- Pull out of the vagina before the penis softens.

- Hold the base of condom snugly against the penis when pulling out.

- Use the condom once and then throw it away. Never reuse a
  condom.

How Effective Is It?

Of 100 women whose partners use male condoms, about 18 may become pregnant. Condoms are more effective at preventing pregnancy when they are used correctly every time you have sex.

Except for abstinence from all sexual contact, latex and polyurethane condoms are the best protection against STDs, including human immunodeficiency virus (HIV). Lambskin condoms do not protect against STDs and HIV.

How Do I Get It?

You can buy condoms at many stores, including pharmacies, grocery, and discount stores. Health departments, clinics, and student health centers may offer free or low-cost condoms as well. You do not need a prescription or personal identification to buy them.

Advantages and Disadvantages of Using a Male Condom

Advantages of the Male Condom

- Male condoms do not require a prescription.

- Anyone may buy them.

- They are safe and easy to use.

- They can be used for vaginal, anal, and oral sex.

- Flavored condoms are available, which may improve the experience when using them for protection against STDs during oral sex.

- Latex and polyurethane condoms offer protection against STDs, including HIV, and they also prevent pregnancy.

Drawbacks of the Male Condom

- Male condoms must be used correctly and consistently to be beneficial.

- You must use a new condom each time you have sex.

- Condoms made from latex can cause irritation or allergic reactions in some people.

- Both partners must agree to use a condom.

Section 35.2

Withdrawal

What Is Withdrawal All About?

Withdrawal, or the pull-out method, has been practiced for centuries to avoid the risk of unwanted pregnancy during sexual intercourse. Scientifically known as *"Coitus interruptus"* (Latin for interrupted intercourse), withdrawal happens when a man removes his penis from the vagina before ejaculating (the moment when semen spurts out of the penis).

What Is the Logic behind Withdrawal?

Withdrawal prevents sperm from entering the woman's vagina, thereby preventing contact between the sperm and the egg.

Why Use Withdrawal?

Withdrawal continues to be a popular birth control method among younger couples. There are a number of factors that make this an attractive option including:

- It can be used when no other method is available.

- It is free

- It has none of the side effects that can be associated with other birth control methods.

Is Withdrawal Fail-Proof?

No. For a number of reasons, withdrawal is an unreliable form of birth control.

The practice of withdrawal requires a lot of trust, self-control, and experience. It requires the male partner to know the sexual responses of his own body so as to know when to pull out. It is generally not recommended for teens and sexually inexperienced men. If done incorrectly and a man is unable to predict, and control the exact moment of his ejaculation, this method could be very ineffective.

What Are the Risks?

Even if the guy pulls out in time, there is still a risk of pregnancy from pre-ejaculate, or precum sperm, that is still in the urinary tract from a previous ejaculation. It is advisable for a guy to urinate, to get rid of all the pre-cum from the urethra before intercourse, and clean properly to get rid of any fluid before having intercourse again.

While withdrawal may prevent unwanted pregnancy if practiced correctly, it does not protect the couple engaged in intercourse from the risk of sexually transmitted diseases (STDs) and human immunodeficiency virus (HIV). It is always wiser to protect yourself from the risk of pregnancy, STDs, and the transmission of HIV by correctly and consistently using male latex condoms and/or other contraceptive methods.

For women who do not want to risk pregnancy due to medical or personal reasons, it is always better to rely on other forms of birth control, such as diaphragms, caps, or a female condom.

References

1. "Withdrawal Method (*Coitus Interruptus*)," Mayo Clinic Staff, March 5, 2015.

2. Dr. David Delvin. "*Coitus Interruptus* (Withdrawal Method)," NetDoctor, December 22, 2014.

Chapter 36

Safer Sex Guidelines

We know a lot about how the human immunodeficiency virus (HIV) is transmitted from person to person. Having safer sex means you take this into account and avoid risky practices.

There are two reasons to practice safer sex: to protect yourself and to protect others.

Protecting Yourself

If you have HIV, you need to protect your health. When it comes to sex, this means practicing safer sex (such as using condoms) to avoid sexually transmitted diseases (STDs) like herpes and hepatitis. HIV makes it harder for your body to fight off diseases. What might be a small health problem for someone without HIV could be big health problem for you.

Protecting Your Partner

Taking care of others means making sure that you do not pass along HIV to them. If your sex partners already have HIV, you should still avoid infecting them with another STD you may be carrying.

Most people would agree that you owe it to your sexual partners to tell them that you have HIV. This is being honest with them. Even though it can be very hard to do, you will probably feel much better about yourself in the long run.

This chapter includes text excerpted from "What Is 'Safer Sex'?" U.S. Department of Veterans Affairs (VA), February 8, 2018.

Some people with HIV have found that people who love them think that condomless sex is a sign of greater love or trust. If someone offers to have condomless sex with you, it is still up to you to protect them by being safe.

"Being safe" usually means protecting yourself and others by using condoms for the highest-risk sex activities, specifically for anal and vaginal sex. When done correctly, condom use is very effective at preventing HIV transmission. In recent years, "being safe" has come to include two other important strategies for reducing HIV infections; these are HIV treatment (ART medications) for HIV-positive people and pre-exposure prophylaxis (PrEP) for HIV negatives. Both of these are very effective at reducing the risk of HIV infection. One or more of them is likely to be appropriate for you—be sure to ask your healthcare provider about them.

What about Antiretroviral Therapy for HIV Prevention

One of the most effective ways you can prevent HIV from passing to an HIV-negative sex partner is to take your antiretroviral therapy (ART) medications every day—if they are working well to suppress the HIV in your body, they also will prevent transmission of HIV.

What about Pre-Exposure Prophylaxis

HIV-negative individuals may, under the supervision of their healthcare providers, take an anti-HIV pill every day to prevent themselves from becoming infected. We call this "pre-exposure prophylaxis" or "PrEP." Usually, these are persons who are at a relatively high risk of becoming infected with HIV (for example, because they have a partner with HIV, they have risky sexual exposures, or they share injection drug equipment). The medication used for PrEP is Truvada, a combination tablet containing tenofovir and emtricitabine. PrEP appears to be extremely effective if it is taken every day, and it is not effective if it is taken irregularly. Your healthcare provider can tell you more about the potential benefits and shortcomings of PrEP for HIV-negative persons.

Talking about Safer Sex

You and your partners will have to decide what you are comfortable doing sexually. If you are not used to talking openly about sex, this could be hard to get used to.

Here are some tips:

- Find a time and place outside the bedroom to talk.

- Decide what are your boundaries, concerns, and desires before you start to talk.

- Make sure you clearly state what you want. Use only "I" statements, for example: "I want to use a condom when we have sex."

- Make sure you do not do, or agree to do, anything that you are not 100 percent comfortable with.

- Listen to what your partner is saying. Acknowledge your partner's feelings and opinions. You will need to come up with solutions that work for both of you.

- Be positive. Use reasons for safer sex that are about you not your partner.

Of course, only you and your partner can decide what level of risk you are willing to take.

Chapter 37

Sexually Transmitted Diseases

Chapter Contents

Section 37.1 — What Are Sexually Transmitted
Diseases?.. 498

Section 37.2 — Chlamydia 507

Section 37.3 — Genital Herpes 509

Section 37.4 — Gonorrhea... 512

Section 37.5 — Hepatitis B.. 516

Section 37.6 — Human Papillomavirus..................... 520

Section 37.7 — Pubic Lice 524

Section 37.8 — Scabies 526

Section 37.9 — Syphilis 533

Section 37.10 — Trichomoniasis 537

Section 37.1

What Are Sexually Transmitted Diseases?

This section includes text excerpted from "Sexually Transmitted Diseases (STDs)," *Eunice Kennedy Shriver* National Institute of Child Health and Human Development (NICHD), January 31, 2017.

Sexually transmitted diseases (STDs), also known as "sexually transmitted infections" (STIs), are typically caused by bacteria or viruses and are passed from person to person during sexual contact with the penis, anus, or mouth. The symptoms of STDs/STIs vary between individuals, depending on the cause, and many people may not experience symptoms at all.

Many STDs/STIs have significant health consequences. For instance, certain STIs can also increase the risk of getting and transmitting human immunodeficiency viruses/acquired immunodeficiency syndrome (HIV/AIDS) and alter the way the disease progresses. STIs can also cause long-term health problems, particularly in women and infants. Some of the health problems that arise from STIs include pelvic inflammatory disease, infertility, cervical cancer, and perinatal or congenital infections in infants.

What Are the Symptoms of Sexually Transmitted Disease/Sexually Transmitted Infections?

People with STDs/STIs may feel ill and notice some of the following signs and symptoms:

- Unusual discharge from the penis

- Sores or warts on the genital area

- Painful or frequent urination

- Itching and redness in the genital area

- Blisters or sores in or around the mouth

- Anal itching, soreness, or bleeding

- Abdominal pain

- Fever

In some cases, people with STIs have no symptoms. Over time, any symptoms that are present may improve on their own. It is also possible for a person to have an STI with no symptoms and then pass it on to others without knowing it.

If you are concerned that you or your sexual partner may have an STI, talk to your healthcare provider. Even if you do not have symptoms, it is possible you may have an STI that needs treatment to ensure your and your partners' sexual health.

What Causes Sexually Transmitted Diseases or Sexually Transmitted Infections

There are three major causes of STDs/STIs are:

- Bacteria, including chlamydia, gonorrhea, and syphilis

- Viruses, including HIV/AIDS, herpes simplex virus, human papillomavirus, hepatitis B virus, cytomegalovirus (CMV), and Zika

- Parasites, such as insects, such as crab lice or scabies mites

Any STI can be spread through sexual activity, including sexual intercourse, and some STIs also are spread through oral sex and other sexual activities. Ejaculation does not have to occur for an STI to pass from person to person.

In addition, sharing contaminated needles, such as those used to inject drugs, or using contaminated body piercing or tattooing equipment also can transmit some infections, such as HIV, hepatitis B, and hepatitis C. A few infections can be sexually transmitted but are also spread through nonsexual, close contact. Some of these infections, such as CMV, are not considered STIs even though they can be transmitted through sexual contact.

Regardless of how a person is exposed, once a person is infected by an STI, he can spread the infection to other people through oral, vaginal, or anal sex, even if he has no symptoms.

What Are Some Types of and Treatments for Sexually Transmitted Diseases or Sexually Transmitted Infections?

Approximately 20 different infections are known to be transmitted through sexual contact. Although the *Eunice Kennedy Shriver* National Institute of Child Health and Human Development (NICHD) does study STIs, their prevention, and their effects on pregnancy and long-term health, the Institute is not the lead agency aiming to under-stand STIs.

Chlamydia

- Caused by the bacterium *Chlamydia* trachomatis

- Can be transmitted during vaginal, oral, or anal sexual contact with an infected partner

- Many infected individuals will not experience symptoms, but chlamydia can cause fever, abdominal pain, and unusual discharge from the penis.

- Can be treated with antibiotics

- Because chlamydia and gonorrhea often occur together, people who have one infection are typically treated for both by their healthcare provider.

- To prevent health complications and sexual transmission, treatment should be provided promptly for all persons testing positive for infection, and recent sexual partners should be treated at the same time to prevent reinfection.

- Infected individuals should follow their healthcare provider's recommendations about how long to abstain from sex after the treatment is completed to avoid passing the infection back and forth.

Gonorrhea

- Caused by the bacterium *Neisseria gonorrhea*, which can grow and multiply rapidly in the warm, moist areas of the reproductive tract

- Most common symptoms include discharge from the penis and painful or difficult urination.

- Can be treated with antibiotics

- In men, gonorrhea can also infect the mouth, throat, eyes, and rectum and can spread to the blood and joints, where it can become a life-threatening illness.

- Because chlamydia and gonorrhea often occur together, people who have one infection are typically treated for both by their healthcare provider.

- To prevent health complications and sexual transmission, treatment should be provided promptly for all persons testing positive for infection, and recent sexual partners should be treated at the same time to prevent reinfection.

- People with gonorrhea can more easily contract HIV, the virus that causes AIDS. HIV-infected people with gonorrhea are also more likely to transmit the virus to someone else.

Genital Herpes

- Caused by the herpes simplex virus (HSV)

- There are two different strains, or types: HSV type 1 (HSV-1) and type 2 (HSV-2). Both can cause genital herpes, although most cases of genital herpes are caused by HSV-2.

- Symptoms of HSV-1 usually appear as fever blisters or cold sores on the lips, but it can also infect the genital region through oral-genital or genital-genital contact. Symptoms of HSV-2 are typically painful, watery skin blisters on or around the genitals or anus. However, substantial numbers of people who carry these viruses have no or only minimal signs or symptoms.

- Genital herpes cannot be cured, but it can be controlled with medication.

- One medication can be taken daily to make it less likely that the infection will pass on to sex partner(s) or to infants during childbirth.

- Periodically, some people will experience outbreaks of symptoms in which new blisters form on the skin in the genital area; at those times, the virus is more likely to be passed on to other people.

Human Immunodeficiency Virus/Acquired Immunodeficiency Syndrome

- Human immunodeficiency virus is the virus that causes AIDS.

- Destroys the body's immune system by killing the blood cells that fight infection. Once HIV destroys a substantial proportion of these cells, the body's ability to fight off and recover from infections is compromised. This advanced stage of HIV infection is known as "AIDS."

501

- People whose HIV infection has progressed to AIDS have a weakened immune system and are very susceptible to opportunistic infections that do not normally make people sick and to certain forms of cancer.

- In people who do not have HIV, the infection can be prevented by many tools, including abstaining from sex, limiting the number of sexual partners, never sharing needles, and using condoms appropriately. Persons who may be at a very high risk of HIV infection may be able to obtain HIV Pre-Exposure Prophylaxis or PrEP, which consists of the HIV medication called "Truvada," from their doctor to take every day so they can prevent HIV infection. PrEP will not work if it is not taken consistently.

- Acquired immunodeficiency syndrome can be prevented in those with HIV infection by early initiation of antiretroviral therapy.

- Transmission of the virus primarily occurs during unprotected sexual activity and by sharing needles used to inject intravenous drugs.

Human Papillomavirus

- Human papillomavirus (HPV) is the most common STI. More than 40 HPV types exist, and all of them can infect both men and women.

- The types of HPVs vary in their ability to cause genital warts; infect other regions of the body, including the mouth and throat; and cause cancers of the cervix, vulva, penis, anus, and mouth.

- It cannot be cured but can be prevented with vaccines and controlled with medications.

- Genital warts caused by the virus can also be treated.

- Regular screening with a Pap smear test can prevent or detect at an early stage most cases of HPV-caused cervical cancer. (A Pap smear test involves a healthcare provider taking samples of cells from the cervix during a standard gynecologic exam; these cells are examined under a microscope for signs of developing cancer).

- Two available vaccines protect against most (but not all) HPV types that cause cervical cancer. A group advising the Centers for Disease Control and Prevention (CDC) recommends this vaccine for boys and girls starting at 11 or 12 years of age.

Syphilis

- Caused by the bacterium *Treponema pallidum*

- Passes from person to person during vaginal, anal, or oral sex through direct contact with syphilis sores

- In 2001, the number of cases of syphilis was at its lowest in 60 years. But the syphilis rate has increased nearly every year up to 2016, the most recent year for which data are available. Rates have increased among both men and women, but men account for a vast majority of syphilis cases.

- The first sign of syphilis is a chancre, a painless genital sore that most often appears on the penis. Chancres typically resolve on their own, but the body does not clear the infection on its own.

- Chancres make a person two to five times more likely to contract an HIV infection. If the person is already infected with HIV, chances also increase the likelihood that the HIV virus will be passed on to a sexual partner.

- Can be treated with antibiotics:

  - If recognized during the early stages, usually within the first year of infection, syphilis can be treated with a single injection of antibiotic.

  - If not recognized early, or not treated immediately, syphilis may need longer treatment with antibiotics.

- Without treatment:

  - Usually spreads to other organs, including the skin, heart, blood vessels, liver, bones, and joints in secondary syphilis

  - Other sores, such as a syphilis rash, can break out in later stages.

  - Tertiary syphilis can develop over a period of years and involve the nerves, eyes, and brain and can potentially cause death.

- Infants who get syphilis infection in the womb may have misshapen bones, very low red blood cell count (called "severe anemia"), enlarged liver and spleen, jaundice (yellowing of the skin or eyes), nerve problems, blindness or deafness, meningitis, and skin rashes.

- Those being treated for syphilis must avoid sexual contact until the syphilis sores are completely healed to avoid infecting other people.

- Persons with syphilis must notify their sex partners so that they also can be tested and receive treatment if necessary.

Trichomoniasis

- Caused by the single-celled parasite *Trichomonas vaginalis*

- Common in young, sexually active women but also infects men, though less frequently

- The parasite can be transmitted between men and women.

- Can cause frequent, painful, or "burning" urination in men, as well as genital soreness. However, it may not cause any symptoms.

- Because the infection can occur without symptoms, a person may be unaware that he is infected and continue to reinfect a sexual partner who is having recurrent signs of infection.

- Can be treated with a single dose of an antibiotic, usually either metronidazole or tinidazole, taken by mouth

- Because of reinfection, it is important to make sure that the diagnosed individual and all sexual partners are treated at the same time.

Viral Hepatitis

- Caused by several different viral strains

- Hepatitis A virus (HAV):

  - Causes a short-term or self-limited liver infection that can be quite serious

  - Does not result in chronic infection

  - Can be transmitted during sexual activity and through oral-anal contact

  - Vaccination can prevent HAV infection

  - May cause abdominal pain, nausea, and vomiting

  - Usually, the infection gets better on its own without requiring treatment. In some cases, however, individuals may have such severe nausea and vomiting that they must be admitted to the hospital or may have lasting damage to their livers.

- Hepatitis B virus (HBV):

  - Causes a serious liver infection that can result in both immediate illness and lifelong infection and disease, leading to permanent liver scarring (cirrhosis), cancer, liver failure, and death

  - Can be treated with antiviral medications

  - Vaccination can prevent HBV infection.

  - Spreads through sexual contact, as well as through contact with other bodily fluids, such as blood; through shared contaminated needles used for injecting intravenous drugs; and through tattooing and piercing

  - People with chronic HBV infection will need to see a liver specialist with experience treating individuals with chronic liver disease. These individuals need to take special care not to pass on the virus to their sexual partners, and sexual partners should receive hepatitis B vaccine if they are not already immune.

- Hepatitis C virus (HCV):

  - Serious infection of the liver that can cause an immediate illness but that, in most people, becomes a silent, chronic infection that leads to liver scarring (cirrhosis), cancer, liver failure, and death.

  - Most infected people may not be aware of their infection because they do not develop symptoms.

  - Most commonly transmitted through sharing needles or exposure to infected blood. Less commonly, it can spread through sexual contact.

  - Can be treated. New medications seem to be more effective and have fewer side effects than previous options. The Food and Drug Administration (FDA) maintains a complete list of approved treatments for hepatitis C.

Zika

- An infection caused by a virus. In most cases, it is spread by mosquitoes, but Zika virus also can be transmitted sexually.

- Zika is usually mild, with symptoms lasting for several days to a week after being infected.

- Zika also was linked to problems with the adult nervous system, including Guillain-Barré syndrome.

- There is currently no specific medication or treatment for Zika infection.

Is There a Cure for Sexually Transmitted Diseases and Sexually Transmitted Infections?

Viruses, such as HIV, genital herpes, human papillomavirus, hepatitis, and cytomegalovirus, cause STDs/STIs that cannot be cured. People with an STI caused by a virus will be infected for life and will always be at risk of infecting their sexual partners. However, treatments for these viruses can significantly reduce the risk of passing on the infection and can reduce or eliminate symptoms. STIs caused by bacteria, yeast, or parasites can be cured using appropriate medication.

What Are the Treatments for Sexually Transmitted Diseases and Sexually Transmitted Infections?

Sexually transmitted diseases and sexually transmitted infections caused by bacteria or parasites can be treated with antibiotics. These antibiotics are most often given by mouth (orally). However, sometimes they are injected or applied directly to the affected area.

The treatments, complications, and outcomes for viral STIs depend on the particular virus (HIV, genital herpes, human papillomavirus, hepatitis, or cytomegalovirus). Treatments can reduce the symptoms and the progression of most of these infections. For example, medications are available to limit the frequency and severity of genital herpes outbreaks while reducing the risk that the virus will be passed on to other people.

Individuals with HIV need to take special antiretroviral drugs that control the amount of virus they carry. These drugs, called "highly active antiretroviral therapy," or "HAART," can help people live longer, healthier lives and can prevent onward transmission of HIV to others.

Whatever the infection, and regardless of how quickly the symptoms resolve after beginning treatment, the infected person and their partner(s) must take all of the medicine prescribed by the healthcare provider to ensure that the STI is completely treated. Likewise, they should follow healthcare provider recommendations about how long to abstain from sex after the treatment is completed to avoid passing the infection back and forth.

Section 37.2

Chlamydia

This section includes text excerpted from "Chlamydia Infections," MedlinePlus, National Institutes of Health (NIH), May 31, 2018.

What Is Chlamydia?

Chlamydia is a common sexually transmitted disease (STD). It is caused by bacteria called *"Chlamydia trachomatis."* It can infect both men and women. Men can get chlamydia in the urethra (inside the penis), rectum, or throat.

How Do You Get Chlamydia?

You can get chlamydia during oral, vaginal, or anal sex with someone who has the infection.

If you have had chlamydia and were treated in the past, you can get reinfected if you have unprotected sex with someone who has it.

Who Is at Risk of Getting Chlamydia?

Chlamydia is more common in young people, especially young women. You are more likely to get it if you do not consistently use a condom or if you have multiple partners.

What Are the Symptoms of Chlamydia?

Chlamydia does not usually cause any symptoms. So you may not realize that you have it. People with chlamydia who have no symptoms can still pass the disease to others. If you do have symptoms, they may not appear until several weeks after you have sex with an infected partner.

Symptoms in men include:

- Discharge from your penis
- A burning sensation when urinating
- Burning or itching around the opening of your penis
- Pain and swelling in one or both testicles (although this is less common)

If the chlamydia infects the rectum, it can cause rectal pain, discharge, and/or bleeding.

How Is Chlamydia Diagnosed?

There are lab tests to diagnose chlamydia. Your healthcare provider may ask you to provide a urine sample.

Who Should Be Tested for Chlamydia?

You should go to your healthcare provider for a test if you have symptoms of chlamydia, or if you have a partner who has an STD.

MSM are at a higher risk and should get checked for chlamydia every year.

What Are the Complications of Chlamydia?

Men often do not have health problems from chlamydia. Sometimes, it can infect the epididymis (the tube that carries sperm). This can cause pain, fever, and, rarely, infertility.

Both women and men can develop reactive arthritis because of a chlamydia infection. Reactive arthritis is a type of arthritis that happens as a "reaction" to an infection in the body.

Untreated chlamydia may also increase your chances of getting or giving human immunodeficiency virus/acquired immunodeficiency syndrome (HIV/AIDS).

What Are the Treatments for Chlamydia?

Antibiotics will cure the infection. You may get a one-time dose of the antibiotics, or you may need to take medicine every day for seven days. Antibiotics cannot repair any permanent damage that the disease has caused.

To prevent spreading the disease to your partner, you should not have sex until the infection has cleared up. If you got a one-time dose of antibiotics, you should wait seven days after taking the medicine to have sex again. If you have to take medicine every day for seven days, you should not have sex again until you have finished taking all of the doses of your medicine.

It is common to get a repeat infection, so you should get tested again about three months after treatment.

Can Chlamydia Be Prevented?

The only sure way to prevent chlamydia is to not have vaginal, anal, or oral sex.

Correct usage of latex condoms greatly reduces, but does not eliminate, the risk of catching or spreading chlamydia.

Section 37.3

Genital Herpes

This section includes text excerpted from "Genital Herpes,"
U.S. Department of Health and Human Services (HHS), April 2, 2019.

What Is Genital Herpes?

Herpes is a common sexually transmitted disease (STD) that any sexually active person can get. Most people with the virus do not have symptoms. It is important to know that even without signs of the disease, it can still spread to sexual partners.

Genital herpes is an STD that appears on the sex organs and can be caused by two types of viruses. The viruses are called "herpes simplex type 1" (HSV-1) and "herpes simplex type 2" (HSV-2).

How Common Is Genital Herpes?

Genital herpes is common in the United States where about 17 out of 100 people between the ages of 14 and 49, have genital herpes.

How Is Genital Herpes Spread?

You can get herpes by having vaginal, anal, or oral sex with someone who has the disease.

Fluids found in a herpes sore carry the virus, and contact with those fluids can cause infection. You can also get herpes from an infected sex partner who does not have a visible sore or who may not know they are infected because the virus can be released through the skin and spread to a sex partner.

What Are the Symptoms of Genital Herpes?

Most people who have herpes have no symptoms or have very mild ones. You may not notice mild symptoms or you may mistake them for another skin condition, such as a pimple or an ingrown hair. Because of this, most people who have herpes do not know they have it.

Genital herpes sores usually appear as one or more blisters on or around the genitals, rectum, or mouth. The blisters break and leave painful sores that may take weeks to heal. These symptoms are sometimes called "having an outbreak." The first time someone has an outbreak, they may also have flu-like symptoms, such as fever, body aches, or swollen glands.

Repeat outbreaks of genital herpes are common, especially during the first year after infection. Repeat outbreaks are usually shorter and less severe than the first outbreak. Although the infection can stay in the body for the rest of your life, the number of outbreaks tends to decrease over a period of years.

You should be examined by your healthcare provider if your partner has an STD or if you or your partner notice symptoms of an STD, such as an unusual sore, smelly discharge, burning when urinating.

What Are the Risk Factors for Genital Herpes?

A risk factor is the chance that something will harm or otherwise affect a person's health.

Risk factors for becoming infected with genital herpes include:

• Engaging in unprotected vaginal, anal, or oral sex. Herpes symptoms can occur in both male and female genital areas that are covered by a latex condom. However, outbreaks can also occur in areas that are not covered by a condom—so condoms may not fully protect you from getting herpes.

- Having sex with multiple partners

- Having a sexual partner who has tested positive for herpes

Have an honest and open talk with your healthcare provider and ask whether you should be tested for herpes or other STDs.

What Is the Link between Genital Herpes and Human Immunodeficiency Viruses?

Genital herpes can cause sores or breaks in the skin or lining of the mouth and rectum. The genital sores caused by herpes can bleed easily. When the sores come into contact with the mouth or rectum during sex, they increase the risk of giving or getting HIV if you or your partner has HIV.

What Is the Link between Genital Herpes and Oral Herpes?

Oral herpes (such as cold sores or fever blisters on or around the mouth) is usually caused by HSV-1. Most people are infected with HSV-1 during childhood from nonsexual contact. For example, people can become infected by a kiss from a relative or friend with oral herpes. More than half of the population in the United States has HSV-1, even if they do not show any signs or symptoms. HSV-1 can also be spread from the mouth to the genitals through oral sex. This is why some cases of genital herpes are caused by HSV-1, although most cases of genital herpes are caused by HSV-2.

Are There Tests for Genital Herpes?

Your healthcare provider often can diagnose genital herpes simply by looking at your symptoms. Laboratory tests can also be done including testing a sample from the sore(s) and a blood test. Ask your healthcare provider if you should be tested for herpes or other STDs.

How Is Genital Herpes Treated?

There is no cure for herpes. However, there are medications that can prevent or shorten outbreaks. One of these herpes medications can be taken daily and makes it less likely that you will pass the infection on to your sex partner(s), in addition to lessening the chance of having an outbreak or shortening the duration of the outbreak if you do have one.

I Was Treated for Genital Herpes. When Can I Have Sex Again?

Having sores or other symptoms of herpes can increase your risk of spreading the virus. Even if you do not have any symptoms, you can still infect your sex partners. Using condoms may help lower this risk, but it will not get rid of the risk completely. If you have herpes, you should tell your sex partner(s) and let them know so they can get tested and treated if necessary.

What Happens If I Do Not Get Treated

Genital herpes can cause painful genital sores and can be severe in people with suppressed immune systems. If you touch your sores or the fluids from the sores, you may transfer herpes to another part of your body, such as your eyes. Do not touch the sores or fluids to avoid spreading herpes to another part of your body. If you touch the sores or fluids, immediately wash your hands thoroughly to help avoid spreading infection.

Some people who get genital herpes have concerns about how it will impact their overall health, sex life, and relationships. It is best for you to talk to a healthcare provider about those concerns, but it also is important to recognize that while herpes is not curable, it can be managed.

Section 37.4

Gonorrhea

This section includes text excerpted from
"Gonorrhea," U.S. Department of Health and
Human Services (HHS), April 2, 2019.

What Is Gonorrhea?

Gonorrhea is a sexually transmitted disease (STD) that can infect both men and women. It can cause an infection in the genitals (sex organs), rectum (the final part of the large intestine, ending at the anus), and throat. It is a very common infection, especially among young people between the ages of 15 and 24. Anyone who is sexually active can get gonorrhea. Gonorrhea can cause very serious complications when not treated, but it can be cured with the right medication.

How Is Gonorrhea Spread?

You can get gonorrhea by having vaginal, anal, or oral sex with someone who has gonorrhea.

What Are the Symptoms of Gonorrhea?

Most people who have gonorrhea have no symptoms. If symptoms are present, they may be mild or may not appear for several days after having sex with an infected partner.

Symptoms include:

- A burning sensation when urinating

- A white, yellow, or green discharge from the penis

- Painful or swollen testicles (although this is less common)

Men and women can also get infected with gonorrhea in their rectum, either through receptive anal sex or from another infected site (such as the vagina). Symptoms can include:

- Discharge

- Anal itching

- Soreness

- Bleeding

- Painful bowel movements

A healthcare provider should be consulted if any of these symptoms are present.

What Are the Risk Factors for Gonorrhea?

A risk factor is the chance that something will harm or otherwise affect a person's health. Any sexually active person can get gonorrhea through unprotected vaginal, anal, or oral sex.

Risk factors include:

- Engaging in unprotected vaginal, anal, or oral sex

- Having sex with new or multiple sex partners
- Being a man who has sex with men
- Having human immunodeficiency virus (HIV)
- Being sexually active and under 25 years of age
- Having a sexual partner who is infected with gonorrhea. Gonorrhea can increase the risk of spreading other STDs, including HIV.

Have an honest and open talk with your healthcare provider, and ask whether you should be tested for gonorrhea or other STDs. If you have any of these risk factors, you should be tested for gonorrhea every year.

How Can I Reduce My Risk of Getting Gonorrhea?

The only way to avoid gonorrhea is to not have vaginal, anal, or oral sex.

If you are sexually active, the following could lower your chances of getting gonorrhea:

- Being in a long-term, mutually monogamous relationship with a partner who has tested as negative for STDs, including gonorrhea
- Using latex condoms correctly every time you have sex

Are There Tests for Gonorrhea?

Most of the time, urine can be used to test for gonorrhea. However, swabs may be used to collect samples from the throat and/or rectum if you have had oral and/or anal sex. In some cases, a swab may be used to collect a sample from a man's urethra (urine canal) or a woman's cervix (opening to the womb).

How Is Gonorrhea Treated?

Gonorrhea can be cured with the right treatment. It is important that you take all of the medication prescribed by a healthcare provider to cure your infection. Medication for gonorrhea should not be shared with anyone. Although medication will stop the infection, it will not undo any permanent damage caused by the disease.

It is becoming harder to treat gonorrhea because drug-resistant strains of gonorrhea are increasing. If symptoms continue for more than a few days after receiving treatment, it will be necessary to return to a healthcare provider to be checked again. Repeat infection with gonorrhea is possible. Repeat testing for gonorrhea three months after treatment ends is recommended, even if sex partners are treated.

I Was Treated for Gonorrhea. When Can I Have Sex Again?

You should wait seven days after finishing all medication used to treat gonorrhea before having sex. To avoid getting infected with gonorrhea again or spreading gonorrhea, you and your sex partner(s) should avoid having sex until you have each completed treatment. If you have had gonorrhea and were treated in the past, you can still get infected again if you have unprotected sex with a person who has gonorrhea.

Even if you do not have any symptoms, you can still infect your sex partners. Using condoms may help lower this risk, but it will not get rid of the risk completely. If you have gonorrhea, you should tell your sex partner(s) and let him know so they can get tested and treated, if necessary.

What Happens If I Do Not Get Treated

Untreated gonorrhea can cause serious and permanent health problems in both women and men.

In men, gonorrhea can cause a painful condition in the tubes attached to the testicles. In rare cases, this may cause a man to be sterile, or prevent him from being able to father a child. Untreated chlamydia in both men can also increase risk for contracting or spreading HIV, the virus that causes acquired immunodeficiency syndrome (AIDS).

Rarely, untreated gonorrhea can also spread to your blood or joints. This condition can be life-threatening.

Section 37.5

Hepatitis B

This section includes text excerpted from
"Hepatitis B," U.S. Department of Health and
Human Services (HHS), March 29, 2019.

What Is Hepatitis B?

Hepatitis B is a viral infection that affects the liver. Hepatitis B begins as an "acute" infection, meaning it is often a short-term illness from which people recover.

In some cases, hepatitis B remains in the body and becomes a long-term or "chronic" infection. The younger a person is when he contracts hepatitis B, the more likely they are to develop a chronic infection.

How Common Is Hepatitis B?

Between 800,000 and 1.4 million people in the United States are living with chronic hepatitis B. There are approximately 43,000 new hepatitis B cases each year in the United States.

How Is Hepatitis B Spread?

Hepatitis B is more infectious than human immunodeficiency virus (HIV) and can be passed through the exchange of bodily fluids, such as semen, vaginal fluids, and blood. Hepatitis B is most commonly transmitted through:

- Sexual contact with an infected partner (this is the most common way adults and adolescents get the virus.)
- Sharing needles and syringes
- Sharing razors and toothbrushes (less common)
- Childbirth, if the mother has the infection

Hepatitis B is not spread through sharing cups and utensils, or through hugging, kissing, shaking hands, or breastfeeding.

What Are the Symptoms of Hepatitis B?

About 70 out of 100 adults with hepatitis B will develop symptoms. Some young children, especially those under 5 years of age, are less likely to have symptoms but are at a greater risk of developing chronic hepatitis B. On average, symptoms appear 90 days (or 3 months) after exposure, but they can appear any time between 6 weeks and 6 months after exposure.

What Are the Symptoms of Acute Hepatitis B?

If present, symptoms of acute hepatitis B might include:

- Jaundice (yellowing of the skin and eyes)
- Nausea and vomiting
- Abdominal pain
- Dark urine
- Joint pain
- Loss of appetite
- Fever
- Malaise (feeling generally ill)
- Fatigue (feeling tired all the time)

What Are the Symptoms of Chronic Hepatitis B?

Some people have symptoms similar to acute hepatitis B, but most with chronic hepatitis B go as long as 20 to 30 years without any signs. Between 15 and 25 of every 100 people with chronic hepatitis B develop serious liver diseases, such as cancer, cirrhosis (scarring of the liver), or liver failure, all of which can be fatal.

What Are the Risk Factors for Hepatitis B?

A risk factor is the chance that something will harm or otherwise affect a person's health.

Risk factors for hepatitis B include:

- Having sex with an infected person
- Having multiple sex partners
- Having a sexually transmitted disease
- Being a man who has sex with other men
- Injecting drugs or sharing needles, syringes, or other drug equipment

- Receiving a body piercing or tattoo with nonsterile instruments
- Living with a person who has chronic hepatitis B
- Being born to an infected mother
- Working in a health field and being exposed to blood
- Receiving hemodialysis
- Traveling to countries with moderate to high rates of hepatitis B

Anyone can get hepatitis B. To protect against infection, a vaccine is available. The hepatitis B vaccine provides excellent protection against infection and is given in a series of 3 to 4 injections over 6 months. After receiving all doses, the hepatitis B vaccine provides greater than 90 percent protection to infants, children, and adults before being exposed to the virus. The vaccine is recommended for:

- Infants and children under the age of 19
- Men who have sex with men
- Sexual partners of those with hepatitis B
- Injection drug users who share needles, syringes, or other equipment
- Healthcare workers
- Travelers to areas where hepatitis B is common
- Patients with chronic liver disease

For unvaccinated individuals with a recent exposure to someone with acute hepatitis B, an injection of hepatitis B immune globulin (HBIG) may prevent illness. An injection can provide protection for about three months.

There are several other things that can lower a person's risk of getting hepatitis B:

- Avoid sharing objects, such as needles, razors, and toothbrushes.
- Always use condoms or another latex barrier (such as a dental dam) during sex (oral, anal, and vaginal). A barrier should be put on before any sexual contact takes place.
- Have sex with only one partner (who only has sex with you).

Are There Tests for Hepatitis B?

There are many tests available for hepatitis B, and they can be done as a single test or a series of several tests. Some tests for hepatitis B look for particles of the virus (antigens), while others look for substances the immune system produces in response to an infection (antibodies) to hepatitis B. Blood tests can also indicate if a person has acute or chronic hepatitis.

How Is Hepatitis B Treated?

How Is Acute Hepatitis B Treated?

There is no medication to treat acute hepatitis B, which is typically an infection of short duration. Healthcare providers often recommend getting rest, drinking plenty of fluids, and eating a healthy diet.

How Is Chronic Hepatitis B Treated?

Anyone with chronic hepatitis B should be referred to a healthcare provider with specialized experience in treating hepatitis and liver diseases. There are several medications available to treat chronic hepatitis B, but not every case requires treatment. It is important that a patient with chronic hepatitis B is checked often to make sure their liver is healthy.

A person with hepatitis B should avoid alcohol and should consult with a healthcare provider before taking any supplements or over-the-counter (OTC) medications (as some of these products can damage the liver).

I Was Treated for Hepatitis B. When Can I Have Sex Again?

After treatment for hepatitis B, there is no waiting period needed to have sex. Because hepatitis B is most commonly spread through sexual contact, all heterosexual and homosexual persons, especially those with concurrent HIV infection, a new partner, or more than one partner, should protect their partners against transmission of hepatitis B by using a condom, even if you have been treated for hepatitis B.

I Was Treated for Hepatitis B. Can I Get It Again?

No, a person who is treated for hepatitis B develops antibodies that provide protection from the virus for life. An antibody is a substance found in the blood that the body produces in response to a virus. Antibodies protect the body from disease by attaching to the virus and destroying it. However, some people, especially those infected during early childhood, may remain infected for life because they never clear the virus from their bodies.

What Happens If I Do Not Get Treated

For most people who are infected with acute hepatitis B, the virus will clear on its own without treatment and they will not develop the chronic infection. For others who develop chronic hepatitis B, lack of treatment could result in liver damage, liver cancer, or, in rare cases, death.

Section 37.6

Human Papillomavirus

This section includes text excerpted from "Human Papillomavirus (HPV)," U.S. Department of Health and Human Services (HHS), February 22, 2019.

What Is Human Papillomavirus?

Genital human papillomavirus (also called "HPV") is the most common sexually transmitted disease (STD) in the United States. Most types of HPV are not harmful to people. There are more than 40 types of HPV that can infect the genital areas, as well as the mouth and throat. Most people who become infected with HPV do not know they are infected.

The same types of HPV that infect the genital areas can infect the mouth and throat. HPV found in the mouth and throat is called "oral HPV." In most cases, HPV infections of all types go away before they cause any health problems.

There are two categories of HPV. These categories are:

1. **Low-risk strains.** Low-risk strains of HPV can cause warts on the genitals. Warts can be itchy, embarrassing, and unpleasant, but these strains do not cause cancer.

2. **High-risk strains.** High-risk strains do not cause warts but can, in some cases, cause oropharyngeal cancer (cancer of the head and neck area).

How Common Is Human Papillomavirus?

Human papillomavirus is one of the most common sexually transmitted infections in the world. More than 75 out of 100 sexually active people will get genital HPV at some point in their life.

How Is Human Papillomavirus Spread?

Human papillomavirus is passed by direct skin-to-skin contact during vaginal, anal, and oral sex with someone who has this infection. Rarely, a partner with HPV on his hands can pass the infection to the genitals. Most cases of HPV are spread by partners who do not have visible signs or symptoms and do not know they have the virus. A person can have HPV for months or even years without knowing it.

Only a few studies have looked at how people get oral HPV, and some of these studies show conflicting results. Some studies suggest that oral HPV may be passed along during oral sex (from mouth-to-genital or mouth-to-anus contact) or open-mouthed ("French") kissing, others have not. The likelihood of getting HPV from kissing or having oral sex with someone who has HPV is not known. We do know that partners who have been together a long time tend to share genital HPV—meaning that they both may have it. More research is needed to understand exactly how people get and give oral HPV infections.

Human Papillomavirus Vaccines

Human papillomavirus vaccines are safe and effective. They can protect males and females against diseases and health problems (including genital warts and some cancers) caused by HPV when given as a series for these recommended age groups:

* All boys and girls 11 or 12 years of age should be vaccinated. A vaccination series can start as early as 9 years of age.

- Boys and girls who are 11 or 12 years of age should receive 2 doses of the HPV vaccine, 6 to 12 months apart. Adolescents who receive their 2 doses of the HPV vaccine less than 5 months apart will require a third dose of the vaccine.

- Catch-up vaccines are recommended for males through the age of 21, and for females through the age of 26, if they were not vaccinated when they were younger. Those who are between 15 and 26 years of age when they first receive the vaccine will need three doses of the HPV vaccine.

The vaccine is also recommended for gay or bisexual men (or any man who has sex with a man) through the age of 26. It is also recommended for men with compromised immune systems (including people living with human immunodeficiency virus/acquired immunodeficiency syndrome (HIV/AIDS) through the age of 26 if they did not get fully vaccinated when they were younger. 3 doses of the vaccine are recommended for people between the ages of 9 and 26 who are living with certain immunocompromising conditions, such as HIV/AIDS.

Human papillomavirus vaccines are effective at blocking infection with the HPV types associated with most cases of cervical cancer. The HPV vaccine works best if a person receives their first dose before having sex for the first time. Talk to your healthcare provider about the HPV vaccine.

What Are the Symptoms of Human Papillomavirus?

Human papillomavirus can cause genital warts, which usually appear as a small bump or group of bumps in the genital area. Warts can be small or large, raised or flat, or shaped like cauliflower.

Human papillomavirus can cause cervical cancer and other cancers, including cancer of the penis, anus, or throat (oropharyngeal cancer).

In most cases, HPV goes away on its own and does not cause any health problems. However, there is no way to know if people who have HPV will develop cancer or other health problems. People with weak immune systems may be less able to fight off HPV and more likely to develop health problems; this includes people with HIV/AIDS.

What Are the Risk Factors for Human Papillomavirus?

A risk factor is the chance that something will harm or otherwise affect a person's health.

Risk factors for HPV include:

- Engaging in unprotected vaginal, anal, or oral sex
- Having sex with multiple partners
- Having HIV
- Having a sexual partner who has HPV

The most reliable way to avoid transmission of STDs is to abstain from oral, vaginal, and anal sex or to be in a long-term, mutually monogamous relationship with a partner known to be uninfected.

Are There Tests for Human Papillomavirus?

Currently, there is not an approved HPV test for males that will detect HPV in the mouth or throat. Talk to your dentist about any symptoms that could suggest early signs of oropharyngeal cancer (persistent sore throat, earaches, hoarseness, enlarged lymph nodes, pain when swallowing, and unexplained weight loss).

How Is Human Papillomavirus Treated?

In most cases, HPV goes away on its own and does not cause any health problems.

There is no treatment for HPV itself. However, there are treatments for the health problems that HPV can cause:

- Genital warts can be treated with prescription medications, freezing with liquid nitrogen, and cauterization (burning or freezing of the tissue).

- Precancer is treated by taking out the cells that are not normal. This is usually done through a short procedure in a healthcare provider's office or a health center.

- Most of the time, cancer, including cervical cancer and oropharyngeal cancer, will be treated with surgery, radiation therapy, or chemotherapy. Sometimes more than one type of treatment is used.

Talk to your healthcare provider to help determine what course of treatment is best.

Even if you do not have any symptoms, you can still infect your sex partners. Using condoms may help lower this risk but it will not get rid of the risk completely.

If you have HPV, you should tell your sex partner(s) so they can make an appointment to discuss their options with a healthcare provider. Because a positive STD diagnosis may affect how you will feel about current or future sexual relationships, it is important to understand how to talk to sexual partners about STDs.

Section 37.7

Pubic Lice

This section includes text excerpted from "Pubic Lice,"
MedlinePlus, National Institutes of Health (NIH), April 18, 2018.

What Are Pubic Lice?

Pubic lice (also called "crabs") are tiny insects which usually live in the pubic or genital area of humans. They are also sometimes found on other coarse body hair, such as hair on the legs, armpits, mustache, beard, eyebrows, or eyelashes. Pubic lice on the eyebrows or eyelashes of children or teens may be a sign of sexual exposure or abuse.

Pubic lice are parasites, and they need to feed on human blood to survive. They are one of the three types of lice that live on humans. The other two types are head lice and body lice. Each type of lice is different, and getting one type does not mean that you will get another type.

How Do Pubic Lice Spread?

Pubic lice move by crawling because they cannot hop or fly. They usually spread through sexual contact. Occasionally, they may spread through physical contact with a person who has pubic lice or through contact with clothing, beds, bed linens, or towels that were used by a person with pubic lice. You cannot get pubic lice from animals.

Who Is at Risk for Pubic Lice?

Since they spread mainly through sexual contact, pubic lice are most common in adults.

What Are the Symptoms of Pubic Lice?

The most common symptom of pubic lice is intense itching in the genital area. You may also see nits (lice eggs) or crawling lice.

How Do You Know If You Have Pubic Lice?

A diagnosis of a pubic lice usually comes from seeing a louse or nit. But, lice and nits can be difficult to find because there may be only a few present. Also, they often attach themselves to more than one hair, and they do not crawl as quickly as head and body lice. Sometimes it takes a magnifying lens to see the lice or nits.

People who have pubic lice should also be checked for other sexually transmitted diseases (STDs), and their sexual partners should also be checked for pubic lice.

What Are the Treatments for Pubic Lice?

The main treatment for pubic lice is a lice-killing lotion. Options include a lotion that contains permethrin or a mousse containing pyrethrins and piperonyl butoxide. These products are available over-the-counter (OTC) without a prescription. They are safe and effective when you use them according to the instructions. Usually, 1 treatment will get rid of the lice. If not, you may need another treatment after 9 to 10 days.

There are other lice-killing medicines that are available with a prescription from your healthcare provider.

You should also wash your clothes, bedding, and towels with hot water, and dry them using the hot cycle of the dryer.

Scabies

This section includes text excerpted from "Scabies
Frequently Asked Questions (FAQs)," Centers for Disease
Control and Prevention (CDC), October 24, 2018.

What Is Scabies?

Scabies is an infestation of the skin by the human itch mite (Sarcoptes scabiei var. hominis). The microscopic scabies mite burrows into the upper layer of the skin where it lives and lays its eggs. The most common symptoms of scabies are intense itching and a pimple-like skin rash. The scabies mite usually is spread by direct, prolonged, skin-to-skin contact with a person who has scabies.

Scabies is found worldwide and affects people of all races and social classes. Scabies can spread rapidly under crowded conditions where close body and skin contact is frequent. Institutions, such as nursing homes, extended-care facilities, and prisons, are often sites of scabies outbreaks. Child care facilities also are a common site of scabies infestations.

What Is Crusted (Norwegian) Scabies?

Crusted scabies is a severe form of scabies that can occur in some persons who are immunocompromised (have a weak immune system), elderly, disabled, or debilitated. It is also called "Norwegian scabies." Persons with crusted scabies have thick crusts of skin that contain large numbers of scabies mites and eggs. Persons with crusted scabies are very contagious to other persons and can spread the infestation easily, both by direct skin-to-skin contact and by contamination of items, such as their clothing, bedding, and furniture. Persons with crusted scabies may not show the usual signs and symptoms of scabies, such as the characteristic rash or itching (pruritus). Persons with crusted scabies should receive quick and aggressive medical treatment for their infestation to prevent outbreaks of scabies.

How Soon after Infestation Do Symptoms of Scabies Begin?

If a person has never had scabies before, symptoms may take as long as four to six weeks to begin. It is important to remember that an infected person can spread scabies during this time, even if he does not have symptoms yet.

In a person who has had scabies before, symptoms usually appear much sooner (one to four days) after exposure.

What Are the Signs and Symptoms of Scabies Infestation?

The most common signs and symptoms of scabies are intense itching (pruritus), especially at night, and a pimple-like (papular) itchy rash. The itching and rash each may affect much of the body or be limited to common sites, such as the wrist, elbow, armpit, webbing between the fingers, nipple, penis, waist, belt-line, and buttocks. The rash also can include tiny blisters (vesicles) and scales. Scratching the rash can cause skin sores; sometimes these sores become infected by bacteria.

Tiny burrows sometimes are seen on the skin; these are caused by the female scabies mite tunneling just beneath the surface of the skin. These burrows appear as tiny raised and crooked (serpiginous) grayish-white or skin-colored lines on the skin surface. Because mites are often few in number (only 10 to 15 mites per person), these burrows may be difficult to find. They are found most often in the webbing between the fingers, in the skin folds on the wrist, elbow, or knee, and on the penis, breast, or shoulder blades.

The head, face, neck, palms, and soles often are involved in infants and very young children, but usually not adults and older children.

Persons with crusted scabies may not show the usual signs and symptoms of scabies, such as the characteristic rash or itching (pruritus).

How Did I Get Scabies?

Scabies usually is spread by direct, prolonged, skin-to-skin contact with a person who has scabies. Contact generally must be prolonged; a quick handshake or hug usually will not spread scabies. Scabies is spread easily to sexual partners and household members. Scabies in adults frequently is sexually acquired. Scabies sometimes is spread indirectly by sharing articles, such as clothing, towels, or bedding used by an infected person; however, such indirect spread can occur much more easily when the infected person has crusted scabies.

527

How Is Scabies Infestation Diagnosed?

Diagnosis of a scabies infestation usually is made based on the customary appearance and distribution of the rash and the presence of burrows. Whenever possible, the diagnosis of scabies should be confirmed by identifying the mite, mite eggs, or mite fecal matter (scybala). This can be done by carefully removing a mite from the end of its burrow using the tip of a needle or by obtaining skin scraping to examine under a microscope for mites, eggs, or mite fecal matter. It is important to remember that a person can still be infected even if mites, eggs, or fecal matter cannot be found; typically fewer than 10 to 15 mites can be present on the entire body of an infected person who is otherwise healthy. However, persons with crusted scabies can be infected with thousands of mites and should be considered highly contagious.

How Long Can Scabies Mites Live?

On a person, scabies mites can live for as long as 1 to 2 months. Off a person, scabies mites usually do not survive more than 48 to 72 hours. Scabies mites will die if exposed to a temperature of 122°F (50°C) for 10 minutes.

Can Scabies Be Treated?

Yes. Products used to treat scabies are called "scabicides" because they kill scabies mites; some also kill eggs. Scabicides to treat human scabies are available only with a doctor's prescription; no "over-the-counter" (OTC) (nonprescription) products have been tested and approved for humans.

Always carefully follow the instructions provided by the doctor and pharmacist, as well as those contained in the box or printed on the label. When treating adults and older children, scabicide cream or lotion is applied to all areas of the body from the neck down to the feet and toes; when treating infants and young children, the cream or lotion also is applied to the head and neck. The medication should be left on the body for the recommended time before it is washed off. Clean clothes should be worn after treatment.

In addition to the infected person, treatment also is recommended for household members and sexual contacts, particularly those who have had prolonged skin-to-skin contact with the infected person. All persons should be treated at the same time in order to prevent reinfection. Retreatment may be necessary if itching continues more than two to four weeks after treatment or if new burrows or rash continue to appear.

Never use a scabicide intended for veterinary or agricultural use to treat humans.

Who Should Be Treated for Scabies?

Anyone who is diagnosed with scabies, as well as his sexual partners and other contacts who have had prolonged skin-to-skin contact with the infected person, should be treated. Treatment is recommended for members of the same household as the person with scabies, particularly those persons who have had prolonged skin-to-skin contact with the infected person. All persons should be treated at the same time to prevent reinfestation.

Retreatment may be necessary if itching continues more than two to four weeks after treatment or if new burrows or rash continue to appear.

How Soon after Treatment Will I Feel Better?

If itching continues more than two to four weeks after initial treatment or if new burrows or rash continue to appear (if initial treatment includes more than one application or dose, then the two to four time period begins after the last application or dose), retreatment with scabicide may be necessary; seek the advice of a physician.

Did I Get Scabies from My Pet?

No. Animals do not spread human scabies. Pets can become infected with a different kind of scabies mite that does not survive or reproduce on humans but causes "mange" in animals. If an animal with "mange" has close contact with a person, the animal mite can get under the person's skin and cause temporary itching and skin irritation. However, the animal mite cannot reproduce on a person and will die on its own in a couple of days. Although the person does not need to be treated, the animal should be treated because its mites can continue to burrow into the person's skin and cause symptoms until the animal has been treated successfully.

Can Scabies Be Spread by Swimming in a Public Pool?

Scabies is spread by prolonged skin-to-skin contact with a person who has scabies. Scabies sometimes also can be spread by contact with items, such as clothing, bedding, or towels that have been used by a person with scabies, but such spread is very uncommon unless the infected person has crusted scabies.

Scabies is very unlikely to be spread by water in a swimming pool. Except for a person with crusted scabies, only about 10–15 scabies mites are present on an infected person; it is extremely unlikely that any would emerge from under wet skin.

Although uncommon, scabies can be spread by sharing a towel or item of clothing that has been used by a person with scabies.

How Can I Remove Scabies Mites from My House or Carpet?

Scabies mites do not survive more than 2 to 3 days away from human skin. Items, such as bedding, clothing, and towels, used by a person with scabies can be decontaminated by machine-washing in hot water and drying using the hot cycle or by dry-cleaning. Items that cannot be washed or dry-cleaned can be decontaminated by removing from any body contact for at least 72 hours.

Because persons with crusted scabies are considered very infectious, careful vacuuming of furniture and carpets in rooms used by these persons is recommended.

Fumigation of living areas is unnecessary.

How Can I Remove Scabies Mites from My Clothes?

Scabies mites do not survive more than 2 to 3 days away from human skin. Items, such as bedding, clothing, and towels used by a person with scabies can be decontaminated by machine-washing in hot water and drying using the hot cycle or by dry-cleaning. Items that cannot be washed or dry-cleaned can be decontaminated by removing from any body contact for at least 72 hours.

My Spouse and I Were Diagnosed with Scabies. after Several Treatments, She/He Still Has Symptoms While I Am Cured. Why?

The rash and itching of scabies can persist for several weeks to a month after treatment, even if the treatment was successful and all the mites and eggs have been killed. Your healthcare provider may prescribe additional medication to relieve itching if it is severe. Symptoms that persist for longer than two weeks after treatment can be due to a number of reasons, including:

- Incorrect diagnosis of scabies. Many drug reactions can mimic the symptoms of scabies and cause a skin rash and itching; the diagnosis of scabies should be confirmed by a skin scraping that includes observing the mite, eggs, or scybala under a microscope. If you are sleeping in the same bed with your spouse and have not become reinfected, and you have not retreated yourself for at least 30 days, then it is unlikely that your spouse has scabies.

- Reinfestation with scabies from a family member or other infected person if all patients and their contacts are not treated at the same time; infected persons and their contacts must be treated at the same time to prevent reinfestation.

- Treatment failure caused by resistance to medication, by faulty application of topical scabicides, or by failure to do a second application when necessary; no new burrows should appear 24 to 48 hours after effective treatment.

- Treatment failure of crusted scabies because of poor penetration of scabicide into thick scaly skin containing large numbers of scabies mites; repeated treatment with a combination of both topical and oral medication may be necessary to treat crusted scabies successfully.

- Reinfestation from items (fomites), such as clothing, bedding, or towels that were not appropriately washed or dry-cleaned (this is mainly of concern for items used by persons with crusted scabies); potentially contaminated items (fomites) should be machine washed in hot water and dried using the hot temperature cycle, dry-cleaned, or removed from skin contact for at least 72 hours

- An allergic skin rash (dermatitis)

- Exposure to household mites that cause symptoms to persist because of cross-reactivity between mite antigens

If itching continues more than two to four weeks or if new burrows or rash continue to appear, seek the advice of a physician; retreatment with the same or a different scabicide may be necessary.

If I Come in Contact with a Person Who Has Scabies, Should I Treat Myself?

No. If a person thinks he might have scabies, he should contact a doctor. The doctor can examine the person, confirm the diagnosis of scabies, and prescribe an appropriate treatment. Products used to treat scabies in humans are available only with a doctor's prescription.

Sleeping with or having sex with any scabies infected person presents a high risk for transmission. The longer a person has skin-to-skin exposure, the greater is the likelihood for transmission to occur. Although briefly shaking hands with a person who has noncrusted scabies could be considered as presenting a relatively low risk, holding the hand of a person with scabies for 5 to 10 minutes could be considered to present a relatively high risk of transmission. However, transmission can occur even after brief skin-to-skin contact, such as a handshake, with a person who has crusted scabies. In general, a person who has skin-to-skin contact with a person who has crusted scabies would be considered a good candidate for treatment.

To determine when prophylactic treatment should be given to reduce the risk of transmission, early consultation should be sought with a healthcare provider who understands:

1. The type of scabies (i.e., noncrusted vs crusted) to which a person has been exposed

2. The degree and duration of skin exposure that a person has had to the infected patient

3. Whether the exposure occurred before or after the patient was treated for scabies

4. Whether the exposed person works in an environment where he would be likely to expose other people during the asymptomatic incubation period. For example, a nurse or caretaker who works in a nursing home or hospital often would be treated prophylactically to reduce the risk of further scabies transmission in the facility.

Section 37.9

Syphilis

This section includes text excerpted from "Syphilis," U.S. Department of Health and Human Services (HHS), March 29, 2019.

What Is Syphilis?

Syphilis is a bacterial sexually transmitted disease (STD) that can cause long-term complications if not treated correctly. In 2015, the United States experienced the highest number and rate of reported syphilis cases in more than 20 years. During 2014 to 2015, syphilis rates increased in every region, in a majority of age groups, and across almost every race/ethnicity.

How Is Syphilis Spread?

Syphilis can be spread by direct contact with a syphilis sore during vaginal, anal, or oral sex. Sores can be found on the penis, anus, in the rectum, or on the lips and in the mouth. Syphilis can be spread during the infection's primary, secondary, and early latent stages. Syphilis can also be spread from an infected mother to the fetus.

What Are the Symptoms of Syphilis?

Syphilis is divided into stages (primary, secondary, latent, and late syphilis), and there are different signs and symptoms associated with each stage. A person with primary syphilis generally has a painless sore or sores at the site of the infection. In the secondary stage, a person may develop a nonitchy body rash that can show up on the palms of the hands and soles of the feet, all over the body, or in just a few places. In the latent/late stage, syphilis can cause severe medical problems affecting the heart, brain, eyes, and other organs. In the latent stage, sometimes also known as the "hidden" stage, there are usually no visible signs or symptoms of syphilis.

Symptoms of syphilis in adults can be divided into stages:

Primary Stage

During the first (primary) stage of syphilis, there may be a single sore or multiple sores. The sore is the location where syphilis entered the body. The sore is usually firm, round, and painless. Because the sore is painless, it can easily go unnoticed. The sore lasts three to six weeks and heals regardless of whether or not you receive treatment. Even though the sore goes away, a person must still receive treatment so the infection does not move to the secondary stage.

Secondary Stage

During the secondary stage, skin rashes and/or sores in the mouth or anus (also called "mucous membrane lesions") may occur. This stage usually starts with a rash on one or more areas of the body. The rash can show up when a primary sore is healing or several weeks after the sore has healed. The rash can look like rough, red, or reddish brown spots on the palms of the hands and/or the bottoms of the feet. The rash usually will not itch and it is sometimes so faint that it will not be noticed. Other symptoms may include fever, swollen lymph glands (also called "lymph nodes," groups of cells that help to fight infection), sore throat, patchy hair loss, headaches, weight loss, muscle aches, and fatigue (feeling very tired). The symptoms from this stage will go away whether or not a person receives treatment. Without the right treatment, the infection will move to the latent and possibly late stages of syphilis.

Latent and Late Stages

The latent stage of syphilis begins when all of the earlier symptoms disappear. Without treatment, a person can continue to have syphilis in their body for years without any signs or symptoms. Most people with untreated syphilis do not develop late-stage syphilis. However, when it does happen, it is very serious and occurs roughly 10 to 30 years after the infection begins. Symptoms of the late stage of syphilis include difficulty coordinating muscle movements, paralysis (not able to move certain parts of your body), numbness, blindness, and dementia (mental disorder). In the late stages of syphilis, the disease damages internal organs and can result in death.

A syphilis infection is called an "early case" if a patient has been infected for a year or less, such as during the primary or secondary stages of syphilis. People who have early syphilis infections can more easily spread the infection to their sex partners. The majority of early syphilis cases are currently found among men who have sex with men.

What Are the Risk Factors for Syphilis?

A risk factor is the chance that something will harm or otherwise affect a person's health.

Risk factors for syphilis include:

- Engaging in unprotected vaginal, anal, or oral sex
- Having sex with multiple partners
- Being a man who has sex with men
- Having human immunodeficiency virus
- Having a sexual partner who has tested positive for syphilis

Have an honest and open talk with your healthcare provider and ask whether you should be tested for syphilis or other STDs.

How Can I Reduce My Risk of Getting Syphilis?

The only way to avoid syphilis completely is to not have vaginal, anal, or oral sex.

If you are sexually active, the following can lower your chances of getting syphilis:

- Being in a long-term, mutually monogamous relationship with a partner who has been tested and has negative STD test results.

- Using latex condoms correctly every time you have sex. Condoms prevent transmission of syphilis by preventing contact with a sore. Sometimes sores occur in areas not covered by a condom. Contact with these sores can still transmit syphilis.

Are There Tests for Syphilis?

Most of the time, a blood test can be used to test for syphilis. Some healthcare providers will diagnose syphilis by testing fluid from a syphilis sore.

You should get tested regularly for syphilis if you are a man who has sex with men, have HIV infection, and/or have partner(s) who have tested positive for syphilis.

How Is Syphilis Treated?

When treated in the early stages, syphilis is easy to cure. The preferred treatment is penicillin, an antibiotic medication. If you are allergic to penicillin, your healthcare provider will suggest another antibiotic. However, treatment will not undo any damage that the infection has already caused.

I Was Treated for Syphilis. When Can I Have Sex Again?

Avoid sexual contact until you have completed the treatment and blood tests indicate the infection is cured.

I Was Treated for Syphilis. Can I Get It Again?

Having syphilis once does not protect you from getting it again. Even after you have been successfully treated, you can still be reinfected. Only laboratory tests can confirm whether you have syphilis. Follow-up testing by your healthcare provider is recommended to make sure that your treatment was successful.

Even if you do not have any symptoms, you can still infect your sex partners. Using condoms may help lower this risk but it will not get rid of the risk completely.

Because syphilis sores can be hidden in the anus, under the foreskin of the penis, or in the mouth, it may not be obvious that a sex partner has syphilis. Unless you know that your sex partner(s) has been tested and treated, you may be at risk of getting syphilis again from an untreated sex partner.

If you have syphilis, you should tell your sex partner(s) and let them know so they can get tested and treated, if necessary.

What Happens If I Do Not Get Treated

Without treatment, syphilis can spread to the brain and nervous system, or the eyes, even causing blindness. Syphilis is serious and should be treated as soon as it is diagnosed.

Section 37.10

Trichomoniasis

This section includes text excerpted from "Trichomoniasis," U.S. Department of Health and Human Services (HHS), April 5, 2019.

What Is Trichomoniasis?

Trichomoniasis (or "trich") is a very common sexually transmitted disease (STD) that is caused by infection with a protozoan parasite called *"Trichomonas vaginalis."* Although symptoms of the disease vary, most women and men who have the parasite cannot tell they are infected.

Trichomoniasis can cause genital inflammation and increase the risk of getting infected with other STDs, including human immunodeficiency virus (HIV).

How Common Is Trichomoniasis?

Trichomoniasis is considered the most common, curable STD. An estimated 3.7 million people have the infection in the United States, but only about 30 out of 100 infected people develop any symptoms of trichomoniasis. Infection is more common in women than in men.

How Is Trichomoniasis Spread?

The parasite is passed from an infected person to an uninfected person during sex. In men, the most commonly infected body part is the inside of the penis (urethra, or urine canal). During sex, the parasite is usually transmitted through vaginal sex.

What Are the Symptoms of Trichomoniasis?

Most people (about 70 out of every 100 people) who have trichomoniasis do not have any signs or symptoms. Infected people without symptoms can still pass the infection on to others.

When trichomoniasis does cause symptoms, they can range from mild irritation to severe inflammation. Some people who develop symptoms get them within 5 to 28 days after being infected, but others do not develop symptoms until much later. Symptoms can come and go.

Men with trichomoniasis may feel itching or irritation inside the penis, burning after urination or ejaculation, or some discharge from the penis.

Having trichomoniasis can make it feel unpleasant to have sex. Without treatment, the infection can last for months or even years.

What Are the Risk Factors for Trichomoniasis?

A risk factor is the chance that something will harm or otherwise affect a person's health.

Risk factors for trichomoniasis include:

- Having sex without a condom. However, condoms do not cover the entire genital region, and it is possible to get or spread this infection even when using a condom.

- Having a history of STDs

- Having a past trichomoniasis infection

- Having multiple sex partners

Are There Tests for Trichomoniasis?

It is not possible to diagnose trichomoniasis based on symptoms alone. Your healthcare provider must do a physical exam and a laboratory test, looking at a sample of urine for men, to diagnose trichomoniasis.

How Is Trichomoniasis Treated?

Trichomoniasis can be cured with a single dose of prescription antibiotic medication (either metronidazole or tinidazole) which can be taken by mouth. Some people who drink alcohol within 24 hours after taking this kind of antibiotic can have uncomfortable side effects.

People who have been treated for trichomoniasis can get it again. About 20 out of 100 people get infected again within three months after treatment. Get checked again if your symptoms come back.

I Was Treated for Trichomoniasis. When Can I Have Sex Again?

Wait to have sex again until all of your symptoms go away (after about a week). To avoid getting reinfected, make sure that all of your sex partners get treated too.

Even if you do not have any symptoms, you can still infect your sex partners. Using condoms may help lower this risk but it will not get rid of the risk completely. If you have trichomoniasis, you should tell your sex partner(s) so they can get tested and treated, if necessary.

What Happens If I Do Not Get Treated

If you do not get treated for trichomoniasis and you have other STDs, it can increase the risk of spreading other STDs, including HIV.

Part Four

Other Medical Issues of Concern to Men

Chapter 38

Male-Linked Genetic Disorders

Chapter Contents

Section 38.1—Color Vision Deficiency 544

Section 38.2—Fragile X Syndrome 549

Section 38.3—Hemophilia 554

Section 38.4—Klinefelter Syndrome 566

Section 38.5—Muscular Dystrophy 578

Section 38.1

Color Vision Deficiency

This section includes text excerpted from "Facts about Color Blindness," National Eye Institute (NEI), February 2015. Reviewed June 2019.

What Is Color Blindness?

Most of us share a common color vision sensory experience. Some people, however, have a color vision deficiency, which means that their perception of colors is different from what most of us see. The most severe forms of these deficiencies are referred to as "color blindness." People with color blindness are not aware of differences among colors that are obvious to the rest of us. People who do not have the more severe types of color blindness may not even be aware of their condition unless they are tested in a clinic or laboratory.

Inherited color blindness is caused by abnormal photopigments. These color-detecting molecules are located in cone-shaped cells within the retina, called "cone cells." In humans, several genes are needed for the body to make photopigments, and defects in these genes can lead to color blindness.

There are three main kinds of color blindness, based on photopigment defects in the three different kinds of cones that respond to blue, green, and red light. Red-green color blindness is the most common, followed by blue-yellow color blindness. A complete absence of color vision—total color blindness—is rare.

Sometimes, color blindness can be caused by physical or chemical damage to the eye, the optic nerve, or parts of the brain that process color information. Color vision can also decline with age, most often because of cataract—a clouding and yellowing of the eye's lens.

Who Gets Color Blindness

As many as 8 percent of men and 0.5 percent of women with Northern European ancestry have the common form of red-green color blindness.

Men are much more likely to be colorblind than women because the genes responsible for the most common inherited color blindness are on the X chromosome. Males only have one X chromosome, while females have two X chromosomes. In females, a functional gene on only one of the X chromosomes is enough to compensate for the loss on the other. This kind of inheritance pattern is called "X-linked," and it primarily affects males. Inherited color blindness can be present at birth, begin in childhood, or not appear until the adult years.

How Do We See Color?

What color is a strawberry? Most of us would say red, but do we all see the same red? Color vision depends on our eyes and brain working together to perceive different properties of light.

We see the natural and artificial light that illuminates our world as white, although it is actually a mixture of colors that, perceived on their own, would span the visual spectrum from deep blue to deep red. You can see this when rain separates sunlight into a rainbow or a glass prism separates white light into a multi-color band. The color of light is determined by its wavelength. Longer wavelength corresponds to red light and shorter wavelength corresponds to blue light.

Strawberries and other objects reflect some wavelengths of light and absorb others. The reflected light we perceive as color. So, a strawberry is red because its surface is only reflecting the long wavelengths we see as red and absorbing the others. An object appears white when it reflects all wavelengths and black when it absorbs all wavelengths.

Vision begins when light enters the eye, and the cornea and lens focus it onto the retina, a thin layer of tissue at the back of the eye that contains millions of light-sensitive cells called "photoreceptors." Some photoreceptors are shaped like rods, and some are shaped like cones. In each eye, there are many more rods than cones—approximately 120 million rods compared to only 6 million cones. Rods and cones both contain photopigment molecules that undergo a chemical change when they absorb light. This chemical change acts like an on-switch, triggering electrical signals that are then passed from the retina to the visual parts of the brain.

Rods and cones are different in how they respond to light. Rods are more responsive to dim light, which makes them useful for night vision. Cones are more responsive to bright light, such as in the daytime when light is plentiful.

Another important difference is that all rods contain only one photopigment, while cones contain one of three different photopigments. This makes cones sensitive to long (red), medium (green), or short (blue) wavelengths of light. The presence of three types of photopigments, each sensitive to a different part of the visual spectrum, is what gives us our rich color vision.

545

Humans are unusual among mammals for our trichromatic vision— named for the three different types of photopigments we have. Most mammals, including dogs, have just two photopigment types. Other creatures, such as butterflies, have more than three. They may be able to see colors we can only imagine.

Most of us have a full set of the three different cone photopigments and so we share a very similar color vision experience, but because the human eye and brain together translate light into color, each of us sees colors differently. The differences may be slight. Your blue may be more blue than someone else's, or in the case of color blindness, your red and green may be someone else's brown.

What Are the Different Types of Color Blindness?

The most common types of color blindness are inherited. They are the result of defects in the genes that contain the instructions for making the photopigments found in cones. Some defects alter the photopigment's sensitivity to color, for example, and it might be slightly more sensitive to deeper red and less sensitive to green. Other defects can result in the total loss of a photopigment. Depending on the type of defect and the cone that is affected problems can arise with red, green, or blue color vision.

Red-Green Color Blindness

The most common types of hereditary color blindness are due to the loss or limited function of red cone (known as "protan") or green cone ("deutran") photopigments. This kind of color blindness is commonly referred to as "red-green color blindness."

- **Protanomaly:** In males with protanomaly, the red cone photopigment is abnormal. Red, orange, and yellow appear greener, and colors are not as bright. This condition is mild and does not usually interfere with daily living. Protanomaly is an X-linked disorder estimated to affect one percent of males.

- **Protanopia:** In males with protanopia, there are no working red cone cells. Red appears as black. Certain shades of orange, yellow, and green all appear as yellow. Protanopia is an X-linked disorder that is estimated to affect one percent of males.

- **Deuteranomaly:** In males with deuteranomaly, the green cone photopigment is abnormal. Yellow and green appear redder, and it is difficult to tell violet from blue. This condition is mild and does not interfere with daily living. Deuteranomaly is the most common form of color blindness and is an X-linked disorder affecting five percent of males.

- **Deuteranopia:** In males with deuteranopia, there are no working green cone cells. They tend to see reds as brownish-yellow and greens as beige. Deuteranopia is an X-linked disorder that affects about one percent of males.

Blue-Yellow Color Blindness

Blue-yellow color blindness is rarer than red-green color blindness. Blue-cone (tritan) photopigments are either missing or have limited function.

- **Tritanomaly:** People with tritanomaly have functionally limited blue cone cells. Blue appears greener, and it can be difficult to tell yellow and red from pink. Tritanomaly is extremely rare. It is an autosomal dominant disorder affecting males and females equally.

- **Tritanopia:** People with tritanopia, also known as "blue-yellow color blindness," lack blue cone cells. Blue appears green, and yellow appears violet or light grey. Tritanopia is an extremely rare autosomal recessive disorder affecting males and females equally.

Complete Color Blindness

People with complete color blindness (monochromacy) do not experience color at all, and the clearness of their vision (visual acuity) may also be affected.

There are two types of monochromacy:

- **Cone monochromacy:** This rare form of color blindness results from a failure of two of the three cone cell photopigments to work. There is red cone monochromacy, green cone monochromacy, and blue cone monochromacy. People with cone monochromacy have trouble distinguishing colors because the brain needs to compare the signals from different types of cones in order to see color. When only one type of cone works, this comparison is not possible. People with blue cone monochromacy, may also have reduced visual acuity; nearsightedness; and uncontrollable eye movements, a condition known as "nystagmus." Cone monochromacy is an autosomal recessive disorder.

- **Rod monochromacy or achromatopsia:** This type of monochromacy is rare and is the most severe form of color blindness. It is present at birth. None of the cone cells have functional photopigments. Lacking all cone vision, people with rod monochromacy see the world in black, white, and gray. And since rods respond to dim light, people with rod monochromacy tend to be photophobic—very uncomfortable in bright environments. They also experience nystagmus. Rod monochromacy is an autosomal recessive disorder.

How Is Color Blindness Diagnosed?

Eye care professionals use a variety of tests to diagnose color blindness. These tests can quickly diagnose specific types of color blindness.

The Ishihara Color Test is the most common test for red-green color blindness. The test consists of a series of colored circles, called "Ishihara plates," each of which contains a collection of dots in different colors and sizes. Within the circle are dots that form a shape clearly visible to those with normal color vision, but it is invisible or difficult to see for those with red-green color blindness.

The newer Cambridge Color Test uses a visual array similar to the Ishihara plates, except displayed on a computer monitor. The goal is to identify a C shape that is different in color from the background. The "C" is presented randomly in one of four orientations. When test-takers see the "C," they are asked to press one of four keys that correspond to the orientation.

The anomaloscope uses a test in which two different light sources have to be matched in color. Looking through the eyepiece, the viewer sees a circle. The upper half is a yellow light that can be adjusted in brightness. The lower half is a combination of red and green lights that can be mixed in variable proportions. The viewer uses one knob to adjust the brightness of the top half, and another to adjust the color of the lower half. The goal is to make the upper and lower halves the same brightness and color.

The HRR Pseudoisochromatic Color Test is another red-green color blindness test that uses color plates to test for color blindness.

The Farnsworth-Munsell 100 Hue Test uses a set of blocks or pegs that are roughly the same color but in different hues (shades of the color). The goal is to arrange them in a line in order of hue. This test measures the ability to discriminate subtle color changes. It is used by industries that depend on the accurate color perception of its employees, such as graphic design, photography, and food quality inspection.

The Farnsworth Lantern Test is used by the U.S. military to determine the severity of color blindness. Those with mild forms pass the test and are allowed to serve in the armed forces.

Are There Treatments for Color Blindness?

There is no cure for color blindness. However, people with red-green color blindness may be able to use a special set of lenses to help them perceive colors more accurately. These lenses can only be used outdoors under bright lighting conditions. Visual aids have also been developed to help people cope with color blindness. There are iPhone and iPad apps, for example, that help people with color blindness discriminate among colors. Some of these apps allow users to snap a photo and tap it anywhere on the image to see the color of that area. More sophisticated apps allow users to find out both color and shades of color. These kinds of apps can be helpful in selecting ripe fruits, such as bananas, or finding complementary colors when picking out clothing.

Section 38.2

Fragile X Syndrome

This section includes text excerpted from "Fragile X Syndrome," *Eunice Kennedy Shriver* National Institute of Child Health and Human Development (NICHD), December 1, 2016.

How Is a Change in the FMR1 *Gene Related to Fragile X and Associated Disorders?*

Fragile X syndrome and its associated conditions are caused by changes (mutations) in the *FMR1* gene found on the X chromosome. This mutation affects how the body makes the fragile X mental retardation protein, or FMRP. The mutation causes the body to make only a little bit or none of the protein, which can cause the symptoms of fragile X.

In a gene, the information for making a protein has two parts: the introduction and the instructions for making the protein itself. Researchers call the introduction "the promoter" because of how it helps to start the process of building the protein.

The promoter part of the *FMR1* gene includes many repeats— repeated instances of a specific deoxyribonucleic acid (DNA) sequence called the "CGG sequence." A normal *FMR1* gene has between 6 and 40 repeats in the promoter; the average is 30 repeats.

People with between 55 and 200 repeats have a premutation of the gene. The premutation may cause the gene to not work properly, but it does not cause intellectual and developmental disability (IDD). The premutation is linked to the disorders fragile X-associated primary ovarian insufficiency (FXPOI) and fragile X-associated tremor/ataxia syndrome (FXTAS). However, not all people with the premutation show symptoms of FXPOI or FXTAS.

People with 200 or more repeats in the promoter part of the gene have a full mutation, meaning the gene might not work at all. People with a full mutation often have fragile X syndrome.

The number of repeats, also called the "size of the mutation," affects the type of symptoms and how serious the symptoms of fragile X syndrome will be.

Inheriting Fragile X Syndrome

Fragile X syndrome is inherited, which means it is passed down from parents to children. Anyone with the *FMR1* gene mutation can pass it to their children. However, a person who inherits the gene mutation may not develop fragile X syndrome. Males will pass it down to all of their daughters and not their sons. Females have a 50/50 chance to pass it along to both their sons and daughters. In some cases, an *FMR1* premutation can change to a full mutation when it is passed from parent to child.

What Causes Fragile X Syndrome

Fragile X results from a change or mutation in the *FMR1* gene, which is found on the X chromosome. The gene normally makes the FMRP protein, which protein is important for creating and maintaining connections between cells in the brain and nervous system. The mutation causes the body to make only a little bit or none of the protein, which often causes the symptoms of fragile X.

Not everyone with the mutated *FMR1* gene has symptoms of fragile X syndrome, because the body may still be able to make FMRP. A few things affect how much FMRP the body can make:

- **The size of the mutation.** Some people have a smaller mutation (a lower number of repeats) in their *FMR1* gene, while others have big mutations (a large number of repeats) in the gene. If the mutation is small, the body may be able to make some of the protein. Having the protein available makes the symptoms milder.

- **The number of cells that have the mutation.** Because not every cell in the body is exactly the same, some cells might have the *FMR1* mutation while others do not. This situation is called "mosaicism." If the mutation is in most of the body's cells, the person will probably have symptoms of fragile X syndrome. If the mutation is in only some of the cells, the person might not have any symptoms at all or only mild symptoms.

- **Being female.** Females have two X chromosomes (XX), while males have only one. In females, if the *FMR1* gene on one X chromosome has the mutation, the *FMR1* gene on the other X chromosome might not have the mutation. Even if one of the female's genes has a very large mutation, the body can usually make at least some FMRP, leading to milder symptoms.

What Are the Symptoms of Fragile X Syndrome?

People with fragile X do not all have the same signs and symptoms, but they do have some things in common. Symptoms are often milder in females than in males.

- **Intelligence and learning.** Many people with fragile X have problems with intellectual functioning.

- These problems can range from the mild, such as learning disorders or problems with mathematics, to the severe, such as an intellectual or developmental disability.

- The syndrome may affect the ability to think, reason, and learn.

- Because many people with fragile X also have attention disorders, hyperactivity, anxiety, and language-processing problems, a person with fragile X may have more capabilities than her or his intelligence quotient (IQ) score suggests.

- **Physical.** Most infants and younger children with fragile X do not have any specific physical features of this syndrome. When these children start to go through puberty, however, many will begin to develop certain features that are typical of those with fragile X.

- These features include a narrow face, large head, large ears, flexible joints, flat feet, and a prominent forehead.

- These physical signs become more obvious with age.

- **Behavioral, social, and emotional.** Most children with fragile X have some behavioral challenges.

- They may be afraid or anxious in new situations.

- They may have trouble making eye contact with other people.

- Boys, especially, may have trouble paying attention or be aggressive.

- Girls may be shy around new people. They may also have attention disorders and problems with hyperactivity.

- **Speech and language.** Most boys with fragile X have some problems with speech and language.

- They may have trouble speaking clearly, may stutter, or may leave out parts of words. They may also have problems understanding other people's social cues, such as tone of voice or specific types of body language.

- Girls usually do not have severe problems with speech or language.

- Some children with fragile X begin talking later than typically developing children. Most will talk eventually, but a few might stay nonverbal throughout their lives.

- **Sensory.** Many children with fragile X are bothered by certain sensations, such as bright light, loud noises or the way certain clothing feels on their bodies.

- These sensory issues might cause them to act out or display behavior problems.

How Do Healthcare Providers Diagnose Fragile X Syndrome?

Healthcare providers often use a blood sample to diagnose fragile X. The healthcare provider will take a sample of blood and will send it to a laboratory, which will determine what form of the *FMR1* gene is present.

Prenatal Testing

Pregnant women who have an *FMR1* premutation or full mutation may pass that mutated gene on to their children. A prenatal test allows healthcare providers to detect the mutated gene in the developing fetus. This important information helps families and providers to prepare for fragile X syndrome and to intervene as early as possible.

Possible types of prenatal tests include:

- **Amniocentesis.** A healthcare provider takes a sample of amniotic fluid, which is then tested for the *FMR1* mutation.

- **Chorionic villus sampling (CVS).** A healthcare provider takes a sample of cells from the placenta, which is then tested for the *FMR1* mutation.

Because prenatal testing involves some risk to the mother and fetus, if you or a family member is considering prenatal testing for fragile X, discuss all the risks and benefits with your healthcare provider.

Prenatal testing is not very common, and many parents do not know they carry the mutation. Therefore, parents usually start to notice symptoms in their children when they are infants or toddlers. The average age at diagnosis is 36 months of age for boys and 42 months of age for girls.

Diagnosis of Children

Many parents first notice symptoms of delayed development in their infants or toddlers. These symptoms may include delays in speech and language skills, social and emotional difficulties, and being sensitive to certain sensations. Children may also be delayed in or have problems with motor skills, such as learning to walk.

A healthcare provider can perform developmental screening to determine the nature of delays in a child. If a healthcare provider suspects the child has fragile X syndrome, she or he can refer parents to a clinical geneticist, who can perform a genetic test for fragile X syndrome.

What Are the Treatments for Fragile X Syndrome?

There is no single treatment for fragile X syndrome, but there are treatments that help minimize the symptoms of the condition.

Individuals with fragile X who receive appropriate education, therapy services, and medications have the best chance of using all of their individual capabilities and skills. Even those with an intellectual or developmental disability can learn to master many self-help skills.

Early intervention is important. Because a young child's brain is still forming, early intervention gives children the best start possible and the greatest chance of developing a full range of skills. The sooner a child with fragile X syndrome gets treatment, the more opportunity there is for learning.

Section 38.3

Hemophilia

This section includes text excerpted from "Hemophilia," National Heart, Lung, and Blood Institute (NHLBI), February 28, 2018.

What Is Hemophilia?

Hemophilia is a rare bleeding disorder in which the blood does not clot normally.

If you have hemophilia, you may bleed for a longer time than others after an injury. You also may bleed inside your body (internally), especially in your knees, ankles, and elbows. This bleeding can damage your organs and tissues, and it may be life-threatening.

Causes of Hemophilia

A defect in one of the genes that determines how the body makes blood clotting factor VIII or IX causes hemophilia. These genes are located on the X chromosomes.

Chromosomes come in pairs. Females have two X chromosomes, while males have one X and one Y chromosome. Only the X chromosome carries the genes related to clotting factors.

A male who has a hemophilia gene on his X chromosome will have hemophilia. When a female has a hemophilia gene on only one of her X chromosomes, she is a "hemophilia carrier" and can pass the gene to her children. Sometimes, carriers have low levels of clotting factor and have symptoms of hemophilia, including bleeding. Clotting factors are proteins in the blood that work together with platelets to stop or control bleeding.

Very rarely, a girl may be born with a very low clotting factor level and have a greater risk for bleeding, similar to boys who have hemophilia and very low levels of clotting factor. There are several hereditary and genetic causes of this much rarer form of hemophilia in females.

Some males who have the disorder are born to mothers who are not carriers. In these cases, a mutation (random change) occurs in the gene as it is passed to the child.

Below are two examples of how the hemophilia gene is inherited.

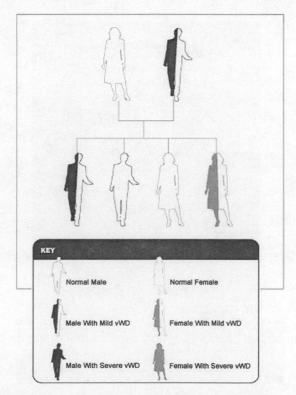

Figure 38.1. *Inheritance Pattern for Hemophilia—Example 1*

The image shows one example of how the hemophilia gene is inherited. In this example, the father does not have hemophilia (that is, he has two normal chromosomes—X and Y). The mother is a carrier of hemophilia (that is, she has one hemophilia gene on one X chromosome and one normal X chromosome).

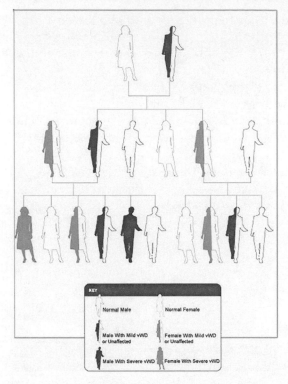

Figure 38.2. *Inheritance Pattern for Hemophilia—Example 2*

The image shows one example of how the hemophilia gene is inherited. In this example, the father has hemophilia (that is, he has the hemophilia gene on the X chromosome). The mother is not a hemophilia carrier (that is, she has two normal X chromosomes).

Signs, Symptoms, and Complications of Hemophilia

The major signs and symptoms of hemophilia are excessive bleeding and easy bruising.

Excessive Bleeding

The extent of bleeding depends on how severe the hemophilia is.

Children who have mild hemophilia may not have signs unless they have excessive bleeding from a dental procedure, an accident, or surgery. Males who have severe hemophilia may bleed heavily after circumcision.

Bleeding can occur on the body's surface (external bleeding) or inside the body (internal bleeding).

Signs of external bleeding may include:

- Bleeding in the mouth from a cut or bite, or from cutting or losing a tooth
- Nosebleeds for no obvious reason
- Heavy bleeding from a minor cut
- Bleeding from a cut that resumes after stopping for a short time

Signs of internal bleeding may include:

- Blood in the urine (from bleeding in the kidneys or bladder)
- Blood in the stool (from bleeding in the intestines or stomach)
- Large bruises (from bleeding into the large muscles of the body)

Bleeding in the Joints

Bleeding in the knees, elbows, or other joints is another common form of internal bleeding in people who have hemophilia. This bleeding can occur without obvious injury.

At first, the bleeding causes tightness in the joint with no real pain or any visible signs of bleeding. The joint then becomes swollen, hot to touch, and painful to bend.

The swelling continues as the bleeding continues. Eventually, movement in the joint is temporarily lost. Pain can be severe. Joint bleeding that is not treated quickly can damage the joint.

Bleeding in the Brain

Internal bleeding in the brain is a very serious complication of hemophilia. It can happen after a simple bump on the head or a more serious injury. The signs and symptoms of bleeding in the brain include:

- Long-lasting, painful headaches or neck pain or stiffness
- Repeated vomiting
- Sleepiness or changes in behavior
- Sudden weakness or clumsiness of the arms or legs or problems walking
- Double vision
- Convulsions or seizures

Diagnosis for Hemophilia

If you or your child appears to have a bleeding problem, your doctor will ask about your personal and family medical histories. This will reveal whether you or your family members, including women and girls, have bleeding problems. However, some people who have hemophilia have no recent family history of the disease.

You or your child also will likely have a physical exam and blood tests to diagnose hemophilia. Blood tests are used to find out:

- How long it takes for your blood to clot

- Whether your blood has low levels of any clotting factors

- Whether any clotting factors are completely missing from your blood

- The test results will show whether you have hemophilia, what type of hemophilia you have, and how severe it is.

Hemophilia A and B are classified as mild, moderate, or severe, depending on the amount of clotting factor VIII or IX in the blood.

Table 38.1. Types of Hemophilia

Mild hemophilia	5 to 40 percent of normal clotting factor
Moderate hemophilia	1 to 5 percent of normal clotting factor
Severe hemophilia	Less than 1 percent of normal clotting factor

The severity of symptoms can overlap between the categories. For example, some people who have mild hemophilia may have bleeding problems almost as often or as severe as some people who have moderate hemophilia.

Severe hemophilia can cause serious bleeding problems in babies. Thus, children who have severe hemophilia usually are diagnosed during the first year of life. People who have milder forms of hemophilia may not be diagnosed until they are adults.

The bleeding problems of hemophilia A and hemophilia B are the same. Only special blood tests can tell which type of the disorder you or your child has. Knowing which type is important because the treatments are different.

Pregnant women who are known hemophilia carriers can have the disorder diagnosed in the fetus as early as 12 weeks into their pregnancies.

Women who are hemophilia carriers also can have a "preimplantation diagnosis" to have children who do not have hemophilia.

For this process, women have their eggs removed and fertilized by sperm in a laboratory. The embryos are then tested for hemophilia. Only embryos without the disorder are implanted in the womb.

Treatment for Hemophilia
Treatment with Replacement Therapy

The main treatment for hemophilia is called "replacement therapy." Concentrates of clotting factor VIII (for hemophilia A) or clotting factor IX (for hemophilia B) are slowly dripped or injected into a vein. These infusions help replace the clotting factor that is missing or low.

Clotting factor concentrates can be made from human blood. The blood is treated to prevent the spread of diseases, such as hepatitis. With the current methods of screening and treating donated blood, the risk of getting an infectious disease from human clotting factors is very small.

To further reduce the risk, you or your child can take clotting factor concentrates that are not made from human blood. These are called "recombinant clotting factors." Clotting factors are easy to store, mix, and use at home—it only takes about 15 minutes to receive the factor.

You may have replacement therapy on a regular basis to prevent bleeding. This is called "preventive therapy" or "prophylactic therapy." Or, you may only need replacement therapy to stop bleeding when it occurs. This use of the treatment, on an as-needed basis, is called "demand therapy."

Demand therapy is less intensive and expensive than preventive therapy. However, there is a risk that bleeding will cause damage before you receive the demand therapy.

Complications of Replacement Therapy

Complications of replacement therapy include:

- Developing antibodies (proteins) that attack the clotting factor

- Developing viral infections from human clotting factors

- Damage to joints, muscles, or other parts of the body resulting from delays in treatment

Antibodies to the clotting factor. Antibodies can destroy the clotting factor before it has a chance to work. This is a very serious problem. It prevents the main treatment for hemophilia (replacement therapy) from working.

These antibodies, also called "inhibitors," develop in about 20 to 30 percent of people who have severe hemophilia A. Inhibitors develop in 2 to 5 percent of people who have hemophilia B.

When antibodies develop, doctors may use larger doses of clotting factor or try different clotting factor sources. Sometimes, the antibodies go away.

Researchers are studying new ways to deal with antibodies to clotting factors.

Viruses from human clotting factors. Clotting factors made from human blood can carry the viruses that cause human immunodeficiency virus (HIV), acquired immunodeficiency syndrome (AIDS), and hepatitis. However, the risk of getting an infectious disease from human clotting factors is very small due to:

- Careful screening of blood donors

- Testing of donated blood products

- Treating donated blood products with a detergent and heat to destroy viruses

- Vaccinating people who have hemophilia for hepatitis A and B

Damage to joints, muscles, and other parts of the body. Delays in treatment can cause damage such as:

- Bleeding into a joint. If this happens many times, it can lead to changes in the shape of the joint and impair the joint's function.

- Swelling of the membrane around a joint

- Pain, swelling, and redness of a joint

- Pressure on a joint from swelling, which can destroy the joint

Home Treatment with Replacement Therapy

You can do both preventive (ongoing) and demand (as-needed) replacement therapy at home. Many people learn to do the infusions at home for their child or for themselves. Home treatment has several advantages:

- You or your child can get quicker treatment when bleeding happens. Early treatment lowers the risk of complications.

- Fewer visits to the doctor or emergency room are needed.

- Home treatment costs less than treatment in a medical care setting.

- Home treatment helps children accept treatment and take responsibility for their own health.

Discuss options for home treatment with your doctor or your child's doctor. A doctor or other healthcare provider can teach you the steps and safety procedures for home treatment.

Doctors can surgically implant vein access devices to make it easier for you to access a vein for treatment with replacement therapy. These devices can be helpful if treatment occurs often. However, infections can be a problem with these devices. Your doctor can help you decide whether this type of device is right for you or your child.

Other Types of Treatment
Desmopressin

Desmopressin (DDAVP) is a human-made hormone used to treat people who have mild hemophilia A. DDAVP is not used to treat hemophilia B or severe hemophilia A.

Desmopressin stimulates the release of stored factor VIII and von Willebrand factor; it also increases the level of these proteins in your blood. Von Willebrand factor carries and binds factor VIII, which can then stay in the bloodstream longer.

Desmopressin usually is given by injection or as nasal spray. Because the effect of this medicine wears off if it is used often, the medicine is given only in certain situations. For example, you may take this medicine prior to dental work or before playing certain sports to prevent or reduce bleeding.

Antifibrinolytic Medicines

Antifibrinolytic medicines (including tranexamic acid and epsilon-aminocaproic acid (EACA)) may be used with replacement therapy. They are usually given as a pill, and they help keep blood clots from breaking down.

These medicines most often are used before dental work, to treat bleeding from the mouth or nose, or for mild intestinal bleeding.

Gene Therapy

Researchers are trying to find ways to correct the faulty genes that cause hemophilia. Gene therapy has not yet developed to the point that it is an accepted treatment for hemophilia. However, researchers continue to test gene therapy in clinical trials.

Treatment of a Specific Bleeding Site

Pain medicines, steroids, and physical therapy may be used to reduce pain and swelling in an affected joint. Talk with your doctor or pharmacist about which medicines are safe for you to take.

Which Treatment Is Best for You?

The type of treatment you or your child receives depends on several things, including how severe the hemophilia is, the activities you will be doing, and the dental or medical procedures you will be having.

- **Mild hemophilia**—Replacement therapy usually is not needed for mild hemophilia. Sometimes though, DDAVP is given to raise the body's level of factor VIII.

- **Moderate hemophilia**—You may need replacement therapy only when bleeding occurs or to prevent bleeding that could occur when doing certain activities. Your doctor also may recommend DDAVP prior to having a procedure or doing an activity that increases the risk of bleeding.

- **Severe hemophilia**—You usually need replacement therapy to prevent bleeding that could damage your joints, muscles, or other parts of your body. Typically, replacement therapy is given at home two or three times a week. This preventive therapy usually is started in patients at a young age and may need to continue for life.

For both types of hemophilia, getting quick treatment for bleeding is important. Quick treatment can limit damage to your body. If you or your child has hemophilia, learn to recognize signs of bleeding.

Other family members also should learn to watch for signs of bleeding in a child who has hemophilia. Children sometimes ignore signs of bleeding because they want to avoid the discomfort of treatment.

Living with Hemophilia

If you or your child has hemophilia, you can take steps to prevent bleeding problems. Thanks to improvements in treatment, a child who has hemophilia is likely to live a normal lifespan.

Hemophilia Treatment Centers

The federal government funds a nationwide network of hemophilia treatment centers (HTCs). These centers are an important resource for people who have hemophilia and their families.

The medical experts at HTCs provide treatment, education, and support. They can teach you or your family members how to do home treatments. Center staff also can provide your doctor with information.

People who get care at HTCs are less likely than those who get care elsewhere to have bleeding complications and hospitalizations. They are also more likely to have a better quality of life. This may be due to the centers' emphasis on bleeding prevention and the education and support provided to patients and their caregivers.

More than 100 federally funded HTCs are located throughout the United States. Many HTCs are located at major university medical and research centers. The hemophilia teams at these centers include:

- Nurse coordinators

- Pediatricians (doctors who treat children) and adult and pediatric hematologists (doctors who specialize in blood disorders)

- Social workers (who can help with financial issues, transportation, mental health, and other issues)

- Physical therapists and orthopedists (doctors who specialize in disorders of the bones and joints)

- Dentists

Many people who have hemophilia go to HTCs for annual checkups, even if it means traveling some distance to do so.

At an HTC, you or your child may be able to take part in clinical research and benefit from the latest hemophilia research findings. The HTC team also will work with your local healthcare providers to help meet your needs or your child's needs.

Ongoing Care

If you have hemophilia, you can take steps to avoid complications. For example:

- Follow your treatment plan exactly as your doctor prescribes.

- Have regular checkups and vaccinations as recommended.

- Tell all of your healthcare providers—such as your doctor, dentist, and pharmacist—that you have hemophilia. You also may want to tell people like your employee health nurse, gym trainer, and sports coach about your condition.

- Have regular dental care. Dentists at the HTCs are experts in providing dental care for people who have hemophilia. If you see another dentist, tell her or him that you have hemophilia. The dentist can provide medicine that will reduce bleeding during dental work.

- Know the signs and symptoms of bleeding in joints and other parts of the body. Know when to call your doctor or go to the emergency room. For example, you will need care if you have:

  - Heavy bleeding that cannot be stopped or a wound that continues to ooze blood

  - Any signs or symptoms of bleeding in the brain. Such bleeding is life-threatening and requires emergency care.

  - Limited motion, pain, or swelling of any joint

It is a good idea to keep a record of all previous treatments. Be sure to take this information with you to medical appointments and to the hospital or emergency room.

Physical Activity and Hemophilia

Physical activity helps keep muscles flexible, strengthens joints, and helps maintain a healthy weight. Children and adults who have hemophilia should be physically active, but they may have limits on what they can do safely.

People who have mild hemophilia can take part in many activities. Those who have severe hemophilia should avoid contact sports and other activities that are likely to lead to injuries that could cause bleeding. Examples of these activities include football, hockey, and wrestling.

Physical therapists at HTCs can develop exercise programs tailored to your needs and teach you how to exercise safely.

Talk with your doctor or physical therapist about recommended types of physical activity and sports. In general, some safe physical activities are swimming, biking (while wearing a helmet), walking, and golf.

To prevent bleeding, you also may be able to take clotting factors prior to exercise or a sporting event.

Medicine Precautions

Some medicines increase the risk of bleeding, such as:

- Aspirin and other medicines that contain salicylates

- Ibuprofen, naproxen, and some other nonsteroidal anti-inflammatory medicines (NSAIDs)

Talk with your doctor or pharmacist about which medicines are safe for you to take.

Treatment at Home and When Traveling

Home treatment with replacement therapy has many benefits. It lets you treat bleeding early, before complications are likely to develop. Home treatment also can prevent frequent trips to the doctor's office or hospital. This can give you more independence and control over your hemophilia.

However, if you are treating yourself or your child with clotting factors at home, you should take some steps for safety:

- Follow instructions for storage, preparation, and use of clotting factors and treatment materials.

- Keep a record of all medical treatment.

- Know the signs and symptoms of bleeding, infection, or an allergic reaction, and know the correct way to respond.

- Have someone with you when you treat yourself.

- Know when to call the doctor or 911.

When you are traveling, be sure to take enough treatment supplies along. You also should carry a letter from your doctor describing your hemophilia and treatment. It is a good idea to find out in advance where to go for care when out of town.

Cost Issues

Clotting factors are very costly. Many health insurance companies will only pay for clotting factors on a case-by-case basis. It is important to know:

- What your insurance covers

- Whether your insurance has a limit on the dollar amount it will cover and what that amount is

- Whether restrictions or waiting periods apply

As children grow, it is important to learn about available options for insurance. Look into what kinds of health insurance are offered when seeking a job.

Section 38.4

Klinefelter Syndrome

This section includes text excerpted from "Klinefelter Syndrome (KS): Condition Information," *Eunice Kennedy Shriver* National Institute of Child Health and Human Development (NICHD) December 1, 2016.

What Is Klinefelter Syndrome?

The term "Klinefelter syndrome," or KS, describes a set of features that can occur in a male who is born with an extra X chromosome in his cells. It is named after Dr. Henry Klinefelter, who identified the condition in the 1940s.

Usually, every cell in a male's body, except sperm and red blood cells (RBCs), contains 46 chromosomes. The 45th and 46th chromosomes— the X and Y chromosomes—are sometimes called "sex chromosomes" because they determine a person's sex. Normally, males have one X and one Y chromosome, making them XY. Males with KS have an extra X chromosome, making them XXY.

KS is sometimes called "47,XXY" (47 refers to total chromosomes) or the "XXY condition." Those with KS are sometimes called "XXY males."

Some males with KS may have both XY cells and XXY cells in their bodies. This is called "mosaic." Mosaic males may have fewer symptoms of KS depending on the number of XY cells they have in their bodies and where these cells are located. For example, males who have normal XY cells in their testes may be fertile.

In very rare cases, males might have two or more extra X chromosomes in their cells, for instance XXXY or XXXXY, or an extra Y, such as XXYY. This is called "poly-X Klinefelter syndrome," and it causes more severe symptoms.

What Causes Klinefelter Syndrome

The extra chromosome results from a random error that occurs when a sperm or egg is formed; this error causes an extra X cell to be included each time the cell divides to form new cells. In very rare cases, more than one extra X or an extra Y is included.

How Many People Are Affected by or at Risk for Klinefelter Syndrome?

Researchers estimate that 1 male in about 500 newborn males has an extra X chromosome, making KS among the most common chromosomal disorders seen in all newborns. The likelihood of a third or fourth X is much rarer.

Table 38.2. Prevalence of Klinefelter Syndrome Variants

Number of Extra X Chromosomes	One (XXY)	Two (XXXY)	Three (XXXXY)
Number of Newborn Males with the Condition	1 in 500	1 in 50,000	1 in 85,000 to 100,000

Scientists are not sure what factors increase the risk of KS. The error that produces the extra chromosome occurs at random, meaning that the error is not hereditary or passed down from parent to child. Research suggests that older mothers might be slightly more likely to have a son with KS. However, the extra X chromosome in KS comes from the father about one-half of the time.

What Are Common Symptoms of Klinefelter Syndrome?

Because XXY males do not really appear different from other males and because they may not have any or have mild symptoms, XXY males often do not know they have KS.

In other cases, males with KS may have mild or severe symptoms. Whether or not a male with KS has visible symptoms depends on many factors, including how much testosterone his body makes, if he is mosaic (with both XY and XXY cells), and his age when the condition is diagnosed and treated.

Klinefelter syndrome symptoms fall into these main categories:

- Physical symptoms

- Language and learning symptoms

- Social and behavioral symptoms

- Symptoms of Poly-X KS

Physical Symptoms

Many physical symptoms of KS result from low testosterone levels in the body. The degree of symptoms differs based on the amount of testosterone needed for a specific age or developmental stage and the amount of testosterone the body makes or has available.

During the first few years of life, when the need for testosterone is low, most XXY males do not show any obvious differences from typical male infants and young boys. Some may have slightly weaker muscles, meaning that they might sit up, crawl, and walk slightly later than average. For example, on average, baby boys with KS do not start walking until 18 months of age.

After 5 years of age, when compared to typically developing boys, boys with KS may be slightly:

- Taller

- Fatter around the belly

- Clumsier

- Slower in developing motor skills, coordination, speed, and muscle strength

Puberty for boys with KS usually starts normally. But because their bodies make less testosterone than non-KS boys, their pubertal development may be disrupted or slow. In addition to being tall, KS boys may have:

- Smaller testes and penis

- Breast growth (about one-third of teens with KS have breast growth)

- Less facial and body hair
- Reduced muscle tone
- Narrower shoulders and wider hips
- Weaker bones, greater risk for bone fractures
- Decreased sexual interest
- Lower energy
- Reduced sperm production

An adult male with KS may have these features:

- Infertility: nearly all men with KS are unable to father a biologically-related child without help from a fertility specialist.
- Small testes, with the possibility of testes shrinking slightly after the teen years
- Lower testosterone levels, which lead to less muscle, hair, and sexual interest and function
- Breasts or breast growth (called "gynecomastia")
- In some cases, breast growth can be permanent, and about 10 percent of XXY males need breast-reduction surgery.

Language and Learning Symptoms

Most males with KS have normal intelligence quotients (IQs) and successfully complete education at all levels. (IQ is a frequently used intelligence measure, but it does not include emotional, creative, or other types of intelligence.) Between 25 percent and 85 percent of all males with KS have some kind of learning or language-related problem, which makes it more likely that they will need some extra help in school. Without this help or intervention, KS males might fall behind their classmates as schoolwork becomes harder.

Klinefelter syndrome males may experience some of the following learning and language-related challenges:

- **A delay in learning to talk.** Infants with KS tend to make only a few different vocal sounds. As they grow older, they may have difficulty saying words clearly. It might be hard for them to distinguish differences between similar sounds.
- **Trouble using language to express their thoughts and needs.** Boys with KS might have problems putting their

thoughts, ideas, and emotions into words. Some may find it hard to learn and remember some words, such as the names of common objects.

- **Trouble processing what they hear.** Although most boys with KS can understand what is being said to them, they might take longer to process multiple or complex sentences. In some cases, they might fidget or "tune out" because they take longer to process the information. It might also be difficult for KS males to concentrate in noisy settings. They might also be less able to understand a speaker's feelings from just speech alone.

- **Reading difficulties.** Many boys with KS have difficulty understanding what they read (called "poor reading comprehension"). They might also read more slowly than other boys.

By adulthood, most males with KS learn to speak and converse normally, although they may have a harder time doing work that involves extensive reading and writing.

Social and Behavioral Symptoms

Many of the social and behavioral symptoms in KS may result from the language and learning difficulties. For instance, boys with KS who have language difficulties might hold back socially and could use help building social relationships.

Boys with KS, when compared to typically developing boys, tend to be:

- Quieter

- Less assertive or self-confident

- More anxious or restless

- Less physically active

- More helpful and eager to please

- More obedient or more ready to follow directions

In the teenage years, boys with KS may feel their differences more strongly. As a result, these teen boys are at higher risk of depression, substance abuse, and behavioral disorders. Some teens might withdraw, feel sad, or act out their frustration and anger.

As adults, most men with KS have lives similar to those of men without KS. They successfully complete high school, college, and other levels of education. They have successful and meaningful careers and professions. They have friends and families.

Contrary to research findings published several decades ago, males with KS are no more likely to have serious psychiatric disorders or to get into trouble with the law.

Symptoms of Poly-X Klinefelter Syndrome 11

Males with poly-X Klinefelter syndrome have more than one extra X chromosome, so their symptoms might be more pronounced than in males with KS. In childhood, they may also have seizures, crossed eyes, constipation, and recurrent ear infections. Poly-KS males might also show slight differences in other physical features.

Some common additional symptoms for several poly-X Klinefelter syndromes are listed below.

48,XXYY

- Long legs
- Little body hair
- Lower IQ, average of 60 to 80 (normal IQ is 90 to 110)
- Leg ulcers and other vascular disease symptoms
- Extreme shyness, but also sometimes aggression and impulsiveness

48,XXXY (Or Tetrasomy)

- Eyes set further apart
- Flat nose bridge
- Arm bones connected to each other in an unusual way
- Short
- Fifth (smallest) fingers curve inward (clinodactyly)
- Lower IQ, average 40 to 60
- Immature behavior

49,XXXXY (Or Pentasomy)

- Low IQ, usually between 20 and 60

- Small head
- Short
- Upward-slanted eyes
- Heart defects, such as when the chambers do not form properly
- High feet arches
- Shy, but friendly
- Difficulty with changing routines

What Are the Treatments for Symptoms in Klinefelter Syndrome?

It is important to remember that because symptoms can be mild, many males with KS are never diagnosed or treated.

The earlier in life that KS symptoms are recognized and treated, the more likely it is that the symptoms can be reduced or eliminated. It is especially helpful to begin treatment by early puberty. Puberty is a time of rapid physical and psychological change, and treatment can successfully limit symptoms. However, treatment can bring benefits at any age.

The type of treatment needed depends on the type of symptoms being treated.

- Treating physical symptoms
- Treating language and learning symptoms
- Treating social and behavioral symptoms

Treating Physical Symptoms
Treatment for Low Testosterone

About one-half of XXY males' chromosomes have low testosterone levels. These levels can be raised by taking supplemental testosterone. Testosterone treatment can:

- Improve muscle mass
- Deepen the voice
- Promote growth of facial and body hair
- Help the reproductive organs to mature

- Build and maintain bone strength and help prevent osteoporosis in later years

- Produce a more masculine appearance, which can also help relieve anxiety and depression

- Increase focus and attention

There are various ways to take testosterone:

- Injections or shots, every two to three weeks

- Pills

- Through the skin, also called "transdermal." Current methods include wearing a testosterone patch or rubbing testosterone gel on the skin.

Males taking testosterone treatment should work closely with an endocrinologist, a doctor who specializes in hormones and their functions, to ensure the best outcome from testosterone therapy.

Not all males with XXY condition benefit from testosterone therapy.

For males whose testosterone level is low to normal, the benefits of taking testosterone are less clear than for when testosterone is very low. Side effects, although generally mild, can include acne, skin rashes from patches or gels, breathing problems (especially during sleep), and a higher risk of an enlarged prostate gland or prostate cancer in older age. In addition, testosterone supplementation will not increase testicular size, decrease breast growth, or correct infertility.

Although the majority of boys with KS grow up to live as males, some develop atypical gender identities. For these males, supplemental testosterone may not be suitable. Gender identity should be discussed with healthcare specialists before starting treatment.

Treatment for Enlarged Breasts

No approved drug treatment exists for this condition of over-developed breast tissue, termed "gynecomastia." Some healthcare providers recommend surgery—called "mastectomy"—to remove or reduce the breasts of XXY males.

When adult men have breasts, they are at higher risk for breast cancer than other men and need to be checked for this condition regularly. The mastectomy lowers the risk of cancer and can reduce the social stress associated with XXY males having enlarged breasts.

Because it is a surgical procedure, mastectomy carries a variety of risks. XXY males who are thinking about mastectomy should discuss all the risks and benefits with their healthcare provider.

Treatment for Infertility

Between 95 percent and 99 percent of XXY men are infertile because they do not produce enough sperm to fertilize an egg naturally. But, sperm are found in more than 50 percent of men with KS.

Advances in assistive reproductive technology (ART) have made it possible for some men with KS to conceive. One type of ART, called "testicular sperm extraction" (TESE) with intracytoplasmic sperm injection (ICSI), has shown success for XXY males. For this procedure, a surgeon removes sperm from the testes and places one sperm into an egg.

Like all ART, TESE-ICSI carries both risks and benefits. For instance, it is possible that the resulting child might have the XXY condition. In addition, the procedure is expensive and often is not covered by health insurance plans. Importantly, there is no guarantee the procedure will work.

Studies suggest that collecting sperm from adolescent XXY males and freezing the sperm until later might result in more pregnancies during subsequent fertility treatments. This is because although XXY males may make some healthy sperm during puberty, this becomes more difficult as they leave adolescence and enter adulthood.

Treating Language and Learning Symptoms

Some, but not all, children with KS have language development and learning delays. They might be slow to learn to talk, read, and write, and they might have difficulty processing what they hear. But various interventions, such as speech therapy and educational assistance, can help to reduce and even eliminate these difficulties. The earlier treatment begins, the better the outcomes.

Parents might need to bring these types of problems to the teacher's attention. Because these boys can be quiet and cooperative in the classroom, teachers may not notice the need for help.

Boys and men with KS can benefit by visiting therapists who are experts in areas, such as coordination, social skills, and coping. XXY males might benefit from any or all of the following:

- **Physical therapists** design activities and exercises to build motor skills and strength and to improve muscle control, posture, and balance.

- **Occupational therapists** help build skills needed for daily functioning, such as social and play skills, interaction and conversation skills, and job or career skills that match interests and abilities.

- **Behavioral therapists** help with specific social skills, such as asking other kids to play and starting conversations. They can also teach productive ways of handling frustration, shyness, anger, and other emotions that can arise from feeling "different."

- **Mental-health therapists** or counselors help males with KS find ways to cope with feelings of sadness, depression, self-doubt, and low self-esteem. They can also help with substance abuse problems. These professionals can also help families deal with the emotions of having a son with KS.

- **Family therapists** provide counseling to a man with KS, his spouse, partner, or family. They can help identify relationship problems and help patients develop communication skills and understand other people's needs.

Parents of XXY males have also mentioned that taking part in physical activities at low-key levels, such as karate, swimming, tennis, and golf, were helpful in improving motor skills, coordination, and confidence.

With regard to education, some boys with KS will qualify to receive state-sponsored special needs services to address their developmental and learning symptoms. But, because these symptoms may be mild, many XXY males will not be eligible for these services. Families can contact a local school district official or special education coordinator to learn more about whether XXY males can receive the following free services:

- The Early Intervention Program for Infants and Toddlers with Disabilities is required by two national laws, the Individuals with Disabilities and Education Improvement Act (IDEIA) and the Individuals with Disabilities Education Act (IDEA). Every state operates special programs for children from birth to age 3, helping them develop in areas, such as behavior, development, communication, and social play.

- An Individualized Education Plan (IEP) for school is created and administered by a team of people, starting with parents and including teachers and school psychologists. The team works together to design an IEP with specific academic, communication, motor, learning, functional, and socialization goals, based on the child's educational needs and specific symptoms.

Treating Social and Behavioral Symptoms

Many of the professionals and methods for treating learning and language symptoms of the XXY condition are similar to or the same as the ones used to address social and behavioral symptoms.

For instance, boys with KS may need help with social skills and interacting in groups. Occupational or behavioral therapists might be able to assist with these skills. Some school districts and health centers might also offer these types of skill-building programs or classes.

In adolescence, symptoms, such as lack of body hair, could make XXY males uncomfortable in school or other social settings, and this discomfort can lead to depression, substance abuse, and behavioral problems or "acting out." They might also have questions about their masculinity or gender identity. In these instances, consulting a psychologist, counselor, or psychiatrist may be helpful.

Contrary to research results released decades ago, research shows that XXY males are no more likely than other males to have serious psychiatric disorders or to get into trouble with the law.

How Do Healthcare Providers Diagnose Klinefelter Syndrome?

The only way to confirm the presence of an extra chromosome is by a karyotype test. A healthcare provider will take a small blood or skin sample and send it to a laboratory, where a technician inspects the cells under a microscope to find the extra chromosome. A karyotype test shows the same results at any time in a person's life.

Tests for chromosome disorders, including KS, may be done before birth. To obtain tissue or liquid for this test, a pregnant woman undergoes chorionic villus sampling (CVS) or amniocentesis. These types of prenatal testing carry a small risk for miscarriage and are not routinely conducted unless the woman has a family history of chromosomal disorders, has other medical problems, or is above 35 years of age.

Factors That Influence When Klinefelter Syndrome Is Diagnosed

Because symptoms can be mild, some males with KS are never diagnosed.

Several factors affect whether and when a diagnosis occurs:

• Few newborns and boys are tested for or diagnosed with KS.

• Although newborns in the United States are screened for some conditions, they are not screened for XXY or other sex-chromosome differences.

• In childhood, symptoms can be subtle and overlooked easily. Only about 1 in 10 males with KS is diagnosed before puberty.

• Sometimes, visiting a healthcare provider will not produce a diagnosis. Some symptoms, such as delayed early speech, might be treated successfully without further testing for KS.

• Most XXY diagnoses occur at puberty or in adulthood.

• Puberty brings a surge in diagnoses as some males (or their parents) become concerned about slow testes growth or breast development and consult a healthcare provider.

• Many men are diagnosed for the first time in fertility clinics. Among men seeking help for infertility, about 15 percent have KS.

Is There a Cure for Klinefelter Syndrome?

Currently, there is no way to remove chromosomes from cells to "cure" the XXY condition.

But many symptoms can be successfully treated, minimizing the impact the condition has on length and quality of life. Most adult XXY men have full independence and have friends, families, and normal social relationships. They live about as long as other men, on average.

Section 38.5

Muscular Dystrophy

This section contains text excerpted from the following sources:
Text beginning with the heading "What Is Muscular Dystrophy?" is
excerpted from "What Is Muscular Dystrophy?" Centers for Disease
Control and Prevention (CDC), February 22, 2019; Text beginning
with the heading "Treatment of Muscular Dystrophy" is excerpted
from "Muscular Dystrophy Information Page," National Institute of
Neurological Disorders and Stroke (NINDS), May 7, 2019.

What Is Muscular Dystrophy?

Muscular dystrophies (MD) are a group of diseases caused by
defects in a person's genes. Over time, this muscle weakness decreases
mobility and makes the tasks of daily living difficult. There are many
muscular dystrophies, and the Centers for Disease Control and Prevention (CDC) studies the major types.

Different types of muscular dystrophy affect specific groups of muscles, have a specific age when signs and symptoms are first seen, vary
in how severe they can be, and are caused by imperfections in different
genes. Muscular dystrophy can run in the family, or a person might
be the first one in their family to have the condition.

Muscular dystrophy is rare, and there is not a lot of data on how
many people are affected by the condition. Much of the information
comes from outside the United States. Scientists at the CDC are working to estimate the number of people with each type of muscular dystrophy in the United States.

Types of Muscular Dystrophy
Duchenne/Becker
How Common Is This Type?

In 2007, 349 out of 2.37 million males between 5 and 24 years of
age were reported to have Duchenne muscular dystrophy (DMD) or
Becker muscular dystrophy (BMD) in the United States. This means
that about 15 out of every 100,000 males between the ages of 5 and
24 years were affected that year.

In 2009, 233 out of 1.49 million males were reported to have DMD
or BMD in Northern England. That is, about 16 out of every 100,000
males were affected that year.

Are Males or Females More Likely to Be Affected?

Males are more likely to be affected.

When Does Muscle Weakness Typically Begin?

DMD: Before 5 years of age
BMD: Between 7 to 12 years of age

Which Muscles Usually Show Weakness First?

Upper arms, upper legs

What Other Parts of the Body Can Be Affected?

Brain, throat, heart, diaphragm/chest muscles, stomach, intestines, spine

Myotonic
How Common Is This Type?

In 2009, 316 out of 2.99 million individuals of all ages were reported to have myotonic muscular dystrophy (MMD) in Northern England. This means that about 11 out of every 100,000 people were affected that year.

Are Males or Females More Likely to Be Affected?

Males and females are equally affected.

When Does Muscle Weakness Typically Begin?

Between 10 to 30 years of age, but it ranges from birth to 70 years of age.

Which Muscles Usually Show Weakness First?

Face, neck, arms, hands, hips, lower legs

What Other Parts of the Body Can Be Affected?

Eyes, throat, heart, stomach, intestines, hormone-producing organs, nerves, skin

Limb-Girdle
How Common Is This Type?

In 2009, 68 out of 2.99 million individuals of all ages were reported to have limb-girdle muscular dystrophy (LGMD) in Northern England. This means that about 2 out of every 100,000 people were affected that year.

Are Males or Females More Likely to Be Affected?

Males and females are equally affected.

When Does Muscle Weakness Typically Begin?

It ranges from early childhood to late adulthood.

Which Muscles Usually Show Weakness First?

Shoulders, hips

What Other Parts of the Body Can Be Affected?

Heart, diaphragm/chest muscles, spine

Facioscapulohumeral
How Common Is This Type?

In 2009, 118 out of 2.99 million individuals of all ages were reported to have facioscapulohumeral (FSH) in Northern England. This means that about 4 out of every 100,000 people were affected that year.

Are Males or Females More Likely to Be Affected?

Males and females are equally affected.

When Does Muscle Weakness Typically Begin?

By 20 years of age (average age in the teens)

Which Muscles Usually Show Weakness First?

Face, shoulders, upper arms, lower legs

What Other Parts of the Body Can Be Affected?

Eyes, ears, heart, trunk

Congenital and Myopathies
How Common Is This Type?

In 2009, 68 out of 2.99 million individuals of all ages were reported to have congenital and myopathies muscular dystrophy (CMD) in Northern England. This means that about 2 out of every 100,000 people were affected that year.

Are Males or Females More Likely to Be Affected?

Males and females are equally affected.

When Does Muscle Weakness Typically Begin?

At birth or in early infancy

Which Muscles Usually Show Weakness First?

Neck, arms, trunk, legs

What Other Parts of the Body Can Be Affected?

Brain, eyes, throat, heart, diaphragm/chest muscles, nerves, spine

Distal
How Common Is This Type?

In 2009, 10 out of 2.99 million individuals of all ages were reported to have Distal muscular dystrophy (DD) in Northern England. This means less than 1 out of every 100,000 people were affected that year.

Are Males or Females More Likely to Be Affected?

Males and females are equally affected.

When Does Muscle Weakness Typically Begin?

Ranges from late teens to adulthood

Which Muscles Usually Show Weakness First?

Lower arms, hands, lower legs, feet

What Other Parts of the Body Can Be Affected?

Nerves, other muscles, depending on the type of DD

Oculopharyngeal
How Common Is This Type?

In 2009, 4 out of 2.99 million individuals of all ages were reported to have oculopharyngeal muscular dystrophy (OPMD) in Northern England. This means that less than 1 out of every 100,000 people were affected that year.

Are Males or Females More Likely to Be Affected?

Males and females are equally affected.

When Does Muscle Weakness Typically Begin?

After 40 years of age.

Which Muscles Usually Show Weakness First?

Face (mostly around the eyes), neck, upper arms, upper legs

What Other Parts of the Body Can Be Affected?

Throat

Emery-Dreifuss
How Common Is This Type?

In 2009, 4 out of 2.99 million individuals of all ages were reported to have Emery-Dreifuss muscular dystrophy (EDMD) in Northern England. This means that less than 1 out of every 100,000 people were affected that year.

Are Males or Females More Likely to Be Affected?

Males are more likely to be affected.

When Does Muscle Weakness Typically Begin?

Between 5 to 15 years of age

Which Muscles Usually Show Weakness First?

Upper arms, lower legs

What Other Parts of the Body Can Be Affected?

Heart, spine

Treatment of Muscular Dystrophy

There is no specific treatment to stop or reverse any form of MD. Treatment may include physical therapy, respiratory therapy, speech therapy, orthopedic appliances used for support, and corrective orthopedic surgery. Drug therapy includes corticosteroids to slow muscle degeneration, anticonvulsants to control seizures and some muscle activity, immunosuppressants to delay some damage to dying muscle cells, and antibiotics to fight respiratory infections. Some individuals may benefit from occupational therapy and assistive technology. Some patients may need assisted ventilation to treat respiratory muscle weakness and a pacemaker for cardiac abnormalities.

Prognosis of Muscular Dystrophy

The prognosis for people with MD varies according to the type and progression of the disorder. Some cases may be mild and progress very slowly over a normal lifespan, while others produce severe muscle weakness, functional disability, and loss of the ability to walk. Some children with MD die in infancy, while others live into adulthood with only moderate disability.

Chapter 39

Breast Concerns in Men

Chapter Contents

Section 39.1—Breast Cancer in Men 586
Section 39.2—Gynecomastia 605

Section 39.1

Breast Cancer in Men

This section includes text excerpted from "Male Breast
Cancer Treatment (PDQ®)—Patient Version," National Cancer
Institute (NCI), April 12, 2019.

General Information about Male Breast Cancer
What Is Male Breast Cancer?

Breast cancer may occur in men. Breast cancer may occur in men
at any age, but it usually occurs in men between 60 and 70 years of
age. Male breast cancer makes up less than 1 percent of all cases of
breast cancer.

The following types of breast cancer are found in men:

- **Infiltrating ductal carcinoma:** Cancer that has spread beyond
  the cells lining ducts in the breast. This is the most common
  type of breast cancer in men.

- **Ductal carcinoma in situ:** Abnormal cells that are found in
  the lining of a duct; also called "intraductal carcinoma."

- **Inflammatory breast cancer:** A type of cancer in which the
  breast looks red and swollen and feels warm.

- **Paget disease of the nipple:** A tumor that has grown from
  ducts beneath the nipple onto the surface of the nipple.

Lobular carcinoma in situ (abnormal cells found in one of the lobes
or sections of the breast), which sometimes occurs in women, has not
been seen in men.

Risks of Breast Cancer

Anything that increases your risk of getting a disease is called a
"risk factor." Having a risk factor does not mean that you will get cancer; not having risk factors does not mean that you will not get cancer.
Talk with your doctor if you think you may be at risk. Risk factors for
breast cancer in men may include the following:

- Treatment with radiation therapy to your breast/chest

- Having a disease linked to high levels of estrogen in the body,
  such as cirrhosis (liver disease) or Klinefelter syndrome (a
  genetic disorder)

- Having one or more female relatives who have had breast cancer

- Having mutations (changes) in genes, such as *BRCA2*

Male Breast Cancer Caused by Inherited Gene Mutations

The genes in cells carry the hereditary information that is received from a person's parents. Hereditary breast cancer makes up about 5 percent to 10 percent of all breast cancer. Some mutated genes related to breast cancer, such as *BRCA2*, are more common in certain ethnic groups. Men who have a mutated gene related to breast cancer have an increased risk of this disease.

There are tests that can detect (find) mutated genes. These genetic tests are sometimes done for members of families with a high risk of cancer.

Men with Breast Cancer Usually Have Lumps That Can Be Felt

Lumps and other signs may be caused by male breast cancer or by other conditions. Check with your doctor if you have any of the following:

- A lump or thickening in or near the breast or in the underarm area

- A change in the size or shape of the breast

- A dimple or puckering in the skin of the breast

- A nipple turned inward into the breast

- Fluid from the nipple, especially if it is bloody

- Scaly, red, or swollen skin on the breast, nipple, or areola (the dark area of skin around the nipple)

- Dimples in the breast that look like the skin of an orange, called "peau d'orange"

Tests to Detect and Diagnose Breast Cancer in Men

The following tests and procedures may be used:

- **Physical exam and history:** An exam of the body to check general signs of health, including checking for signs of disease, such as lumps or anything else that seems unusual. A history of the patient's health habits and past illnesses and treatments will also be taken.

- **Clinical breast exam (CBE):** An exam of the breast by a doctor or other health professional. The doctor will carefully feel the breasts and under the arms for lumps or anything else that seems unusual.

- **Mammogram:** An X-ray of the breast

- **Ultrasound exam:** A procedure in which high-energy sound waves (ultrasound) are bounced off internal tissues or organs and make echoes. The echoes form a picture of body tissues called a "sonogram." The picture can be printed to be looked at later.

- **Magnetic resonance imaging (MRI):** A procedure that uses a magnet, radio waves, and a computer to make a series of detailed pictures of both breasts. This procedure is also called "nuclear magnetic resonance imaging" (NMRI).

- **Blood chemistry studies:** A procedure in which a blood sample is checked to measure the amounts of certain substances released into the blood by organs and tissues in the body. An unusual (higher or lower than normal) amount of a substance can be a sign of disease.

- **Biopsy:** The removal of cells or tissues so they can be viewed under a microscope by a pathologist to check for signs of cancer. There are four types of biopsies to check for breast cancer:

  - **Excisional biopsy:** The removal of an entire lump of tissue

  - **Incisional biopsy:** The removal of part of a lump or a sample of tissue

  - **Core biopsy:** The removal of tissue using a wide needle

  - **Fine-needle aspiration (FNA) biopsy:** The removal of tissue or fluid using a thin needle

Tests to Study the Cancer Cells

Decisions about the best treatment are based on the results of these tests. The tests give information about:

- How quickly the cancer may grow

- How likely it is that the cancer will spread through the body

- How well certain treatments might work

- How likely the cancer is to recur (come back)

Tests include the following:

- **Estrogen and progesterone receptor test:** A test to measure the amount of estrogen and progesterone (hormones) receptors in cancer tissue. If there are more estrogen and progesterone receptors than normal, the cancer is called "estrogen receptor positive" and/or "progesterone receptor positive." This type of breast cancer may grow more quickly. The test results show whether treatment to block estrogen and progesterone may stop the cancer from growing.

- **HER2 test:** A laboratory test to measure how many HER2/neu genes there are and how much HER2/neu protein is made in a sample of tissue. If there are more HER2/neu genes or higher levels of HER2/neu protein than normal, the cancer is called "HER2/neu positive." This type of breast cancer may grow more quickly and is more likely to spread to other parts of the body. The cancer may be treated with drugs that target the HER2/neu protein, such as trastuzumab and pertuzumab.

Survival for Men with Breast Cancer

Survival for men with breast cancer is similar to that for women with breast cancer when their stage at diagnosis is the same. Breast cancer in men, however, is often diagnosed at a later stage. Cancer found at a later stage may be less likely to be cured.

Factors Affecting Prognosis and Treatment Options

The prognosis (chance of recovery) and treatment options depend on the following:

- The stage of the cancer (the size of the tumor and whether it is in the breast only or has spread to lymph nodes or other places in the body)

- The type of breast cancer

- Estrogen-receptor and progesterone-receptor levels in the tumor tissue

- Whether the cancer is also found in the other breast

- The man's age and general health

- Whether the cancer has just been diagnosed or has recurred

Stages of Male Breast Cancer
Staging

After breast cancer has been diagnosed, tests are done to find out if cancer cells have spread within the breast or to other parts of the body. This process is called "staging." The information gathered from the staging process determines the stage of the disease. It is important to know the stage in order to plan treatment. Breast cancer in men is staged the same as it is in women. The spread of cancer from the breast to lymph nodes and other parts of the body appears to be similar in men and women.

The following tests and procedures may be used in the staging process:

- **Sentinel lymph node biopsy:** The removal of the sentinel lymph node during surgery. The sentinel lymph node is the first lymph node in a group of lymph nodes to receive lymphatic drainage from the primary tumor. It is the first lymph node the cancer is likely to spread to from the primary tumor. A radioactive substance and/or blue dye is injected near the tumor. The substance or dye flows through the lymph ducts to the lymph nodes. The first lymph node to receive the substance or dye is removed. A pathologist views the tissue under a microscope to look for cancer cells. If cancer cells are not found, it may not be necessary to remove more lymph nodes. Sometimes, a sentinel lymph node is found in more than one group of nodes.

- **Chest X-ray:** An X-ray of the organs and bones inside the chest. An X-ray is a type of energy beam that can go through the body and onto film, making a picture of areas inside the body.

- **Computed tomography (CT) scan:** A procedure that makes a series of detailed pictures of areas inside the body, taken from different angles. The pictures are made by a computer linked to an X-ray machine. A dye may be injected into a vein or swallowed to help the organs or tissues show up more clearly. This procedure is also called "computed tomography," "computerized tomography," or "computerized axial tomography."

- **Bone scan:** A procedure to check if there are rapidly dividing cells, such as cancer cells, in the bone. A very small amount of radioactive material is injected into a vein and travels through the bloodstream. The radioactive material collects in the bones with cancer and is detected by a scanner.

- **Positron emission tomography (PET) scan:** A procedure to find malignant tumor cells in the body. A small amount of radioactive glucose (sugar) is injected into a vein. The PET scanner rotates around the body and makes a picture of where glucose is being used in the body. Malignant tumor cells show up brighter in the picture because they are more active and take up more glucose than normal cells do.

Ways Cancer Spreads

Cancer can spread through tissue, the lymph system, and the blood:

- **Tissue.** The cancer spreads from where it began by growing into nearby areas.

- **Lymph system.** The cancer spreads from where it began by getting into the lymph system. The cancer travels through the lymph vessels to other parts of the body.

- **Blood**. The cancer spreads from where it began by getting into the blood. The cancer travels through the blood vessels to other parts of the body.

When cancer spreads to another part of the body, it is called "metastasis." Cancer cells break away from where they began (the primary tumor) and travel through the lymph system or blood.

- **Lymph system.** The cancer gets into the lymph system, travels through the lymph vessels, and forms a tumor (metastatic tumor) in another part of the body.

- **Blood.** The cancer gets into the blood, travels through the blood vessels, and forms a tumor (metastatic tumor) in another part of the body.

The metastatic tumor is the same type of cancer as the primary tumor. For example, if breast cancer spreads to the bone, the cancer cells in the bone are actually breast cancer cells. The disease is metastatic breast cancer, not bone cancer.

In breast cancer, stage is based on the size and location of the primary tumor, the spread of cancer to nearby lymph nodes or other parts of the body, tumor grade, and whether certain biomarkers are present.

To plan the best treatment and understand your prognosis, it is important to know the breast cancer stage.

There are 3 types of breast cancer stage groups:

- **Clinical prognostic stage** is used first to assign a stage for all patients based on health history, physical exam, imaging tests (if done), and biopsies. The clinical prognostic stage is described by the tumor-node-metastasis (TNM) system, tumor grade, and biomarker status (ER, PR, HER2). In clinical staging, mammography or ultrasound is used to check the lymph nodes for signs of cancer.

- **Pathological prognostic stage** is then used for patients who have surgery as their first treatment. The pathological prognostic stage is based on all clinical information, biomarker status, and laboratory test results from breast tissue and lymph nodes removed during surgery.

- **Anatomic stage** is based on the size and the spread of cancer as described by the TNM system. The anatomic stage is used in parts of the world where biomarker testing is not available. It is not used in the United States.

For breast cancer, the TNM system describes the tumor as follows:

Tumor (T)

- **TX:** Primary tumor cannot be assessed.

- **T0:** No sign of a primary tumor in the breast.

  - **Tis:** Carcinoma in situ. There are 2 types of breast carcinoma in situ:

  - **Tis (DCIS):** DCIS is a condition in which abnormal cells are found in the lining of a breast duct. The abnormal cells have not spread outside the duct to other tissues in the breast. In some cases, DCIS may become invasive breast cancer that is able to spread to other tissues. At this time, there is no way to know which lesions can become invasive.

- **Tis (Paget disease):** Paget disease of the nipple is a condition in which abnormal cells are found in the skin cells of the nipple and may spread to the areola. It is not staged according to the TNM system. If Paget disease and an invasive breast cancer are present, the TNM system is used to stage the invasive breast cancer.

- **T1:** The tumor is 20 millimeters or smaller. There are 4 subtypes of a T1 tumor depending on the size of the tumor:

  - **T1mi:** The tumor is 1 millimeter or smaller.

  - **T1a:** The tumor is larger than 1 millimeter but not larger than 5 millimeters.

  - **T1b:** The tumor is larger than 5 millimeters but not larger than 10 millimeters.

  - **T1c:** The tumor is larger than 10 millimeters but not larger than 20 millimeters.

- **T2:** The tumor is larger than 20 millimeters but not larger than 50 millimeters.

- **T3:** The tumor is larger than 50 millimeters.

- **T4:** The tumor is described as one of the following:

  - **T4a:** The tumor has grown into the chest wall.

  - **T4b:** The tumor has grown into the skin—an ulcer has formed on the surface of the skin on the breast, small tumor nodules have formed in the same breast as the primary tumor, and/or there is swelling of the skin on the breast.

  - **T4c:** The tumor has grown into the chest wall and the skin.

  - **T4d:** Inflammatory breast cancer—one-third or more of the skin on the breast is red and swollen (called "peau d'orange").

Lymph Node (N)

When the lymph nodes are removed by surgery and studied under a microscope by a pathologist, pathologic staging is used to describe the lymph nodes. The pathologic staging of lymph nodes is described below.

- **NX:** The lymph nodes cannot be assessed.

- **N0:** No sign of cancer in the lymph nodes, or tiny clusters of cancer cells not larger than 0.2 millimeters in the lymph nodes.

- **N1:** Cancer is described as one of the following:

  - **N1mi:** Cancer has spread to the axillary (armpit area) lymph nodes, and it is larger than 0.2 millimeters but not larger than 2 millimeters.

  - **N1a:** Cancer has spread to one to three axillary lymph nodes, and the cancer in at least one of the lymph nodes is larger than two millimeters.

  - **N1b:** Cancer has spread to lymph nodes near the breastbone on the same side of the body as the primary tumor, and the cancer is larger than 0.2 millimeters and is found by sentinel lymph node biopsy. Cancer is not found in the axillary lymph nodes.

  - **N1c:** Cancer has spread to one to three axillary lymph nodes, and the cancer in at least one of the lymph nodes is larger than two millimeters. Cancer is also found by sentinel lymph node biopsy in the lymph nodes near the breastbone on the same side of the body as the primary tumor.

- **N2:** Cancer is described as one of the following:

  - **N2a:** Cancer has spread to four to nine axillary lymph nodes, and the cancer in at least one of the lymph nodes is larger than two millimeters.

  - **N2b:** Cancer has spread to lymph nodes near the breastbone, and the cancer is found by imaging tests. Cancer is not found in the axillary lymph nodes by sentinel lymph node biopsy or lymph node dissection.

- **N3:** Cancer is described as one of the following:

  - **N3a:** Cancer has spread to 10 or more axillary lymph nodes, and the cancer in at least one of the lymph nodes is larger than 2 millimeters, or cancer has spread to lymph nodes below the collarbone.

  - **N3b:** Cancer has spread to one to nine axillary lymph nodes, and the cancer in at least one of the lymph nodes is larger than two millimeters. Cancer has also spread to lymph nodes near the breastbone, and the cancer is found by imaging tests.

or

- Cancer has spread to 4 to 9 axillary lymph nodes, and cancer in at least one of the lymph nodes is larger than 2 millimeters. Cancer has also spread to lymph nodes near the breastbone on the same side of the body as the primary tumor, and the cancer is larger than 0.2 millimeters and is found by sentinel lymph node biopsy.

- **N3c:** Cancer has spread to lymph nodes above the collarbone on the same side of the body as the primary tumor.

When the lymph nodes are checked using mammography or ultrasound, it is called "clinical staging." The clinical staging of lymph nodes is not described here.

Metastasis (M)

- **M0:** There is no sign that cancer has spread to other parts of the body.

- **M1:** Cancer has spread to other parts of the body, most often the bones, lungs, liver, or brain. If cancer has spread to distant lymph nodes, the cancer in the lymph nodes is larger than 0.2 millimeters.

Breast Cancer Grading System

The grading system describes a tumor based on how abnormal the cancer cells and tissue look under a microscope and how quickly the cancer cells are likely to grow and spread. Low-grade cancer cells look more like normal cells and tend to grow and spread more slowly than high-grade cancer cells. To describe how abnormal the cancer cells and tissue are, the pathologist will assess the following three features:

- How much of the tumor tissue has normal breast ducts

- The size and shape of the nuclei in the tumor cells

- How many dividing cells are present, which is a measure of how fast the tumor cells are growing and dividing

For each feature, the pathologist assigns a score of 1 to 3; a score of "1" means that the cells and tumor tissue look the most like normal cells and tissue, and a score of "3" means that the cells and tissue look the most abnormal. The scores for each feature are added together to get a total score between 3 and 9.

Three grades are possible:

- Total score of 3 to 5: G1 (Low grade or well differentiated)

- Total score of 6 to 7: G2 (Intermediate grade or moderately differentiated)

- Total score of 8 to 9: G3 (High grade or poorly differentiated)

Biomarker Testing

Healthy breast cells, and some breast cancer cells, have receptors that attach to the hormones estrogen and progesterone. These hormones are needed for healthy cells, and some breast cancer cells, to grow and divide. To check for these biomarkers, samples of tissue containing breast cancer cells are removed during a biopsy or surgery. The samples are tested in a laboratory to see whether the breast cancer cells have estrogen or progesterone receptors.

Another type of receptor that is found on the surface of all breast cancer cells is called "HER2." HER2 receptors are needed for the breast cancer cells to grow and divide.

For breast cancer, biomarker testing includes the following:

- **Estrogen receptor (ER).** If the breast cancer cells have estrogen receptors, the cancer cells are called "ER-positive" (ER+). If the breast cancer cells do not have estrogen receptors, the cancer cells are called "ER-negative" (ER-).

- **Progesterone receptor (PR).** If the breast cancer cells have progesterone receptors, the cancer cells are called "PR-positive" (PR+). If the breast cancer cells do not have progesterone receptors, the cancer cells are called "PR-negative" (PR-).

- **Human epidermal growth factor type 2 receptor (HER2/ neu or HER2).** If the breast cancer cells have larger than normal amounts of HER2 receptors on their surface, the cancer cells are called "HER2-positive" (HER2+). If the breast cancer cells have a normal amount of HER2 on their surface, the cancer cells are called "HER2-negative" (HER2-). HER2+ breast cancer is more likely to grow and divide faster than HER2- breast cancer.

Sometimes, the breast cancer cells will be described as triple negative or triple positive.

- **Triple negative.** If the breast cancer cells do not have estrogen receptors, progesterone receptors, or a larger than normal amount of HER2 receptors, the cancer cells are called "triple negative."

- **Triple positive.** If the breast cancer cells do have estrogen receptors, progesterone receptors, and a larger than normal amount of HER2 receptors, the cancer cells are called "triple positive."

It is important to know the estrogen receptor, progesterone receptor, and HER2 receptor status to choose the best treatment. There are drugs that can stop the receptors from attaching to the hormones estrogen and progesterone and stop the cancer from growing. Other drugs may be used to block the HER2 receptors on the surface of the breast cancer cells and stop the cancer from growing.

Tumor-Node-Metastasis System, the Grading System, and Biomarker Status

Here are three examples that combine the TNM system, the grading system, and the biomarker status to find out the pathological prognostic breast cancer stage for a woman whose first treatment was surgery:

If the tumor size is 30 millimeters (T2), has not spread to nearby lymph nodes (N0), has not spread to distant parts of the body (M0), and is:

- Grade 1
- HER2+
- ER-
- PR-

The cancer is stage IIA.

If the tumor size is 53 millimeters (T3), has spread to 4 to 9 axillary lymph nodes (N2), has not spread to other parts of the body (M0), and is:

- Grade 2
- HER2+

- ER+
- PR-

The tumor is stage IIIA.

If the tumor size is 65 millimeters (T3), has spread to 3 axillary lymph nodes (N1a), has spread to the lungs (M1), and is:

- Grade 1
- HER2+
- ER-
- PR-

The cancer is stage IV.

Talk to Your Doctor

After surgery, your doctor will receive a pathology report that describes the size and location of the primary tumor, the spread of cancer to nearby lymph nodes, tumor grade, and whether certain biomarkers are present. The pathology report and other test results are used to determine your breast cancer stage.

You are likely to have many questions. Ask your doctor to explain how staging is used to decide the best options to treat your cancer and whether there are clinical trials that might be right for you.

Treatment Options Overview
Different Types of Treatment for Breast Cancer

Different types of treatment are available for men with breast cancer. Some treatments are standard (the currently used treatment), and some are being tested in clinical trials. A treatment clinical trial is a research study meant to help improve current treatments or obtain information on new treatments for patients with cancer. When clinical trials show that a new treatment is better than the standard treatment, the new treatment may become the standard treatment.

For some patients, taking part in a clinical trial may be the best treatment choice. Many of today's standard treatments for cancer are based on earlier clinical trials. Patients who take part in a clinical trial may receive the standard treatment or be among the first to receive a new treatment.

Patients who take part in clinical trials also help improve the way cancer will be treated in the future. Even when clinical trials do not lead to effective new treatments, they often answer important questions and help move research forward.

Some clinical trials only include patients who have not yet received treatment. Other trials test treatments for patients whose cancer has not gotten better. There are also clinical trials that test new ways to stop cancer from recurring or to reduce the side effects of cancer treatment.

Types of Standard Treatments
Surgery

Surgery for men with breast cancer is usually a modified radical mastectomy (removal of the breast, many of the lymph nodes under the arm, the lining over the chest muscles, and sometimes part of the chest wall muscles).

Breast-conserving surgery, an operation to remove the cancer but not the breast itself, is also used for some men with breast cancer. A lumpectomy is done to remove the tumor (lump) and a small amount of normal tissue around it. Radiation therapy is given after surgery to kill any cancer cells that are left.

Chemotherapy

Chemotherapy is a cancer treatment that uses drugs to stop the growth of cancer cells, either by killing the cells or by stopping them from dividing. When chemotherapy is taken by mouth or injected into a vein or muscle, the drugs enter the bloodstream and can reach cancer cells throughout the body (systemic chemotherapy). When chemotherapy is placed directly into the cerebrospinal fluid; an organ or a body cavity, such as the abdomen, the drugs mainly affect cancer cells in those areas (regional chemotherapy).

The way the chemotherapy is given depends on the type and stage of the cancer being treated. Systemic chemotherapy is used to treat breast cancer in men.

Hormone Therapy

Hormone therapy is a cancer treatment that removes hormones or blocks their action and stops cancer cells from growing. Hormones are substances made by glands in the body and circulated in the bloodstream. Some hormones can cause certain cancers to grow. If tests show that the cancer cells have places where hormones can attach (receptors), drugs, surgery, or radiation therapy is used to reduce the production of hormones or block them from working.

599

Hormone therapy with tamoxifen is often given to patients with estrogen-receptor and progesterone-receptor-positive breast cancer and to patients with metastatic breast cancer.

Hormone therapy with an aromatase inhibitor is given to some men who have metastatic breast cancer. Aromatase inhibitors decrease the body's estrogen by blocking an enzyme called "aromatase" from turning androgen into estrogen. Anastrozole, letrozole, and exemestane are types of aromatase inhibitors.

Hormone therapy with a luteinizing hormone-releasing hormone (LHRH) agonist is given to some men who have metastatic breast cancer. LHRH agonists affect the pituitary gland, which controls how much testosterone is made by the testicles. In men who are taking LHRH agonists, the pituitary gland tells the testicles to make less testosterone. Leuprolide and goserelin are types of LHRH agonists.

Other types of hormone therapy include megestrol acetate or anti-estrogen therapy, such as fulvestrant.

Radiation Therapy. Radiation therapy is a cancer treatment that uses high-energy X-rays or other types of radiation to kill cancer cells or keep them from growing. There are two types of radiation therapy:

- External radiation therapy uses a machine outside the body to send radiation toward the cancer.

- Internal radiation therapy uses a radioactive substance sealed in needles, seeds, wires, or catheters that are placed directly into or near the cancer.

The way the radiation therapy is given depends on the type and stage of the cancer being treated. External radiation therapy is used to treat male breast cancer.

Targeted Therapy. Targeted therapy is a type of treatment that uses drugs or other substances to identify and attack specific cancer cells without harming normal cells. Monoclonal antibody therapy, tyrosine kinase inhibitors, cyclin-dependent kinase inhibitors, and mammalian target of rapamycin (mTOR) inhibitors are types of targeted therapies used to treat men with breast cancer.

Monoclonal antibody therapy uses antibodies made in the laboratory from a single type of immune system cell. These antibodies can identify substances on cancer cells or normal substances that may help cancer cells grow. The antibodies attach to the substances and kill the cancer cells, block their growth, or keep them from spreading. Monoclonal antibodies are given by infusion. They may be used alone or to carry drugs, toxins, or radioactive material directly to cancer cells. Monoclonal antibodies are also used with chemotherapy as adjuvant therapy (treatment given after surgery to lower the risk that the cancer will come back).

Types of monoclonal antibody therapy include the following:

- Trastuzumab is a monoclonal antibody that blocks the effects of the growth factor protein HER2.

- Pertuzumab is a monoclonal antibody that may be combined with trastuzumab and chemotherapy to treat breast cancer.

- Ado-trastuzumab emtansine is a monoclonal antibody linked to an anticancer drug. This is called an "antibody-drug conjugate." It may be used to treat men with hormone receptor-positive breast cancer that has spread to other parts of the body.

Tyrosine kinase inhibitors are targeted therapy drugs that block signals needed for tumors to grow. Lapatinib is a tyrosine kinase inhibitor that may be used to treat men with metastatic breast cancer.

Cyclin-dependent kinase inhibitors are targeted therapy drugs that block proteins called "cyclin-dependent kinases," which cause the growth of cancer cells. Palbociclib is a cyclin-dependent kinase inhibitor used to treat men with metastatic breast cancer.

Mammalian target of rapamycin (mTOR) inhibitors block a protein called "mTOR," which may keep cancer cells from growing and prevent the growth of new blood vessels that tumors need to grow.

Treatment of Male Breast Cancer

For treatment options for stage I, stage II, stage IIIA, and operable stage IIIC breast cancer:

Early/Localized/Operable Male Breast Cancer

Treatment of early, localized, or operable breast cancer may include the following:

Initial Surgery

Treatment for men diagnosed with breast cancer is usually modified radical mastectomy.

Breast-conserving surgery with lumpectomy followed by radiation therapy may be used for some men.

Adjuvant Therapy

Therapy given after an operation when cancer cells can no longer be seen is called "adjuvant therapy." Even if the doctor removes all the cancer that can be seen at the time of the operation, the patient may be given radiation therapy, chemotherapy, hormone therapy, and/or targeted therapy after surgery to try to kill any cancer cells that may be left.

- **Node-negative:** For men whose cancer is node-negative (cancer has not spread to the lymph nodes), adjuvant therapy should be considered on the same basis as for a woman with breast cancer because there is no evidence that response to therapy is different for men and women.

- **Node-positive:** For men whose cancer is node-positive (cancer has spread to the lymph nodes), adjuvant therapy may include the following:

  - Chemotherapy

  - Hormone therapy with tamoxifen (to block the effect of estrogen)or, less often, aromatase inhibitors (to reduce the amount of estrogen in the body)

  - Targeted therapy with a monoclonal antibody (trastuzumab or pertuzumab)

These treatments appear to increase survival in men as they do in women. The patient's response to hormone therapy depends on whether there are hormone receptors (proteins) in the tumor. Most breast cancers in men have these receptors. Hormone therapy is usually recommended for male breast cancer patients, but it can have many side effects, including hot flashes and impotence (the inability to have an erection adequate for sexual intercourse).

For treatment options for cancer that has recurred near the area where it first formed:

Locoregional Recurrent Male Breast Cancer

For men with locally recurrent disease (cancer that has come back in a limited area after treatment), treatment options include:

- Surgery

- Radiation therapy combined with chemotherapy

For treatment options for stage IV breast cancer or breast cancer that has recurred in other parts of the body.

Metastatic Breast Cancer in Men

Treatment options for metastatic breast cancer (cancer that has spread to distant parts of the body) may include the following:

Hormone Therapy

In men who have just been diagnosed with metastatic breast cancer that is hormone receptor positive or if the hormone receptor status is not known, treatment may include:

- Tamoxifen therapy

- Aromatase inhibitor therapy (anastrozole, letrozole, or exemestane) with or without an LHRH agonist. Sometimes cyclin-dependent kinase inhibitor therapy (palbociclib) is also given.

In men whose tumors are hormone receptor positive or hormone receptor unknown, with spread to the bone or soft tissue only, and who have been treated with tamoxifen, treatment may include:

- Aromatase inhibitor therapy with or without LHRH agonist

- Other hormone therapy, such as megestrol acetate, estrogen or androgen therapy, or anti-estrogen therapy, such as fulvestrant

Targeted Therapy

In men with metastatic breast cancer that is hormone receptor positive and has not responded to other treatments, options may include targeted therapy, such as:

- Trastuzumab, lapatinib, pertuzumab, or mTOR inhibitors

- Antibody-drug conjugate therapy with ado-trastuzumab emtansine

- Cyclin-dependent kinase inhibitor therapy (palbociclib) combined with letrozole

603

In men with metastatic breast cancer that is HER2/neu positive, treatment may include:

- Targeted therapy, such as trastuzumab, pertuzumab, ado-trastuzumab emtansine, or lapatinib.

Chemotherapy

In men with metastatic breast cancer that is hormone receptor negative, has not responded to hormone therapy, has spread to other organs, or has caused symptoms, treatment may include:

- Chemotherapy with one or more drugs

Surgery

- Total mastectomy for men with open or painful breast lesions. Radiation therapy may be given after surgery.

- Surgery to remove cancer that has spread to the brain or spine. Radiation therapy may be given after surgery.

- Surgery to remove cancer that has spread to the lung.

- Surgery to repair or help support weak or broken bones. Radiation therapy may be given after surgery.

- Surgery to remove fluid that has collected around the lungs or heart

Radiation Therapy

- Radiation therapy to the bones, brain, spinal cord, breast, or chest wall to relieve symptoms and improve quality of life

- Strontium-89 (a radionuclide) to relieve pain from cancer that has spread to bones throughout the body

Other Treatment Options

Other treatment options for metastatic breast cancer include:

- Drug therapy with bisphosphonates or denosumab to reduce bone disease and pain when cancer has spread to the bone

- Clinical trials testing new anticancer drugs, new drug combinations, and new ways of giving treatment

Inflammatory Male Breast Cancer

In inflammatory breast cancer, cancer has spread to the skin of the breast, and the breast looks red and swollen and feels warm. The redness and warmth occur because the cancer cells block the lymph vessels in the skin. The skin of the breast may also show the dimpled appearance called "peau d'orange." There may not be any lumps in the breast that can be felt. Inflammatory breast cancer may be stage IIIB, stage IIIC, or stage IV.

Recurrent Male Breast Cancer

Recurrent breast cancer is cancer that has come back after it has been treated. The cancer may come back in the breast, in the chest wall, or in other parts of the body.

Section 39.2

Gynecomastia

"Gynecomastia," © 2017 Omnigraphics.
Reviewed June 2019.

What Is Gynecomastia?

Gynecomastia is the enlargement of male breast tissue, most often due to an imbalance of the hormones estrogen and testosterone. The condition can affect one or both breasts and can make the breast tender. It is usually not permanent or dangerous; however, affected males can experience a considerable amount of social embarrassment and psychological distress. Pseudogynecomastia (false gynecomastia) can sometimes be confused with gynecomastia; but, the former is caused by an excessive amount of fat tissue on the chest, while the latter is an above-average growth of the breast tissue itself.

Prevalence of Gynecomastia

Gynecomastia can occur at any stage of a man's life, depending on the degree of hormonal change. Newborn babies often have this condition for a short time immediately after birth when the mother's estrogen remains in their bloodstreams. In infants, it usually disappears within the first year of life. Teenage boys may experience gynecomastia during puberty starting from as early as the age of 10, with aggressive growth between the ages of 13 and 14, and slowly regressing in the later teen years. Statistically, only about 4 percent of males between the ages of 10 and 19 are found to have gynecomastia. The condition is most prevalent among older adults between the ages of 50 and 80. 1 in every 4 men in this age group is affected, and in these cases, there may be other medical problems associated with the condition.

Causes and Risk Factors of Gynecomastia

The exact cause of gynecomastia is unclear; however, in most cases, it is thought to be the result of an imbalance between estrogen and testosterone. These hormones are responsible for the development and control of sex characteristics in both males and females. In general, testosterone helps create typically male characteristics, such as facial hair, muscle mass, body hair, and a deep voice. Estrogen aids in the development of what are commonly regarded as feminine characteristics, including breast development. Since men have both hormones in their systems, if an imbalance favors estrogen, gynecomastia can result.

Some other causes and risk factors of gynecomastia include:

- Medication, such as antibiotics, anti-anxiety drugs, anabolic steroids, heart medications, anti-androgens, tricyclic antidepressants, gastric motility medications, and ulcer medications

- Cancer and acquired immunodeficiency syndrome (AIDS) treatments

- The use of substances, such as alcohol, heroin, methadone, marijuana, and amphetamines

- A variety of physical conditions, including hypogonadism, tumors, kidney failure, liver failure, cirrhosis, malnutrition, and starvation

- The use of tea tree oil or lavender oil, herbal products that contain natural estrogen

- Obesity or the lack of a proper diet and nutrition

Diagnosis of Gynecomastia

To begin evaluating a patient for gynecomastia, a healthcare provider will ask for a medical history, including such information as the symptoms being experienced, how long they have persisted, if tenderness is present around the breast area, type of medication being taken, general health condition, drug history, and family health history. The healthcare provider will then perform a careful examination of the breast tissue, genitals, and abdomen.

Tests a doctor may order to help confirm a diagnosis of gynecomastia include:

- Computerized tomography (CT) scans

- Blood tests

- Mammograms

- Magnetic resonance imaging (MRI) scans

- Tissue biopsies

- Testicular ultrasounds

Treatment of Gynecomastia

In young patients, treatment is often not necessary, since in such cases, gynecomastia usually resolves on its own. For older individuals, a number of treatment methods can be recommended by healthcare providers. For example, medications may be prescribed to help restore hormone balance. Certain medications, such as tamoxifen, aromatase inhibitors (Arimidex), and raloxifene (Evista)—while not specifically approved for the treatment of gynecomastia—may help in some cases. If any health condition is causing the gynecomastia, it will need to be addressed through specific treatment. If gynecomastia has been resulted from the use of certain drugs, doctors may prescribe a different medication that may help improve the condition.

In rare cases, surgery may be an option if medication and other treatment prove to be ineffective. Surgical options include liposuction, a procedure that removes the breast fat but not the breast gland tissue, and mastectomy, a procedure that removes the breast gland tissue.

In order to make good decisions and ensure the best possible outcome, before beginning any treatment, the patient should ask the following questions of the healthcare provider:

- Is the breast enlargement likely to resolve on its own?

- What types of treatments are available?

- How long will treatment last?

- Are there any health conditions that are triggering the gynecomastia?

- Should I avoid any particular substance or medication to improve the condition?

- Should I be tested for breast cancer?

- If my breasts are hurting, what can I do to stop the pain?

Treatment options also include getting psychological counseling, as well as help and support from family. The condition can cause stress and embarrassment; therefore, counseling, group therapy, and help explaining the condition to family and friends can have a major impact on the recovery process.

References

1. Booth, Stephanie. "Enlarged Breasts in Men: Causes and Treatments," WebMD, December 13, 2015.

2. "Enlarged Breasts in Men (Gynecomastia)," Mayo Clinic, August 29, 2017.

3. "Gynecomastia," Cleveland Clinic, n.d.

4. "Gynecomastia," Familydoctor.org, March 2014.

5. Lemaine, Valerie, M.D., Cenk Cayci, M.D., Patricia S. Simmons, M.D., and Paul Petty, M.D. "Gynecomastia in Adolescent Males," U.S. National Library of Medicine (NLM), February 27, 2013.

Chapter 40

Osteoporosis in Men

Bone across the Lifespan

Bone is constantly changing—that is, old bone is removed and replaced by new bone. During childhood, more bone is produced than removed, so the skeleton grows in both size and strength. For most people, bone mass peaks during the third decade of life. By this age, men typically have accumulated more bone mass than women. After this point, the amount of bone in the skeleton typically begins to decline slowly as the removal of old bone exceeds the formation of new bone.

Men in their fifties do not experience the rapid loss of bone mass that women do in the years following menopause. By the age of 65 or 70, however, men and women lose bone mass at the same rate, and the absorption of calcium, an essential nutrient for bone health throughout life, decreases in both sexes. Excessive bone loss causes bone to become fragile and more likely to fracture.

Fractures resulting from osteoporosis most commonly occur in the hip, spine, and wrist, and they can be permanently disabling. Hip fractures are especially dangerous. Perhaps because such fractures tend to occur at older ages in men than in women, men who sustain hip fractures are more likely to die from complications than women.

This chapter includes text excerpted from "Osteoporosis in Men," NIH Osteoporosis and Related Bone Diseases—National Resource Center (NIH ORBD—NRC), October 2018.

Primary and Secondary Osteoporosis

There are two main types of osteoporosis: primary and secondary. In cases of primary osteoporosis, either the condition is caused by age-related bone loss (sometimes called "senile osteoporosis"), or the cause is unknown (idiopathic osteoporosis). The term "idiopathic osteoporosis" is typically used only for men younger than 70 years of age; in older men, age-related bone loss is assumed to be the cause.

The majority of men with osteoporosis have at least one (sometimes more than one) secondary cause. In cases of secondary osteoporosis, the loss of bone mass is caused by certain lifestyle behaviors, diseases, or medications. Some of the most common causes of secondary osteoporosis in men include exposure to glucocorticoid medications, hypogonadism (low levels of testosterone), alcohol abuse, smoking, gastrointestinal disease, hypercalciuria, and immobilization.

Some Causes of Osteoporosis in Men

Glucocorticoid medications: Glucocorticoids are steroid medications used to treat diseases, such as asthma and rheumatoid arthritis. Bone loss is a very common side effect of these medications. The bone loss that these medications cause may be due to their direct effect on bone, muscle weakness or immobility, reduced intestinal absorption of calcium, a decrease in testosterone levels, or, most likely, a combination of these factors.

When glucocorticoid medications are used on an ongoing basis, bone mass often decreases quickly and continuously, with most of the bone loss in the ribs and vertebrae. Therefore, people taking these medications should talk to their doctor about having a bone mineral density (BMD) test. Men should also be tested to monitor testosterone levels, as glucocorticoids often reduce testosterone in the blood.

A treatment plan to minimize loss of bone during long-term glucocorticoid therapy may include using the minimal effective dose and discontinuing the drug or administering it through the skin, if possible. Adequate calcium and vitamin D intake is important, as these nutrients help reduce the impact of glucocorticoids on the bones. Other possible treatments include testosterone replacement and osteoporosis medication.

Hypogonadism: Hypogonadism refers to abnormally low levels of sex hormones. It is well known that the loss of estrogen causes osteoporosis in women. In men, reduced levels of sex hormones may also cause osteoporosis.

Although it is natural for testosterone levels to decrease with age, there should not be a sudden drop in this hormone that is comparable to the drop in estrogen experienced by women at menopause. However, medications, such as glucocorticoids (discussed above); cancer treatments (especially for prostate cancer); and many other factors can affect testosterone levels. Testosterone replacement therapy may be helpful in preventing or slowing bone loss. Its success depends on numerous factors, such as age and how long testosterone levels have been reduced. Also, it is not yet clear how long any beneficial effect of testosterone replacement will last. Therefore, doctors usually treat the osteoporosis directly, using medications approved for this purpose.

Research suggests that estrogen deficiency may also be a cause of osteoporosis in men. For example, estrogen levels are low in men with hypogonadism and may play a part in bone loss. Osteoporosis has been found in some men who have rare disorders involving estrogen. Therefore, the role of estrogen in men is under active investigation.

Alcohol abuse: There is a wealth of evidence that alcohol abuse may decrease bone density and lead to an increase in fractures. Low bone mass is common in men who seek medical help for alcohol abuse.

In cases where bone loss is linked to alcohol abuse, the first goal of treatment is to help the patient stop, or at least reduce, his consumption of alcohol. More research is needed to determine whether bone lost to alcohol abuse will rebuild once drinking stops, or even whether further damage will be prevented. It is clear, though, that alcohol abuse causes many other health and social problems, so quitting is ideal. A treatment plan may also include a balanced diet with lots of calcium- and vitamin D-rich foods, a program of physical exercise, and smoking cessation.

Smoking: Bone loss is more rapid, and rates of hip and vertebral fracture are higher, among men who smoke; although, more research is needed to determine exactly how smoking damages bone. Tobacco, nicotine, and other chemicals found in cigarettes may be directly toxic to bone, or they may inhibit absorption of calcium and other nutrients needed for bone health. Quitting is the ideal approach, as smoking is harmful in so many ways. As with alcohol, it is not known whether quitting smoking leads to reduced rates of bone loss or to a gain in bone mass.

Gastrointestinal disorders: Several nutrients, including amino acids, calcium, magnesium, phosphorous, and vitamins D and K, are important for bone health. Diseases of the stomach and intestines can lead to bone disease when they impair absorption of these nutrients. In such cases, treatment for bone loss may include taking supplements to replenish these nutrients.

Hypercalciuria: Hypercalciuria is a disorder that causes too much calcium to be lost through the urine, which makes the calcium unavailable for building bone. Patients with hypercalciuria should talk to their doctor about having a BMD test and, if bone density is low, discuss treatment options.

Immobilization: Weight-bearing activity is essential for maintaining healthy bones. Without it, bone density may decline rapidly. Prolonged bed rest (following fractures, surgery, spinal cord injuries, or illness) or immobilization of some part of the body often results in significant bone loss. It is crucial to resume weight-bearing activities (such as walking, jogging, and dancing) as soon as possible after a period of prolonged bed rest. If this is not possible, you should work with your doctor to minimize other risk factors for osteoporosis.

How Is Osteoporosis Diagnosed in Men?

Osteoporosis can be effectively treated if it is detected before significant bone loss has occurred. A medical workup to diagnose osteoporosis can include a complete medical history, X-rays, and urine and blood tests. The doctor may also order a BMD test. This test can identify osteoporosis, determine your risk for fractures (broken bones), and measure your response to osteoporosis treatment. The most widely recognized BMD test is called a "central dual-energy X-ray absorptiometry," or "central DXA test." It is painless—a bit like having an X-ray, but with much less exposure to radiation. It can measure bone density at your hip and spine.

It is increasingly common for women to be diagnosed with osteoporosis or low bone mass using a BMD test, often at midlife when doctors begin to watch for signs of bone loss. In men, however, the diagnosis is often not made until a fracture occurs or a man complains of back pain and sees his doctor. This makes it especially important for men to inform their doctors about risk factors for developing osteoporosis, loss of height or change in posture, a fracture, or sudden back pain.

What Treatments Are Available?

Once a man has been diagnosed with osteoporosis, his doctor may prescribe one of the medications approved by the U.S. Food and Drug

Administration (FDA) for this disease. The treatment plan will also likely include the nutrition, exercise, and lifestyle guidelines for preventing bone loss.

If bone loss is due to glucocorticoid use, the doctor may prescribe a medication approved to prevent or treat glucocorticoid-induced osteoporosis, monitor bone density, and testosterone levels, and suggest using the minimum effective dose of glucocorticoid.

Other possible prevention or treatment approaches include calcium and/or vitamin D supplements and regular physical activity.

If osteoporosis is the result of another condition (such as testosterone deficiency) or exposure to certain other medications, the doctor may design a treatment plan to address the underlying cause.

How Can Osteoporosis Be Prevented?

There have been fewer research studies on osteoporosis in men than in women. However, experts agree that all people should take the following steps to preserve their bone health:

- Avoid smoking, reduce alcohol intake, and increase your level of physical activity.

- Ensure a daily calcium intake that is adequate for your age.

- Ensure an adequate intake of vitamin D. Dietary vitamin D intake should be 600 IU (International Units) per day up to the age of 70. Men over the age of 70 should increase their uptake to 800 IU daily (see table 40.1). The amount of vitamin D found in 1 quart of fortified milk and most multivitamins is 400 IU.

- Engage in a regular regimen of weight-bearing exercises in which bones and muscles work against gravity. This might include walking, jogging, racquet sports, climbing stairs, and team sports. Resistance exercises, such as lifting weights and using resistance machines, are also important. A doctor should evaluate the exercise program of anyone already diagnosed with osteoporosis to determine if twisting motions and impact activities, such as those used in golf, tennis, or basketball, need to be curtailed.

- Discuss with your doctor the use of medications that are known to cause bone loss, such as glucocorticoids.

- Recognize and seek treatment for any underlying medical conditions that affect bone health.

Table 40.1. Recommended Calcium and Vitamin D Intakes

Life-Stage Group	Calcium mg/day	Vitamin D (IU/day)
Infants 0 to 6 months	200	400
Infants 6 to 12 months	260	400
1 to 3 years old	700	600
4 to 8 years old	1,000	600
9 to 13 years old	1,300	600
14 to 18 years old	1,300	600
19 to 30 years old	1,000	600
31 to 50 years old	1,000	600
51- to 70-year-old males	1,000	600
51- to 70-year-old females	1,200	600
70 years old	1,200	800
14 to 18 years old, pregnant/lactating	1,300	600
19 to 50 years old, pregnant/lactating	1,000	600

(Source: Food and Nutrition Board (FNB), Institute of Medicine (IOM), National Academy of Sciences (NAS), 2010.)

Chapter 41

Sleep Apnea

Sleep apnea is a common disorder that causes your breathing to stop or get very shallow. Breathing pauses can last from a few seconds to minutes. They may occur 30 times or more an hour.

The most common type is obstructive sleep apnea (OSA). It causes your airway to collapse or become blocked during sleep. Normal breathing starts again with a snort or choking sound. People with sleep apnea often snore loudly. However, not everyone who snores has sleep apnea.

You are more at risk for sleep apnea if you are overweight, male, or have a family history or small airways.

Screening and Prevention of Sleep Apnea

To screen for sleep apnea, your doctor will review your medical history and symptoms. To prevent sleep apnea, your doctor may recommend healthy lifestyle changes.

Screening for Sleep Apnea

To screen for sleep apnea or other sleep disorders, your doctor may ask you about common signs and symptoms of this condition, such as

---

This chapter contains text excerpted from the following sources: Text in this chapter begins with excerpts from "Sleep Apnea," MedlinePlus, National Institutes of Health (NIH), February 10, 2016; Text beginning with the heading "Screening and Prevention of Sleep Apnea" is excerpted from "Sleep Apnea," National Heart, Lung, and Blood Institute (NHLBI), December 10, 2018.

how sleepy you feel during the day or when driving, and whether you or your partner has noticed that you snore, stop breathing, or gasp during your sleep. Your doctor may ask questions to assess your risk for developing this condition and take your physical measurements. Your doctor will also want to see whether you have any complications of undiagnosed sleep apnea, such as high blood pressure that is difficult to control. If the screening suggests a sleep breathing disorder, you may get a referral to a sleep specialist to help confirm a diagnosis.

Healthy Lifestyle Changes to Prevent Sleep Apnea

If you are concerned about having risk factors for developing sleep apnea, ask your doctor to recommend healthy lifestyle changes, including eating a heart-healthy diet, aiming for a healthy weight, quitting smoking, and limiting alcohol intake. Your doctor may recommend that you sleep on your side and adopt healthy sleep habits such as getting the recommended amount of sleep.

Signs, Symptoms, and Complications of Sleep Apnea

Common sleep apnea signs and symptoms are snoring or gasping during sleep; reduced or absent breathing, called "apnea events"; and sleepiness. Undiagnosed or untreated sleep apnea prevents restful sleep and can cause complications that may affect many parts of your body.

Signs and Symptoms

Common signs of sleep apnea:

- Apnea events
- Frequent loud snoring
- Gasping for air during sleep

Common symptoms of sleep apnea:

- Excessive daytime sleepiness and fatigue
- Decreases in attention, vigilance, concentration, motor skills, and verbal and visuospatial memory
- Dry mouth or headaches when waking
- Sexual dysfunction or decreased libido
- Waking up often during the night to urinate

Did you know that sleep apnea symptoms may be different for women and children when compared with men?

Women who have sleep apnea more often report headache, fatigue, depression, anxiety, insomnia, and sleep disruption. Children may experience bedwetting, asthma exacerbations, hyperactivity, and learning and academic performance issues.

Complications

Sleep apnea may increase your risk of the following disorders:

- Asthma

- Atrial fibrillation

- Cancers, such as pancreatic, renal, and skin cancers

- Chronic kidney disease

- Cognitive and behavioral disorders, such as decreases in attention, vigilance, concentration, motor skills, and verbal and visuospatial memory, as well as dementia in older adults. In children, sleep apnea has been associated with learning disabilities.

- Diseases of the heart and blood vessels, such as atherosclerosis, heart attacks, heart failure, difficult-to-control high blood pressure, and stroke

- Eye disorders, such as glaucoma, dry eye, or keratoconus

- Metabolic disorders, including glucose intolerance and type 2 diabetes

- Pregnancy complications, including gestational diabetes and gestational high blood pressure, as well as having a baby with low birth weight

Did you know that sleep apnea can cause inflammation and lead to complications?

When blood oxygen levels drop due to OSA, your body and brain trigger the "fight or flight" response. This increases your blood pressure and heart rate and wakes you from sleep so that your upper airway can open. These cycles of decreased and increased blood oxygen levels can cause inflammation that may contribute to atherosclerosis, the buildup of plaque in blood vessels, which can increase the risk of heart attack or stroke. Chronic inflammation can also damage the pancreas and lead to type 2 diabetes.

Diagnosis of Sleep Apnea

Your doctor may diagnose sleep apnea based on your medical history, a physical exam, and results from a sleep study. Before diagnosing you with sleep apnea, your doctor will rule out other medical reasons or conditions that may be causing your signs and symptoms.

Medical History

To help diagnose sleep apnea, your doctor may consider the following:

- Information that you provide, such as signs and symptoms that you are experiencing

- Whether you have a family history of sleep apnea or another sleep disorder

- Whether you have risk factors for sleep apnea

- Whether you have complications of undiagnosed or untreated sleep apnea, such as atrial fibrillation, type 2 diabetes, or hard-to-control high blood pressure

Physical Exam

During the physical exam, your doctor will look for signs of other conditions that can increase your risk for sleep apnea, such as obesity, large tonsils, narrowing of the upper airway, or a large neck circumference. A neck circumference greater than 17 inches for men or 16 inches for women is considered large. Your doctor may also look at your jaw size and structure, the size of your tongue, and your tongue's position in your mouth. Your doctor will check your lungs, heart, and neurological systems to see whether you have any common complications of sleep apnea.

Sleep Studies

To diagnose sleep apnea or another sleep disorder, your doctor may refer you to a sleep specialist or a center for a sleep study. Sleep studies can be done in a special center or at home. Studies at a sleep center can:

- Detect apnea events, which are times when your breathing stops or slows during sleep

- Detect low or high levels of activity in muscles that control breathing
- Monitor blood oxygen levels during sleep
- Monitor brain and heart activity during sleep

Your doctor may be able to diagnose mild, moderate, or severe sleep apnea based on the number of sleep apnea events you have in an hour during the sleep study.

- **Mild:** 5 to 14 apnea events in an hour
- **Moderate:** 15 to 29 apnea events in an hour
- **Severe:** 30 or more apnea events in an hour

Did you know that sleep studies can help determine which type of sleep apnea you have?

Sleep studies can monitor the movement of your muscles and help determine breathing patterns and whether you have obstructive or central sleep apnea. Sleep studies of patients with OSA often show an increase in breathing muscle activity when muscles try to open an obstructed upper airway. In contrast, sleep studies of patients with central sleep apnea tend to show decreased activity in chest muscles, which can lead to periods of slowed or no breathing.

Ruling Out Other Medical Reasons or Conditions

Your doctor may order the following tests to help rule out other medical conditions that can cause sleep apnea:

- Blood tests to check the levels of certain hormones and to rule out endocrine disorders that could be contributing to sleep apnea. Thyroid hormone can rule out hypothyroidism. Growth hormone tests can rule out acromegaly. Total testosterone and dehydroepiandrosterone sulfate (DHEAS) tests can help rule out polycystic ovary syndrome (PCOS) in women.

- Pelvic ultrasound to examine the ovaries and detect cysts in women. This can rule out PCOS.

Your doctor will also want to know whether you are using medicines, such as opioids, that could be affecting your sleep or causing breathing symptoms of sleep apnea. Your doctor may want to know whether you have traveled recently to altitudes greater than 6,000 feet because these low-oxygen environments can cause symptoms of sleep apnea for a few weeks after traveling.

Treatment for Sleep Apnea

If you are diagnosed with sleep apnea, your doctor may make recommendations to help you maintain an open airway during sleep. These could include healthy lifestyle changes or a breathing device such as a positive airway pressure (PAP) machine, mouthpiece, or implant. Talk to your doctor. Depending on the type and severity of your sleep apnea and your needs and preferences, other treatments may be possible.

Healthy Lifestyle Changes

To help control or treat your sleep apnea, your doctor may recommend that you adopt lifelong healthy lifestyle changes.

- **Make heart-healthy eating choices.** This also includes limiting your alcohol intake, especially before bedtime.
- **Get regular physical activity.**
- **Aim for a healthy weight.** Research has shown that losing weight can reduce sleep apnea in people who were also diagnosed with obesity.
- **Develop healthy sleeping habits.** Your doctor may recommend general healthy sleep habits, which include getting the recommended amount of sleep based on your age.

Breathing Devices

A breathing device, such as a continuous positive airway pressure (CPAP) machine, is the most commonly recommended treatment for patients with sleep apnea. If your doctor prescribes a CPAP or other breathing device, be sure to continue your doctor-recommended healthy lifestyle changes.

Mouthpieces

Mouthpieces, or oral appliances, are typically custom-fit devices that you wear while you sleep. There are two types of mouthpieces that work differently to open the upper airway. Some hybrid mouthpieces have features of both types.

- Mandibular repositioning mouthpieces are devices that cover the upper and lower teeth and hold the jaw in a position that prevents it from blocking the upper airway.

- Tongue retaining devices are mouthpieces that hold the tongue in a forward position to prevent it from blocking the upper airway.

Your doctor may prescribe a mouthpiece if you have mild sleep apnea or if your apnea occurs only when you are lying on your back. To get your mouthpiece, your doctor may recommend that you visit a dentist or an orthodontist, a type of dentist who specializes in correcting teeth or jaw problems. These specialists will ensure that the oral appliance is custom fit to your mouth and jaw.

Implants

Implants can benefit some people with sleep apnea. Some devices treat both obstructive and central sleep apnea. You must have surgery to place an implant in your body. The U.S. Food and Drug Administration (FDA) has approved one implant as a treatment for sleep apnea. The device senses breathing patterns and delivers mild stimulation to certain muscles that open the airways during sleep. More research is needed to determine how effective the implant is in treating central sleep apnea.

A nerve stimulator can also treat sleep apnea. This treatment also involves surgery. A surgeon will insert a stimulator for the hypoglossal nerve, which controls tongue movement. Increasing stimulation of this nerve helps position the tongue to keep the upper airway open.

Therapy for Mouth and Facial Muscles

Children and adults with sleep apnea may benefit from therapy for mouth and facial muscles, known as orofacial therapy. This therapy helps improve tongue positioning and strengthen muscles that control the lips, tongue, soft palate, lateral pharyngeal wall, and face.

Surgical Procedures

You may need surgery if you have severe OSA that does not respond to breathing devices such as a CPAP machine, or that is caused by visible obstruction to the upper airway, perhaps due to large tonsils. Possible surgical procedures include:

- **Tonsillectomy:** a surgery to remove the tonsils, which are organs at the back of your throat
- **Maxillary or jaw advancement:** a surgery to move the upper jaw (maxilla) and lower jaw (mandible) forward to enlarge the upper airway

- **Tracheostomy:** a surgery to make a hole through the front of your neck into your trachea, or windpipe. A breathing tube, called a "trach tube," is placed through the hole and directly into your windpipe to help you breathe.

If surgery is considered as a possible treatment, talk to your doctor about the different types of surgical procedures, the risks and benefits of the procedures, potential discomfort, and the recovery time you will need after surgery.

Living with Sleep Apnea

If you have been diagnosed with sleep apnea, it is important that you adopt and maintain healthy lifestyle habits and use your prescribed treatment.

Using and Caring for Your Breathing Device or Mouthpiece

It is important that you properly use and care for your prescribed breathing device or mouthpiece. If your doctor prescribed a breathing device or CPAP machine:

- Be patient with your breathing device or CPAP machine. It may take time to adjust to breathing with the help of a CPAP machine.

- Use your breathing device or CPAP machine for all sleep, including naps. To benefit fully from your treatment, you should wear your device whenever and wherever you sleep. If you are traveling, be sure to bring your breathing device with you. Call your doctor or sleep specialist right away if your device stops working correctly.

- Talk to your doctor or supplier if you experience discomfort or have difficulty using your prescribed breathing device. Let the team or supplier know if you are having irritation from the mask, if your mask is not staying on or fitting well, if it leaks air, if you are having difficulty falling or staying asleep, if you wake with dry mouth, or if you have a stuffy or runny nose. Your doctor can explore options to improve the treatment, such as trying different masks or nasal pillows, adjusting the machine's pressure timing and settings, or trying a different breathing device that has a humidifier chamber or provides bi-level or auto-adjusting pressure settings. Cleaning the mask and washing your face before putting your mask on can help make a better seal between the mask and your skin.

- Properly care for your breathing device or CPAP machine. Know how to set up and properly clean all parts of your machine. Be sure to refill prescriptions on time for all of the device's replaceable parts, including the tubes, masks, and air filters.

- Properly care for your mouthpiece. If you were prescribed a mouthpiece, ask your dentist how to properly care for it. If it does not fit right or your signs and symptoms do not improve, let your dentist know so that she or he can adjust the device. It is common to feel some discomfort after a device is adjusted until your mouth and facial muscles get used to the new fit.

Monitor Your Condition

You should visit your doctor to monitor your response to treatment and see whether you have any complications that, if left untreated, can be life-threatening. Your doctor may do any of the following to monitor your condition.

- If your doctor prescribed a breathing device, your doctor and possibly your insurance company will want to check the data card from the machine. The data card shows how often you use the breathing device and whether the device and its pressure settings are helping to reduce or eliminate apnea events while you sleep. Your doctor may also check to see whether you still experience excessive sleepiness during the day, how you feel about your quality of life, whether you are still snoring, or whether you have experienced weight loss or changes in your lifestyle.

- If you were prescribed a mouthpiece, you should follow up with your dental specialist after six months and then at least every year. This is to see whether the mouthpiece is working correctly, whether it needs adjustment, and whether a replacement device is needed.

Repeat Sleep Studies

Sometimes, repeat sleep studies are necessary. Your doctor may have you repeat a sleep study to monitor your response to the treatment, especially if your sleep symptoms continue, if you are using a mouthpiece, if your weight changes significantly, or if your employer requires these tests.

Learn the Warning Signs of Some Continuous Positive Airway Pressure Side Effects

Side effects of CPAP treatment may include congestion, runny nose, dry mouth, dry eyes, or nosebleeds. If you experience stomach discomfort or bloating, you should stop using your CPAP machine and contact your doctor.

Learn about Other Precautions to Help You Stay Safe

Sleep apnea can increase your risks of complications if you are having surgery, and it can affect your ability to drive.

- **Before surgery.** If you are having any type of surgery that requires medicine to put you to sleep or for pain management, let your surgeon and doctors know that you have sleep apnea. They might have to take extra steps to make sure that your upper airway stays open during the surgery and when selecting your pain medicines.

- **Driving precautions.** Undiagnosed and untreated sleep apnea can decrease learning capabilities, slow down decision making, and decrease attention span, which can result in drowsy driving.

Chapter 42

Male-Pattern Baldness

Androgenetic alopecia is a common form of hair loss in both men and women. In men, this condition is also known as "male-pattern baldness." Hair is lost in a well-defined pattern, beginning above both temples. Over time, the hairline recedes to form a characteristic "M" shape. Hair also thins at the crown (near the top of the head), often progressing to partial or complete baldness.

Androgenetic alopecia in men has been associated with several other medical conditions including coronary heart disease and enlargement of the prostate. Additionally, prostate cancer, disorders of insulin resistance (such as diabetes and obesity), and high blood pressure (hypertension) have been related to androgenetic alopecia.

Frequency of Male-Pattern Baldness

Androgenetic alopecia is a frequent cause of hair loss in both men and women. This form of hair loss affects an estimated 50 million men and 30 million women in the United States. Androgenetic alopecia can start as early as a person's teens and risk increases with age; more than 50 percent of men over age 50 have some degree of hair loss.

This chapter includes text excerpted from "Androgenetic Alopecia," Genetics Home Reference (GHR), National Institutes of Health (NIH), August 2015. Reviewed June 2019.

Causes of Male-Pattern Baldness

A variety of genetic and environmental factors likely play a role in causing androgenetic alopecia. Although researchers are studying risk factors that may contribute to this condition, most of these factors remain unknown. Researchers have determined that this form of hair loss is related to hormones called "androgens," particularly an androgen called "dihydrotestosterone." Androgens are important for normal male sexual development before birth and during puberty. Androgens also have other important functions in both males and females, such as regulating hair growth and sex drive.

Hair growth begins under the skin in structures called "follicles." Each strand of hair normally grows for 2 to 6 years, goes into a resting phase for several months, and then falls out. The cycle starts over when the follicle begins growing a new hair. Increased levels of androgens in hair follicles can lead to a shorter cycle of hair growth and the growth of shorter and thinner strands of hair. Additionally, there is a delay in the growth of new hair to replace strands that are shed.

Although researchers suspect that several genes play a role in androgenetic alopecia, variations in only one gene, AR, have been confirmed in scientific studies. The *AR* gene provides instructions for making a protein called an "androgen receptor." Androgen receptors allow the body to respond appropriately to dihydrotestosterone and other androgens. Studies suggest that variations in the *AR* gene lead to increased activity of androgen receptors in hair follicles. It remains unclear, however, how these genetic changes increase the risk of hair loss in men.

Researchers continue to investigate the connection between androgenetic alopecia and other medical conditions, such as coronary heart disease and prostate cancer in men. They believe that some of these disorders may be associated with elevated androgen levels, which may help explain why they tend to occur with androgen-related hair loss. Other hormonal, environmental, and genetic factors that have not been identified also may be involved.

Inheritance Pattern of Male-Pattern Baldness

The inheritance pattern of androgenetic alopecia is unclear because many genetic and environmental factors are likely to be involved. This condition tends to cluster in families, however, and having a close relative with patterned hair loss appears to be a risk factor for developing the condition.

Chapter 43

Mental-Health Concerns in Men

Chapter Contents

Section 43.1—Men and Mental Health...................................... 628

Section 43.2—Depression 629

Section 43.3—Posttraumatic Stress Disorder 637

Section 43.4—Schizophrenia... 640

Section 43.1

Men and Mental Health

This section includes text excerpted from "Men and
Mental Health," National Institute of Mental
Health (NIMH), June 2019.

Many mental illnesses affect both men and women. However, men
may be less likely to talk about their feelings and seek help. Recognizing the signs that someone may have a mood or mental disorder is the
first step toward getting treatment and living a better life.

Warning Signs

Men and women experience many of the same mental disorders, but
their willingness to talk about their feelings may be very different. This
is one of the reasons that their symptoms may be very different as well.
For example, some men with depression or an anxiety disorder hide
their emotions and may appear to be angry or aggressive, while many
women will express sadness. Some men may turn to drugs or alcohol
to try to cope with their emotional issues. Sometimes, mental-health
symptoms appear to be physical issues. For example, a racing heart,
tightening chest, ongoing headaches, and digestive issues can be a
sign of an emotional problem.

Warning signs include:

- Anger, irritability, or aggressiveness

- Noticeable changes in mood, energy level, or appetite

- Difficulty sleeping or sleeping too much

- Difficulty concentrating, feeling restless, or on edge

- Increased worry or feeling stressed

- A need for alcohol or drugs

- Sadness or hopelessness

- Suicidal thoughts

- Feeling flat or having trouble feeling positive emotions

- Engaging in high-risk activities

- Ongoing headaches, digestive issues, or pain

- Obsessive thinking or compulsive behavior

- Thoughts or behaviors that interfere with work, family, or social life

- Unusual thinking or behaviors that concern other people

Section 43.2

Depression

This section includes text excerpted from "Men and Depression,"
National Institute of Mental Health (NIMH), June 13, 2017.

Men and women both experience depression, but their symptoms can be very different. Because men who are depressed may appear to be angry or aggressive instead of sad, their families, friends, and even their doctors may not always recognize the anger or aggression as depression symptoms. In addition, men are less likely than women to recognize, talk about, and seek treatment for depression. Yet, depression affects a large number of men.

What Is Depression?

Everyone feels sad or irritable and has trouble sleeping once in a while. But, these feelings and troubles usually pass after a couple of days. Depression is a common but serious mood disorder that may cause severe symptoms. Depression affects the ability to feel, think, and handle daily activities. Also known as "major depressive disorder" or "clinical depression," a man must have symptoms for at least two weeks to be diagnosed with depression.

Both men and women get depression, but their willingness to talk about their feelings may be very different. This is one of the reasons that depression symptoms for men and women may be very different as well.

For example, some men with depression hide their emotions and may seem to be angry, irritable, or aggressive, while many women seem sad or express sadness. Men with depression may feel very tired and lose interest in work, family, or hobbies. They may be more likely to have difficulty sleeping than women who have depression. Sometimes mental-health symptoms appear to be physical issues. For example, a racing heart, tightening chest, ongoing headaches, or digestive issues can be signs of a mental-health problem. Many men are more likely to see their doctor about physical symptoms than emotional symptoms.

Some men may turn to drugs or alcohol to try to cope with their emotional symptoms. Also, while women with depression are more likely to attempt suicide, men are more likely to die by suicide because they tend to use more lethal methods.

Depression can affect any man at any age. With the right treatment, most men with depression can get better and gain back their interest in work, family, and their hobbies.

What Are the Signs and Symptoms of Depression in Men?

Different men have different symptoms, but some common depression symptoms include:

- Anger, irritability, or aggressiveness

- Feeling anxious, restless, or "on the edge"

- Loss of interest in work, family, or once-pleasurable activities

- Problems with sexual desire and performance

- Feeling sad, "empty," flat, or hopeless

- Not being able to concentrate or remember details

- Feeling very tired, not being able to sleep, or sleeping too much

- Overeating or not wanting to eat at all

- Thoughts of suicide or suicide attempts

- Physical aches or pains, headaches, cramps, or digestive problems

- Inability to meet the responsibilities of work, caring for family, or other important activities

- Engaging in high-risk activities

- A need for alcohol or drugs

- Withdrawing from family and friends or becoming isolated

Not every man who is depressed experiences every symptom. Some men experience only a few symptoms, while others may experience many.

What Are the Different Types of Depression?

The most common types of depression are:

- **Major depression**—depressive symptoms that interfere with a man's ability to work, sleep, study, eat, and enjoy most aspects of life. An episode of major depression may occur only once in a person's lifetime. But, it is common for a person to have several episodes. Special forms (subtypes) of major depression include:

  - **Psychotic depression**—severe depression associated with delusions (false, fixed beliefs) or hallucinations (hearing or seeing things that are not really there). These psychotic symptoms are depression-themed. For example, a man may believe he is sick or poor when he is not, or he may hear voices that are not real that say that he is worthless.

  - **Seasonal affective disorder**—characterized by depression symptoms that appear every year during the winter months when there is less natural sunlight.

  - **Persistent depressive disorder** (also called "dysthymia")—depressive symptoms that last a long time (two years or longer) but are less severe than those of major depression.

  - **Minor depression**—similar to major depression and persistent depressive disorder, but symptoms are less severe and may not last as long.

- **Bipolar disorder** is different from depression. It is included in this list because a person with bipolar disorder experiences episodes of extreme low moods (depression). But, a person with

631

bipolar disorder also experiences extreme high moods (called "mania").

What Causes Depression in Men

Depression is one of the most common mental disorders in the U.S. Current research suggests that depression is caused by a combination of risk factors including:

- **Genetic factors**—men with a family history of depression may be more likely to develop it than those whose family members do not have the illness.

- **Environmental stress**—financial problems, loss of a loved one, a difficult relationship, major life changes, work problems, or any stressful situation may trigger depression in some men.

- **Illness**—depression can occur with other serious medical illnesses, such as diabetes, cancer, heart disease, or Parkinson disease (PD). Depression can make these conditions worse and vice versa. Sometimes, medications taken for these illnesses may cause side effects that trigger or worsen depression.

How Is Depression Treated?

Men often avoid addressing their feelings and, in many cases, friends and family members are the first to recognize that their loved one is depressed. It is important that friends and family support their loved one and encourage him to visit a doctor or mental-health professional for an evaluation. A health professional can do an exam or lab tests to rule out other conditions that may have symptoms that are like those of depression. She or he also can tell if certain medications are affecting the depression.

The doctor needs to get a complete history of symptoms, such as when they started, how long they have lasted, how bad they are, whether they have occurred before, and if so, how they were treated. It is important that the man seeking help be open and honest about any efforts at "self-medication" with alcohol, nonprescribed drugs, gambling, or high-risk activities. A complete history should include information about a family history of depression or other mental disorders.

After a diagnosis, depression is usually treated with medications, psychotherapy, or a combination of the two. The increasingly-popular "collaborative care" approach combines physical and behavioral healthcare. Collaborative care involves a team of healthcare providers and managers, including a primary care doctor and specialists.

Medication

Medications called "antidepressants" can work well to treat depression, but they can take several weeks to be effective. Often with medication, symptoms—such as sleep, appetite, and concentration problems—improve before mood lifts, so it is important to give medication a chance before deciding whether it is effective or not.

Antidepressants can have side effects including:

- Headache

- Nausea or feeling sick to your stomach

- Difficulty sleeping and nervousness

- Agitation or restlessness

- Sexual problems

Most side effects lessen over time, but it is important to talk with your doctor about any side effects that you may have. Starting antidepressant medication at a low dose and gradually increasing to a full therapeutic dose may help minimize adverse effects.

It is important to know that although antidepressants can be safe and effective for many people, they may present serious risks to some, especially children, teens, and young adults. A "black box" warning—the most serious type of warning that a prescription drug can have—has been added to the labels of antidepressant medications to warn people that antidepressants may cause some young people to have suicidal thoughts or may increase the risk for suicide attempts. This is especially true for those who become agitated when they first start taking the medication and before it begins to work. Anyone taking antidepressants should be monitored closely, especially when they first start taking them.

For most people, though, the risks of untreated depression far outweigh those of taking antidepressant medications under a doctor's supervision. Careful monitoring by a health professional will also minimize any potential risks.

For reasons that are not well understood, many people respond better to some antidepressants than to others. If a man does not respond to one medication, his doctor may suggest trying another. Sometimes, a medication may be only partially effective. In that case, another medication might be added to help make the antidepressant more effective.

If you begin taking antidepressants, do not stop taking them without the help of a doctor. Sometimes, people taking antidepressants feel better and then stop taking the medication on their own, and the depression returns. When it is time to stop the medication, usually after a course of 6 to 12 months, the doctor will help you slowly and safely decrease your dose. Stopping them abruptly can cause withdrawal symptoms.

Some people who relapse back into depression after stopping an antidepressant benefit from staying on medication for additional months or years.

Psychotherapy

Several types of psychotherapy or "talk therapy" can help treat depression. Some therapies are just as effective as medications for certain types of depression. Therapy helps by teaching new ways of thinking and behaving, and changing habits that may be contributing to the depression. Therapy can also help men understand and work through difficult situations or relationships that may be causing their depression or making it worse.

Cognitive behavioral therapy (CBT), interpersonal therapy (IPT), and problem-solving therapy are examples of evidence-based talk therapy treatments for depression.

Treatment for depression should be personalized. Some men might try therapy first and add antidepressant medication later if it is needed. Others might start treatment with both medication and psychotherapy.

How Can I Help a Loved One Who Is Depressed?

It is important to remember that a person with depression cannot simply "snap out of it." It is also important to know that he may not recognize his symptoms and may not want to get professional treatment.

If you think someone has depression, you can support him by helping him find a doctor or mental-health professional and then helping him make an appointment. Even men who have trouble recognizing that they are depressed may agree to seek help for physical symptoms, such as feeling tired or run down. They may be willing to talk with their regular health professional about a new difficulty they are having at work or losing interest in doing things they usually enjoy. Talking with a primary care provider may be a good first step toward learning about and treating possible depression.

Other ways to help include:

- Offering him support, understanding, patience, and encouragement

- Listening carefully and talking with him

- Never ignoring comments about suicide, and alerting his therapist or doctor

- Helping him increase his level of physical and social activity by inviting him out for hikes, games, and other events. If he says, "no," keep trying, but do not push him to take on too much too soon.

- Encouraging him to report any concerns about medications to his healthcare provider

- Ensuring that he gets to his doctor's appointments

- Reminding him that with time and treatment, the depression will lift

How Can I Help Myself If I Am Depressed?

- Spending time with other people and talking with a friend or relative about your feelings

- Increasing your level of physical activity. Regular exercise can help people with mild to moderate depression and may be one part of a treatment plan for those with severe depression. Talk with your healthcare professional about what kind of exercise is right for you.

- Breaking up large tasks into small ones, and tackling what you can as you can. Do not try to do too many things at once.

- Delaying important decisions until you feel better. Discuss decisions with others who know you well.

- Keeping stable daily routines. For example, eating and going to bed at the same time every day.

- Avoiding alcohol

As you continue treatment, gradually you will start to feel better. Remember that if you are taking an antidepressant, it may take several weeks for it to start working. Try to do things that you used to enjoy before you had depression. Go easy on yourself.

Where Can I Go for Help?

If you are unsure of where to go for help, ask your family doctor or healthcare provider. You can also find resources online, including the National Institute of Mental Health (NIMH) website at (www. nimh.nih.gov/FindHelp), or check with your insurance carrier to find someone who participates in your plan. Hospital doctors can help in an emergency.

What If I or Someone I Know Is in Crisis?

Men with depression are at risk for suicide. If you or someone you know is in crisis, get help quickly.

- Call your doctor.
- Call 911 for emergency services.
- Go to the nearest hospital emergency room.
- Call the toll-free, 24-hour hotline of the National Suicide Prevention Lifeline at 800-273-TALK (800-273-8255); TTY: 800-799-4TTY (800-799-4889).
- Veterans can call the Veterans Crisis Line at 800-273-8255.

In many instances, a crisis can be avoided when friends or family members are involved in the treatment and can recognize crisis warning signs. Crisis warning signs are different for different people. One person may have more trouble sleeping and become more agitated. Another person may sleep more, stop eating, and focus on disturbing thoughts. Creating a plan that lists the loved one's warning signs—those actions that usually occur before a crisis—and the healthcare provider's contact information may help avoid a crisis.

Section 43.3

Posttraumatic Stress Disorder

This section includes text excerpted from "PTSD Basics,"
National Center for Posttraumatic Stress Disorder (NCPTSD),
U.S. Department of Veterans Affairs (VA), April 29, 2019.

Posttraumatic stress disorder (PTSD) is a mental-health problem that some people develop after experiencing or witnessing a life-threatening event, such as combat, a natural disaster, a car accident, or sexual assault.

It is normal to have upsetting memories, feel on edge, or have trouble sleeping after a traumatic event. At first, it may be hard to do normal daily activities, such as go to work, go to school, or spend time with people you care about. But most people start to feel better after a few weeks or months.

If it is been longer than a few months and you are still having symptoms, you may have PTSD. For some people, PTSD symptoms may start later on, or they may come and go over time.

Who Develops Posttraumatic Stress Disorder

Anyone can develop PTSD at any age. A number of factors can increase the chance that someone will have PTSD, many of which are not under that person's control. For example, having a very intense or long-lasting traumatic event or getting injured during the event can make it more likely that a person will develop PTSD. PTSD is also more common after certain types of trauma, such as combat and sexual assault.

Personal factors, such as previous traumatic exposure, age, and sex, can affect whether or not a person will develop PTSD. What happens after the traumatic event is also important. Stress can make PTSD more likely, while social support can make it less likely.

What Are the Symptoms of Posttraumatic Stress Disorder?

Posttraumatic stress disorder symptoms usually start soon after the traumatic event, but they may not appear until months or years later. They also may come and go over many years. If the symptoms last longer than four weeks, cause you great distress, or interfere with your work or home life, you might have PTSD.

There are four types of PTSD symptoms, but they may not be exactly the same for everyone. Each person experiences symptoms in their own way.

1. **Reliving the event (also called "re-experiencing symptoms").** Memories of the traumatic event can come back at any time. You may feel the same fear and horror you did when the event took place. For example:

    • You may have nightmares.

    • You may feel like you are going through the event again. This is called a "flashback."

    • You may see, hear, or smell something that causes you to relive the event. This is called a "trigger." News reports, seeing an accident, or hearing a car backfire are examples of triggers.

2. **Avoiding situations that remind you of the event.** You may try to avoid situations or people that trigger memories of the traumatic event. You may even avoid talking or thinking about the event. For example:

    • You may avoid crowds because they feel dangerous.

    • You may avoid driving if you were in a car accident or if your military convoy was bombed.

    • If you were in an earthquake, you may avoid watching movies about earthquakes.

    • You may keep very busy or avoid seeking help because it keeps you from having to think or talk about the event.

3. **Negative changes in beliefs and feelings.** The way you think about yourself and others changes because of the trauma. This symptom has many aspects, including the following:

    • You may not have positive or loving feelings toward other people and may stay away from relationships.

    • You may forget about parts of the traumatic event or not be able to talk about them.

- You may think the world is completely dangerous, and no one can be trusted.

4. **Feeling keyed up (also called "hyperarousal").** You may be jittery or always alert and on the lookout for danger. You might suddenly become angry or irritable. This is known as "hyperarousal." For example:

- You may have a hard time sleeping.

- You may have trouble concentrating.

- You may be startled by a loud noise or surprise.

- You might want to have your back to a wall in a restaurant or waiting room.

Will People with Posttraumatic Stress Disorder Get Better?

After a traumatic event, it is normal to think, act, and feel differently than usual, but most people start to feel better after a few weeks or months. Talk to a doctor or mental-health care provider (such as a psychiatrist, psychologist, or social worker) if your symptoms:

- Last longer than a few months

- Are very upsetting

- Disrupt your daily life

"Getting better" means different things for different people. There are many different treatment options for PTSD. For many people, these treatments can get rid of symptoms altogether. Others find that they have fewer symptoms or feel that their symptoms are less intense. Your symptoms do not have to interfere with your everyday activities, work, and relationships.

What Treatments Are Available?

There are two main types of treatment, psychotherapy (sometimes called "counseling" or "talk therapy") and medication. Sometimes, people combine psychotherapy and medication.

Psychotherapy for Posttraumatic Stress Disorder

Psychotherapy involves meeting with a therapist.

Trauma-focused psychotherapy, which focuses on the memory of the traumatic event or its meaning, is the most effective treatment for PTSD. There are different types of trauma-focused psychotherapy, such as:

- **Cognitive processing therapy (CPT)**, where you learn skills to understand how trauma changed your thoughts and feelings. Changing how you think about the trauma can change how you feel.

- **Prolonged exposure (PE)**, where you talk about your trauma repeatedly until memories are no longer upsetting. This will help you get more control over your thoughts and feelings about the trauma. You also go to places or do things that are safe but you have been staying away from because they remind you of the trauma.

- **Eye movement desensitization and reprocessing (EMDR)**, which involves focusing on sounds or hand movements while you talk about the trauma. This helps your brain work through the traumatic memories.

Medications for Posttraumatic Stress Disorder

Medications can be effective too. Some specific selective serotonin reuptake inhibitors (SSRIs) and serotonin-norepinephrine reuptake inhibitors (SNRIs), which are used for depression, also work for PTSD. These include sertraline, paroxetine, fluoxetine, and venlafaxine.

Section 43.4

Schizophrenia

This section includes text excerpted from "Schizophrenia,"
National Institute of Mental Health (NIMH), February 2016.

Schizophrenia is a chronic and severe mental disorder that affects how a person thinks, feels, and behaves. People with schizophrenia may seem as if they have lost touch with reality. Although schizophrenia is not as common as other mental disorders, the symptoms can be very disabling.

Signs and Symptoms of Schizophrenia

Symptoms of schizophrenia usually start between the ages of 16 and 30. In rare cases, children have schizophrenia too.

The symptoms of schizophrenia fall into three categories: positive, negative, and cognitive.

Positive symptoms: Positive symptoms are psychotic behaviors not generally seen in healthy people. People with positive symptoms may "lose touch" with some aspects of reality. Symptoms include:

- Hallucinations
- Delusions
- Thought disorders (unusual or dysfunctional ways of thinking)
- Movement disorders (agitated body movements)

Negative symptoms: Negative symptoms are associated with disruptions to normal emotions and behaviors. Symptoms include:

- "Flat affect" (reduced expression of emotions via facial expression or voice tone)
- Reduced feelings of pleasure in everyday life
- Difficulty beginning and sustaining activities
- Reduced speaking

Cognitive symptoms: For some patients, the cognitive symptoms of schizophrenia are subtle, but for others, they are more severe and patients may notice changes in their memory or other aspects of thinking. Symptoms include:

- Poor "executive functioning" (the ability to understand information and use it to make decisions)
- Trouble focusing or paying attention
- Problems with "working memory" (the ability to use information immediately after learning it)

Risk Factors of Schizophrenia

There are several factors that contribute to the risk of developing schizophrenia.

Genes and environment: Scientists have long known that schizophrenia sometimes runs in families. However, there are many people who have schizophrenia who do not have a family member with the disorder, and conversely, many people with one or more family members with the disorder who do not develop it themselves.

Scientists believe that many different genes may increase the risk of schizophrenia but that no single gene causes the disorder by itself. It is not yet possible to use genetic information to predict who will develop schizophrenia.

Scientists also think that interactions between genes and aspects of the individual's environment are necessary for schizophrenia to develop. Environmental factors may involve:

- Exposure to viruses
- Malnutrition before birth
- Problems during birth
- Psychosocial factors

Different brain chemistry and structure: Scientists think that an imbalance in the complex, interrelated chemical reactions of the brain involving the neurotransmitters (substances that brain cells use to communicate with each other) dopamine and glutamate, and possibly others, plays a role in schizophrenia.

Some experts also think problems during brain development before birth may lead to faulty connections. The brain also undergoes major changes during puberty, and these changes could trigger psychotic symptoms in people who are vulnerable due to genetics or brain differences.

Treatments and Therapies of Schizophrenia

Because the causes of schizophrenia are still unknown, treatments focus on eliminating the symptoms of the disease. Treatments include:

Antipsychotics

Antipsychotic medications are usually taken daily in pill or liquid form. Some antipsychotics are injections that are given once or twice a month. Some people have side effects when they start taking medications, but most side effects go away after a few days. Doctors and patients can work together to find the best medication or medication combination and the right dose.

Psychosocial Treatments

These treatments are helpful after patients and their doctor find a medication that works. Learning and using coping skills to address the everyday challenges of schizophrenia helps people to pursue their life goals, such as attending school or work. Individuals who participate in regular psychosocial treatment are less likely to have relapses or be hospitalized.

Coordinated Specialty Care

This treatment model integrates medication, psychosocial therapies, case management, family involvement, and supported education and employment services, all aimed at reducing symptoms and improving quality of life. The NIMH Recovery After an Initial Schizophrenia Episode (RAISE) research project seeks to fundamentally change the trajectory and prognosis of schizophrenia through coordinated specialty care treatment in the earliest stages of the disorder. RAISE is designed to reduce the likelihood of long-term disability that people with schizophrenia often experience and help them lead productive, independent lives.

How Can I Help Someone I Know with Schizophrenia?

Caring for and supporting a loved one with schizophrenia can be hard. It can be difficult to know how to respond to someone who makes strange or clearly false statements. It is important to understand that schizophrenia is a biological illness.

Here Are Some Things You Can Do to Help Your Loved One:

- Get them treatment, and encourage them to stay in treatment.
- Remember that their beliefs or hallucinations seem very real to them.
- Tell them that you acknowledge that everyone has the right to see things their own way.

- Be respectful, supportive, and kind without tolerating dangerous or inappropriate behavior.

- Check to see if there are any support groups in your area.

Chapter 44

Alcohol, Tobacco, and Drug Use in Men

Chapter Contents

Section 44.1—Alcohol, Tobacco, and Other Drugs 646

Section 44.2—Excessive Alcohol Use and Risks to
Men's Health 647

Section 44.3—Men's Health and Smoking 648

Section 44.4—Anabolic Steroid Use 650

Section 44.1

Alcohol, Tobacco, and Other Drugs

This section includes text excerpted from "Alcohol, Tobacco, and
Other Drugs," Substance Abuse and Mental Health Services
Administration (SAMHSA), January 30, 2019.

Misusing alcohol; tobacco; and drugs, such as opioids, can have both
immediate and long-term health effects.

The misuse and abuse of alcohol, tobacco, illicit drugs, and prescription medications affect the health and well-being of millions of
Americans.

- Excessive alcohol use can increase a person's risk of developing
  serious health problems, in addition to those issues associated
  with intoxication behaviors and alcohol withdrawal symptoms.

- Tobacco use and smoking do damage to nearly every organ in the
  human body, often leading to lung cancer, respiratory disorders,
  heart disease, stroke, and other illnesses.

- Marijuana has not only immediate effects, such as distorted
  perception, difficulty problem solving, and a loss of motor
  coordination, but it also has effects with long-term use, such as
  respiratory infection, impaired memory, and exposure to cancer-
  causing compounds.

- Opioids reduce the perception of pain but can also produce
  drowsiness, mental confusion, euphoria, nausea, and
  constipation, and—depending upon the amount of drug taken—
  they can depress respiration.

Opioid misuse represents a unique challenge. According to the Centers for Disease Control and Prevention (CDC), an average of 130 Americans die every day from an opioid overdose. Opioids include prescription drugs, such as hydrocodone, oxycodone, morphine, and codeine.
While many people benefit from using these medications to manage
pain, prescription drugs are frequently diverted for improper use.

As people use opioids repeatedly, their tolerance increases and they
may not be able to maintain the source for the drugs. This can cause
them to turn to the black market for these drugs and even switch from
prescription drugs to cheaper and riskier substitutes, such as heroin.
These substances vary in purity and strength, which increases the
risk of serious medical complications or overdose.

Section 44.2

Excessive Alcohol Use and Risks to Men's Health

This section includes text excerpted from "Fact
Sheets—Excessive Alcohol Use and Risks to Men's Health,"
Centers for Disease Control and Prevention (CDC), March 7, 2016.

Men are more likely than women to drink excessively. Excessive drinking is associated with significant increases in short-term risks to health and safety, and the risk increases as the amount of drinking increases. Men are also more likely than women to take other risks (e.g., driving fast or without a safety belt) when combined with excessive drinking, further increasing their risk of injury or death.

Drinking Levels among Men

- Approximately 58 percent of adult men report drinking alcohol in the last 30 days.

- Approximately 23 percent of adult men report binge drinking 5 times a month, averaging 8 drinks per binge.

- Men are almost two times more likely to binge drink than women.

- Most (90%) people who binge drink are not alcoholics or alcohol dependent.

- About 4.5 percent of men and 2.5 percent of women met the diagnostic criteria for alcohol dependence in the past year.

Injuries and Deaths as a Result of Excessive Alcohol Use

- Men consistently have higher rates of alcohol-related deaths and hospitalizations than women.

- Among drivers in fatal motor-vehicle traffic crashes, men are almost twice as likely as women to have been intoxicated (i.e., a blood alcohol concentration of 0.08% or greater).

- Excessive alcohol consumption increases aggression and, as a result, can increase the risk of physically assaulting another person.

- Men are more likely than women to commit suicide, and they are more likely to have been drinking prior to committing suicide.

Reproductive Health and Sexual Function

Excessive alcohol use can interfere with testicular function and male hormone production, resulting in impotence; infertility; and a reduction of male secondary sex characteristics, such as facial and chest hair.

Excessive alcohol use is commonly involved in sexual assault. Also, alcohol use by men increases the chances of engaging in risky sexual activity, including unprotected sex, sex with multiple partners, or sex with a partner at risk for sexually transmitted diseases (STDs).

Section 44.3

Men's Health and Smoking

This section includes text excerpted from "Men's Health and Smoking," U.S. Food and Drug Administration (FDA), August 28, 2018.

Smoking continues to have a profound impact on the health and well-being of men and their families in the United States.

- Almost 16 percent (15.8%) of men smoke cigarettes.

- Each day in the United States, about 1,050 boys under 18 years of age smoke their first cigarette.

- 7.6 percent of high-school-aged boys smoke cigarettes.

Impacts of Men Smoking

There is abundant research about the many harms of smoking— whether it is the dangerous chemicals, the addictive properties, or the damage smoking causes to the lungs, the heart, and nearly every organ in the body. For men who smoke, these effects can have a profound impact on your body and your life, including diminished overall health, increased absenteeism from work, and increased healthcare needs and costs. Smoking also exposes your family to the harmful effects of secondhand smoke. Here are some facts about smoking's effects to you and those around you.

For Men

- Smoking causes heart disease, cancer, and stroke—the first, second, and fifth leading causes of death among men in the United States.

- Smoking cigarettes causes chronic obstructive pulmonary disease (COPD). People with COPD have trouble breathing and slowly start to die from lack of air. Approximately 80 percent of COPD deaths are caused by smoking. Smokers are 12 to 13 times more likely to die from COPD than nonsmokers.

- Smokers are up to 20 times more likely to develop lung cancer than nonsmokers.

- Life expectancy for smokers is at least a decade less than for nonsmokers.

- Smokers with prostate cancer may be more likely to die from the disease than nonsmokers.

- Smoking can damage deoxyribonucleic acid (DNA) in men's sperm, which can cause an increased risk of infertility.

For Families

- Secondhand smoke causes disease and premature death in nonsmoking adults and children.

- The U.S. Surgeon General estimates that living with a smoker increases a nonsmoker's risk of developing lung cancer by 20 to 30 percent.

- Exposure to secondhand smoke increases school children's risk for ear infections, lower respiratory illnesses, more frequent and more severe asthma attacks, and slowed lung growth, and it can cause coughing, wheezing, phlegm, and breathlessness.

- Teens are more likely to smoke if they have friends or family who smoke.

Next Steps

The good news is that you can do something about it now—smoking is what the Centers for Disease Control and Preventions (CDC) terms a "modifiable" risk factor.

Encourage the men in your life—the fathers, sons, brothers, and friends—to take a moment to care for themselves and put their own health first by finding a quit method that works for them.

Section 44.4

Anabolic Steroid Use

This section contains text excerpted from the following sources:
Text beginning with the heading "What Are Anabolic Steroids?"
is excerpted from "Anabolic Steroids," National Institute on Drug
Abuse (NIDA), August 2018; Text under the heading "Who Uses
Anabolic Steroids" is excerpted from "Steroids and Other Appearance
and Performance Enhancing Drugs (APEDS)," National
Institute on Drug Abuse (NIDA), February 2018.

What Are Anabolic Steroids?

Anabolic steroids are synthetic, or human-made, variations of the male sex hormone testosterone. The proper term for these compounds is anabolic-androgenic steroids (AASs). "Anabolic" refers to muscle building, and "androgenic" refers to increased male sex characteristics. Some common names for anabolic steroids are "Gear," "Juice," "Roids," and "Stackers."

Healthcare providers can prescribe steroids to treat hormonal issues, such as delayed puberty. Steroids can also treat diseases that cause muscle loss, such as cancer and acquired immunodeficiency syndrome (AIDS). But, some athletes and bodybuilders misuse these drugs in an attempt to boost performance or improve their physical appearance.

The majority of people who misuse steroids are male weightlifters in their 20s or 30s. Anabolic steroid misuse is much less common in women. It is difficult to measure steroid misuse in the United States because many national surveys do not measure it. However, use among teens is generally minimal. The 2016 National Institute on Drug Abuse (NIDA)-funded Monitoring the Future study has shown that the past-year misuse of steroids has declined among 8th and 10th graders, while holding steady for 12th graders.

How Do People Misuse Anabolic Steroids?

People who misuse anabolic steroids usually take them orally, inject them into their muscles, or apply them to the skin as a gel or cream. These doses may be 10 to 100 times higher than doses prescribed to treat medical conditions.

Commons patterns for misusing steroids include:

- **Cycling**—taking multiple doses for a period of time, stopping for a time, and then restarting

- **Stacking**—combining two or more different steroids and mixing oral and/or injectable types

- **Pyramiding**—slowly increasing the dose or frequency of steroid misuse, reaching a peak amount, and then gradually tapering off to zero

- **Plateauing**—alternating, overlapping, or substituting with another steroid to avoid developing a tolerance

There is no scientific evidence that any of these practices reduce the harmful medical consequences of these drugs.

Who Uses Anabolic Steroids

The vast majority of people who misuse steroids are male nonathlete weightlifters in their 20s or 30s. Contrary to popular belief, only about 22 percent of anabolic steroid users started as teenagers. Anabolic steroid use is less common among females since fewer women desire extreme muscularity and the masculinizing effects of steroids.

Males who are more likely to use steroids tend to have poor self-esteem, higher rates of depression, more suicide attempts, poor knowledge and attitudes about health, greater participation in sports emphasizing weight and shape, greater parental concern about weight, and higher rates of eating disorders and substance use. Steroid misuse is associated with muscle dysmorphia, a behavioral disorder in which men think that they look small and weak, even if they are large and muscular.

Some people who misuse steroids have experienced physical or sexual abuse. In a study of 506 male users and 771 male nonusers of anabolic steroids, users were significantly more likely than nonusers to report being sexually abused in the past. Similarly, female weightlifters who had been raped were found to be twice as likely to report use of anabolic steroids or another purported muscle-building drug when compared with those who had not been raped. Moreover, almost all females who had been raped reported that they markedly increased their bodybuilding activities after the attack. They believed that being bigger and stronger would discourage further attacks because men would find them either intimidating or unattractive.

It is difficult to estimate the true prevalence of steroid misuse in the United States because many surveys that ask about illicit drug use do not include questions about steroids. However, the annual Monitoring the Future study shows that the past-year use of steroids has generally declined among 8th and 10th graders, after peaking in 2000. Past-year steroid use among 12th graders increased from 2011 to 2015; although, use significantly declined from 2015 to 2016. The 2017 rate of use among 12th graders holds relatively steady.

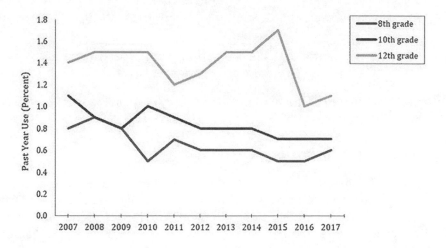

Figure 44.1. *Anabolic Steroid Use among Middle and High School Students, 2007 to 2017*

Data are from the 2017 Monitoring the Future survey, funded by the National Institute on Drug Abuse and conducted annually by the University of Michigan's Institute for Social Research.

Chapter 45

Violence against Men

Chapter Contents

Section 45.1—Myths and Realities of Domestic
            Abuse against Men.. 654

Section 45.2—Sexual Assault of Men 657

Section 45.1

Myths and Realities of Domestic Abuse against Men

"Myths and Realities of Domestic Abuse against Men,"
© 2017 Omnigraphics. Reviewed June 2019.

Domestic or intimate partner abuse can be defined as a pattern of behaviors—including physical and sexual violence, verbal and emotional abuse, or stalking—used by one partner in a relationship to coerce, intimidate, and gain power and control over the other partner. When most people think about domestic violence or intimate partner abuse, they envision a male perpetrating abuse against a female victim. This is the scenario that is most often presented in the media.

In reality, however, domestic abuse can and does affect men, as well as women. Studies have shown that 1 in every 7 men in the United States has been the victim of physical violence by an intimate partner, while 1 in every 10 men has experienced rape or stalking by an intimate partner. Experts believe that these figures underrepresent the true extent of the problem, though, because male victims are less likely to report incidents of domestic violence or seek support for intimate partner abuse.

The topic of domestic abuse against men is surrounded by cultural myths and stereotypes. It is important to examine these myths with a critical eye in order to understand the reality of the problem and ensure that services and support are available for men who need help. Some of the common myths of domestic abuse against men include the following:

- **Any man who allows himself to be the victim of abuse must be weak.**

  The cultural image of manliness leads many people to believe that a "real" man would fight back rather than submit to abuse, especially from a woman. In reality, male victims of domestic abuse often have many reasons for not defending themselves against an intimate partner's assaults. Some have been taught that it is wrong for a man to strike a woman, no matter the circumstances. Others restrain themselves because they realize that their superior size and strength means that they could cause serious physical harm to their partner if they fought back. Finally, some men worry that any actions taken to protect themselves could be misinterpreted and cause them to be arrested as the perpetrator of the abuse.

- **In a domestic dispute, the bigger, stronger person is always the aggressor.**

Many people assume that women cannot be perpetrators of domestic abuse because they are usually smaller and weaker than their male partners. In reality, though, physical size and strength has no bearing on whether a person will be an abuser or a victim of abuse. Many strong people are nonviolent, while even small, frail people can use threats, intimidation, or weapons to coerce or gain power over an intimate partner.

- **Men should not express feelings or share details of their personal lives.**

From an early age, many boys are taught that it is not "manly" to cry, express emotions, or talk openly about their problems. As a result, they grow up believing that their only choice in confronting a difficult situation is to "suck it up" and deal with it on their own. For men who find themselves in abusive relationships, this ingrained attitude may prevent them from acknowledging the abuse or seeking help.

- **Domestic abuse against men is not as serious as domestic abuse against women.**

Some people tend to treat domestic abuse against men as a joke or fail to take it seriously. While the media tends to portray female victims sympathetically, male victims are often treated with scorn, sarcasm, or snide remarks. But domestic abuse is no laughing matter in any situation, and it can have serious consequences for victims. In fact, studies show that male victims of intimate partner violence are significantly more likely to report physical and mental-health problems than nonvictims.

- **Intimate partner abuse does not impact children in the home.**

Some people believe that children do not notice domestic abuse or at least do not suffer lasting effects from it. But domestic violence is a learned behavior, and witnessing abuse in the home increases the likelihood that children will eventually choose violent partners or become abusers themselves. In addition, intimate partner abuse creates a climate of fear and insecurity in the home that may lead children to develop behavioral problems or addiction issues as they get older.

- **If a man is really being abused, he can simply leave the relationship.**

  Many people assume that men face fewer obstacles to leaving an abusive relationship than women, who are more likely to be financially dependent on their abusive partners. But leaving an abusive relationship can be extremely difficult, and it requires money, transportation, housing, and support. Male victims may have many concerns that prevent them from leaving, including fear for the safety of their children, worry that they will be prevented from seeing their children, love and commitment to their partner, a belief that their partner will change, embarrassment about their situation, or confusion about where to go or how to get help. Some men worry that trying to leave will only make the situation worse, since incidents of domestic violence tend to become more severe if the victim attempts to get out of the relationship.

- **There are plenty of shelters and support services available for male victims.**

  Although domestic violence programs must provide services to all victims of abuse in order to receive federal funding, many organizations and shelters are focused on helping women. In fact, some male victims of intimate partner abuse are turned away from women's shelters and referred to local homeless shelters. In addition, few support groups are available to male survivors of domestic violence, and those that are available tend to be aimed at gay, lesbian, bisexual, and transsexual people rather than straight men. Support groups are an important part of the healing process, offering survivors an opportunity to share information and experiences with one another. Men who experience domestic violence need access to such services in order to understand that, despite cultural myths and stereotypes to the contrary, they are not alone.

References

1. "Common Myths about Intimate Partner Abuse against Men," Domestic Abuse Hotline for Men and Women, 2012.

2. "Men Can Be Victims of Abuse Too," National Domestic Violence Hotline, July 22, 2014.

Section 45.2

Sexual Assault of Men

This section includes text excerpted from "Sexual Assault: Males," National Center for Posttraumatic Stress Disorder (NCPTSD), U.S. Department of Veterans Affairs (VA), September 24, 2018.

At least 1 out of every 10 (or 10%) of men in the United States has suffered from trauma as a result of sexual assault. Similar to women, men who experience sexual assault may suffer from depression, posttraumatic stress disorder (PTSD), and other emotional problems as a result. However, because women and men have different life experiences due to their different gender roles, emotional symptoms following trauma can look different in men than they do in women.

Who Are the Perpetrators of Male Sexual Assault?

- Those who sexually assault men or boys differ in a number of ways from those who assault only females.

- Boys are more likely than girls to be sexually abused by strangers or by authority figures in organizations, such as schools, the church, or athletics programs.

- Those who sexually assault males usually choose young men and male adolescents (the average age is 17 years old) as their victims and are more likely to assault many victims when compared to those who sexually assault females.

- Perpetrators often assault young males in isolated areas where help is not readily available. For instance, a perpetrator who assaults males may pick up a teenage hitchhiker on a remote road or find some other way to isolate his intended victim.

- As is true about those who assault and sexually abuse women and girls, most perpetrators of males are men. Specifically, men are perpetrators in about 86 out of every 100 (or 86%) of male victimization cases.

- Despite popular belief that only gay men would sexually assault men or boys, most male perpetrators identify themselves as heterosexuals and often have consensual sexual relationships with women.

What Are Some Symptoms Related to Sexual Trauma in Boys and Men?

Particularly when the assailant is a woman, the impact of sexual assault upon men may be downplayed by professionals and the public. However, men who have early sexual experiences with adults report problems in various areas at a much higher rate than those who do not.

Emotional Disorders

Men and boys who have been sexually assaulted are more likely to suffer from PTSD, anxiety disorders, and depression than those who have never been abused sexually.

Substance Abuse

Men who have been sexually assaulted have a high incidence of alcohol and drug use. For example, the probability for alcohol problems in adulthood is about 80 out of every 100 (or 80%) for men who have experienced sexual abuse, as compared to 11 out of every 100 (or 11%) for men who have never been sexually abused.

Risk-Taking Behavior

Exposure to sexual trauma can lead to risk-taking behavior during adolescence, such as running away and other delinquent behaviors. Having been sexually assaulted also makes boys more likely to engage in behaviors that put them at risk for contracting human immunodeficiency virus (HIV), such as having sex without using condoms.

Help for Men Who Have Been Sexually Assaulted

Men who have been assaulted often feel stigmatized, which can be the most damaging aspect of the assault. It is important for men to discuss the assault with a caring and unbiased support person, whether that person is a friend, clergyman, or clinician. However, it is vital that this person be knowledgeable about sexual assault and men.

A local rape crisis center may be able to refer men to mental-health practitioners who are well-informed about the needs of male sexual assault victims. If you are a man who has been assaulted and you suffer from any of these difficulties, please seek help from a mental-health professional who has expertise working with men who have been sexually assaulted.

Chapter 46

Body Image and Eating Disorders in Men

Chapter Contents

Section 46.1—Eating Disorders in Men...................................... 662

Section 46.2—Muscle Dysmorphic Disorder 667

Section 46.1

Eating Disorders in Men

This section contains text excerpted from the following
sources: Text in this section begins with excerpts from "Eating
Disorders among Men," Substance Abuse and Mental Health Services
Administration (SAMHSA), April 19, 2016; Text beginning with the
heading "Anorexia Nervosa" is excerpted from "Eating Disorders,"
Substance Abuse and Mental Health Services
Administration (SAMHSA), March 21, 2019.

Significant numbers of men are developing eating disorders based on unrealistic body images, and the health results are life-threatening.

"Body dysmorphic disorder (BDD) is a chronic mental illness, wherein the afflicted individual is concerned with body image, manifested as excessive concern about and preoccupation with a perceived defect of their physical appearance. An individual with BDD has perpetual negative thoughts about their appearance," said Leigh Cohn, the editor-in-chief of *Eating Disorders: The Journal of Treatment and Prevention.*

"Men have anorexia. Men have bulimia. Both are just as life-threatening for men as they are for women. There are specific challenges in identifying and treating men for eating disorders, but the biggest challenge is getting men to admit they have a problem because they do not recognize the behavior or understand how much damage it can do," said Cohn.

Eating disorders in men are multi-dimensional. They are the result of genetic factors; peer pressure; family issues; cultural messages; and possible trauma, such as the death or serious illness of the father, according to Cohn.

"The incidence is higher in gay males, but we are seeing eating disorders cross the cultural line into the straight population," Cohn said.

The drivers for men's eating disorders are similar to those for women: an unrealistic ideal in body type, coupled with the notion that looking right will bring success in unrelated areas, such as getting a good job and finding the right partner. This is tied to the cultural notion that men need to be in control, an impulse displaced onto the bodies of those with eating disorders. Some sports, such as wrestling, boxing, and horse racing, foster behaviors of eating disorders due to strict weight restrictions.

Brian Cuban, an attorney, author, and addiction recovery advocate, discussed his own eating disorder, which was coupled with drug and alcohol use that pushed him to a very dangerous bottom.

"I probably became anorexic and bulimic when I was a freshman at Penn State. When I was young, I was heavy and my mother used fat-shaming behaviors. I was the victim of a weight-related assault in junior high school when I was stripped of my pants on a public street and forced to walk home in my underwear. No one helped. I was brought very low by substance abuse but was able to recover with help from my family. However, I still could not admit to the eating disorders. In fact, I first admitted my behavior on a blog before I was able to talk about it with my psychiatrist and my family. I really thought I was the only man out there with this. Then I Googled it and found some message boards: I was not the only one! Writing the blog was my coming out."

"People should remember that words do damage," Cuban continued. "It was when I understood how my mother was raised that I was able to forgive her and understand my body issue, my body dysmorphia." The use of social media and connecting with other men impacted by eating disorders virtually has begun to embolden advocates seeking more nuanced treatment options to overcome discrimination associated with these disorders.

Cohn notes that treating males with eating disorders may require a unique approach.

"One of the biggest challenges is getting men to show up. Men are unaware they are engaging in odd behaviors, such as excessive exercise without enough nutrition. There is also comorbidity with alcohol abuse, getting calories from alcohol. But once a male enters treatment, they can be the better patients because they want to fix things. 'Explain it to me, and I will work on it' is how they approach it. Once they get past the stigma, they can get better," Cohn said.

"Eventually there will not be a stigma for male eating disorders, same as for females now. There are excellent information resources out there, including the National Eating Disorders Association (NEDA). Things are slow to change."

Anorexia Nervosa

Anorexia nervosa is an eating disorder that makes people lose more weight than is considered healthy for their age and height.

Persons with this disorder may have an intense fear of weight gain, even when they are underweight. They may diet or exercise too much, or they use other methods to lose weight.

Causes of Anorexia Nervosa

The exact causes of anorexia nervosa are not known. Many factors probably are involved. Genes and hormones may play a role. Social attitudes that promote very thin body types may also be involved.

Family conflicts are no longer thought to contribute to this or other eating disorders.

Risk factors for anorexia include:

- Being more worried about, or paying more attention to, weight and shape

- Having an anxiety disorder as a child

- Having a negative self-image

- Having eating problems during infancy or early childhood

- Having certain social or cultural ideas about health and beauty

- Trying to be perfect or overly focused on rules

Anorexia usually begins during the teen years or young adulthood. It is more common in females, but it may also be seen in males. The disorder is seen mainly in White women who are high academic achievers and who have a goal-oriented family or personality.

Symptoms of Anorexia Nervosa

To be diagnosed with anorexia, a person must:

- Have an intense fear of gaining weight or becoming fat, even when they are underweight

- Refuse to keep their weight at what is considered normal for their age and height (15 percent or more below the normal weight)

- Have a body image that is very distorted, be very focused on body weight or shape, and refuse to admit the seriousness of weight loss

People with anorexia may severely limit the amount of food they eat, or they may eat and then make themselves throw up. Other behaviors include:

- Cutting food into small pieces or moving them around the plate instead of eating

- Exercising all the time, even when the weather is bad, they are hurt, or their schedule is busy
- Going to the bathroom right after meals
- Refusing to eat around other people
- Using pills to make themselves urinate (water pills or diuretics), have a bowel movement (enemas and laxatives), or decrease their appetite (diet pills)

Other symptoms of anorexia may include:

- Blotchy or yellow skin that is dry and covered with fine hair
- Confused or slow thinking, along with poor memory or judgment
- Depression
- Dry mouth
- Extreme sensitivity to cold (wearing several layers of clothing to stay warm)
- Loss of bone strength
- Wasting away of muscle and loss of body fat

Binge Eating

Binge eating is when a person eats a much larger amount of food in a shorter period of time than she or he normally would. During binge eating, the person also feels a loss of control.

Considerations

A binge eater often:

- Eats 5,000 to 15,000 calories in one sitting
- Often snacks, in addition to eating three meals a day
- Overeats throughout the day

Binge eating by itself usually leads to becoming overweight.

Binge eating may occur on its own or with another eating disorder, such as bulimia. People with bulimia typically eat large amounts of high-calorie foods, usually in secret. After this binge eating they often force themselves to vomit or take laxatives.

Causes of Binge Eating

The cause of binge eating is unknown. However, binge eating often begins during or after strict dieting.

Bulimia

Bulimia is an illness in which a person binges on food or has regular episodes of overeating and feels a loss of control. The person then uses different methods—such as vomiting or abusing laxatives—to prevent weight gain.

Many (but not all) people with bulimia also have anorexia nervosa.

Causes of Bulimia

Many more women than men have bulimia. The disorder is most common in adolescent girls and young women. The affected person is usually aware that their eating pattern is abnormal and may feel fear or guilt with the binge-purge episodes.

The exact cause of bulimia is unknown. Genetic, psychological, trauma, family, society, or cultural factors may play a role. Bulimia is likely due to more than one factor.

Symptoms of Bulimia

In bulimia, eating binges may occur as often as several times a day for many months.

People with bulimia often eat large amounts of high-calorie foods, usually in secret. People can feel a lack of control over their eating during these episodes.

Binges lead to self-disgust, which causes purging to prevent weight gain. Purging may include:

- Forcing yourself to vomit

- Excessive exercise

- Using laxatives, enemas, or diuretics

Purging often brings a sense of relief.

People with bulimia are often at a normal weight, but they may see themselves as being overweight. Because the person's weight is often normal, other people may not notice this eating disorder.

Symptoms that other people can see include:

- Compulsive exercise

- Suddenly eating large amounts of food or buying large amounts of food that disappear right away

- Regularly going to the bathroom right after meals

- Throwing away packages of laxatives, diet pills, emetics (drugs that cause vomiting), or diuretics

Section 46.2

Muscle Dysmorphic Disorder

"Muscle Dysmorphic Disorder,"
© 2019 Omnigraphics. Reviewed June 2019.

What Is Muscle Dysmorphic Disorder?

Muscle dysmorphic disorder (MDD), also known as "reverse anorexia" or "bigorexia," is a subtype of body dysmorphic disorder (BDD) and is when a person obsesses about being too small or under-developed (lean). MDD is a mental disorder in which you keep on thinking about your physique and muscle mass.

Causes of Muscle Dysmorphic Disorder

Muscle dysmorphic disorder is generally underdiagnosed, but it occurs more commonly in men than women. However, bodybuilders and frequent gym-goers are more popular candidates for developing MDD. Biological, social, and psychological factors can cause MDD. It has been found that some men develop this disorder because of their genetics. Also, people who are with low self-esteem have more of a tendency to develop MDD.

Signs and Symptoms of Muscle Dysmorphic Disorder

To determine the presence of this disorder, look for the following signs and symptoms:

- A strong belief that your body is not muscular enough
- Comparing yourself with others' physiques
- Compulsively and frequently looking at yourself in the mirror
- Experiencing eagerness to check your weight often
- Feeling a sense of disappointment in your physical appearance
- Using steroids or other bodybuilding products, such as supplementary foods
- Feeling anxious or depressed because of a missed workout
- Experiencing distress in publicly exposing your body

Because of the tendency to panic over one's physique, a person with MDD often over-trains or over-exercises their muscles, even after an injury.

Consequences of Muscle Dysmorphic Disorder

Constant thinking about muscle insufficiency may interfere with your daily activities, and it also can affect friendships and other close relationships. Some of the risks involved in MDD are as follows:

- Injuries due to over-exercising
- Damage to muscles and joints
- Heart problems
- Kidney damage
- Liver damage
- Mental problems

Diagnosis of Muscle Dysmorphic Disorder

Muscle dysmorphic disorder is very difficult to diagnose, and it is likely underreported. The diagnosis of MDD primarily consists of:

- A psychological evaluation that assesses thoughts, risk factors, behaviors, and feelings related to a negative self-esteem

- A medical history review, including personal, social, and family history

Treatment of Muscle Dysmorphic Disorder

Muscle dysmorphic disorder is curable, and individuals who are suffering from this disorder can overcome the illness with appropriate treatment. It can be done with the help of a psychiatrist, counselor, or an experienced clinician. Cognitive behavioral therapy (CBT) is one of the treatment methods that can be used to treat MDD. CBT involves eradicating negative and destructive behaviors and replacing them with good behaviors. Muscle dysmorphic disorder can also be treated with certain antidepressant medications, such as serotonin-re-uptake inhibitors (SRIs). Both CBT and SRIs help to prevent negative thoughts and behaviors. They also reduce anxiety or depression caused by MDD.

Living with MDD, without treating it, may affect your life and cause problems with your mental and physical health. When you begin to detect symptoms of MDD, consult your doctor.

References

1. "Body Dysmorphic Disorder," Mayo Clinic, April 28, 2016.

2. "Muscle Dysmorphic Disorder (Bigorexia)," ANRED, February 1, 2001.

3. Muhlheim, Lauren. "Muscle Dysmorphia," Mirror-Mirror, June 30, 2014.

4. "Muscle Dysmorphia," McCallum Place, March 10, 2011.

Chapter 47

Male Menopause

What Is Male Menopause?

Male menopause refers to a decline in male hormone levels that occurs due to the aging process. Since men 50 years of age or older often undergo a drop in testosterone production, this condition is also known as "androgen decline," "andropause," or simply "low testosterone."

Testosterone is a hormone that is found in both men and women. In men, it is produced in the testes and is responsible for the development of male sex organs before birth, brings about changes during puberty, plays a role in sex drive and sperm production, fuels physical and mental energy, and helps maintain muscle mass.

Although menopause affects men at about the same age as women, it is not the same as female menopause. In women, menopause occurs as ovulation ends, and hormone production drops off quickly. In men, however, hormone production declines at a slower rate, and this may lead to only slight changes in the way the testes function.

What Are Its Symptoms?

Male menopause can lead to physical, sexual, and psychological problems that may worsen as the person ages.

"Male Menopause," © 2017 Omnigraphics. Reviewed June 2019.

These problems can include:

- Lack of energy

- Decreased muscle mass

- Feelings of physical weakness

- Insomnia or other sleep disorders

- Increased body fat

- Decreased libido

- Erectile dysfunction (ED)

- Infertility

- Lowered self-confidence

- Decreased motivation

- Difficulty concentrating

- Depression

Other less common symptoms may include reduced testicle size, tender or enlarged breasts, hot flashes, loss of body hair, and, in rare cases, osteoporosis.

How Is It Diagnosed?

A doctor will generally diagnose male menopause by asking about symptoms and performing a physical examination. During this conversation, it is vital that the patient informs the doctor fully about issues like sexual problems. Blood tests may be ordered to measure testosterone levels, and in some cases, other tests may be required to rule out medical issues that may contribute to this condition.

How Is It Treated?

Symptoms of male menopause are commonly treated through lifestyle changes, such as eating a healthier diet, getting more sleep and regular exercise, and reducing stress. Antidepressants and therapy may be prescribed if the individual is suffering from depression.

Testosterone replacement therapy may also be suggested to help alleviate such symptoms as fatigue, decreased libido, and depression. Much like hormone replacement therapy for women, treatment using synthetic hormones is controversial and comes with potential risks and side effects. For instance, in an individual with prostate cancer, synthetic hormones may cause an increase in the growth of cancer cells. If a doctor suggests hormone replacement therapy, it is advisable to consider both the positives and negatives of this treatment option thoroughly before making a decision.

References

1. Krans, Brian. "What Is Male Menopause?" Healthline Media, March 8, 2016.

2. Derrer, David T. "Male Menopause," WebMD, LLC, August 17, 2014.

Part Five

Additional Help and Information

Chapter 48

Glossary of Men's Health Terms

abdominal ultrasound: A procedure used to examine the organs in the abdomen.

ablation: The removal or destruction of a body part or tissue or its function.

abstinence: Not having sexual intercourse.

active surveillance: Closely watching a patient's condition but not giving treatment unless there are changes in test results.

addiction: A chronic, relapsing disease, characterized by compulsive drug seeking and use accompanied by neurochemical and molecular changes in the brain.

adjuvant therapy: Treatment given after the main treatment to help cure a disease.

allergy: An abnormally high sensitivity to certain substances, such as pollens or foods.

alopecia: The lack or loss of hair from areas of the body where hair is usually found.

anemia: A condition in which the number of red blood cells is less than normal, resulting in less oxygen carried to the body's cells.

This glossary contains terms excerpted from documents produced by several sources deemed reliable.

aneurysm: A weak or thin spot on an artery wall that has stretched or ballooned out from the wall and filled with blood, or damage to an artery leading to pooling of blood between the layers of the blood vessel walls.

antiandrogen: A substance that prevents cells from making or using androgens (hormones that play a role in the formation of male sex characteristics).

antibiotic: A drug that can destroy or prevent the growth of bacteria.

antiretroviral therapy: The recommended treatment for human immunodeficiency virus (HIV) infection.

artery: Any of the thick-walled blood vessels that carry blood away from the heart to other parts of the body.

atherosclerosis: A blood vessel disease characterized by deposits of lipid material on the inside of the walls of large to medium-sized arteries which make the artery walls thick, hard, brittle, and prone to breaking.

axillary lymph node: A lymph node in the armpit region that drains lymph from the breast and nearby areas.

basal cell: A small, round cell found in the lower part (or base) of the epidermis, the outer layer of the skin.

biopsy: To remove cells or tissues from the body for testing and examination under a microscope.

calories: The energy provided by food/nutrients.

carcinoma: Cancer that begins in the skin or in tissues that line or cover internal organs.

chlamydia: A common sexually transmitted disease caused by the bacterium Chlamydia trachomatis.

cholesterol: A waxy substance, produced naturally by the liver and also found in foods, that circulates in the blood and helps maintain tissues and cell membranes.

cocaine: A highly addictive stimulant drug derived from the coca plant that produces profound feelings of pleasure.

condom: A thin rubber sheath worn on a man's penis during sexual intercourse to block semen from coming in contact with the inside of the vagina.

depression: A disorder marked by sadness, inactivity, difficulty with thinking and concentration, significant increase or decrease in appetite and time spent sleeping, feelings of dejection and hopelessness, and, sometimes, suicidal thoughts or an attempt to commit suicide.

diabetes: A condition characterized by high blood glucose, resulting from the body's inability to use blood glucose for energy.

dialysis: The process of filtering wastes from the blood artificially.

diuretic: A chemical that stimulates the production of urine.

dopamine: A neurotransmitter present in regions of the brain that regulate movement, emotion, motivation, and the feeling of pleasure.

edema: The swelling of a cell that results from the influx of large amounts of water or fluid into the cell.

emphysema: A disease that affects the tiny air sacs in the lungs.

gallstone: Solid material that forms in the gallbladder or common bile duct. Gallstones are made of cholesterol or other substances found in the gallbladder.

gene: The basic unit of heredity. Genes play a role in how high a person's risk is for certain diseases.

gene therapy: Treatment that changes a gene. Gene therapy is used to help the body fight cancer. It also can be used to make cancer cells more sensitive to treatment.

genital warts: A sexually transmitted disease caused by the human papillomavirus.

germ cell tumor: A type of tumor that begins in the cells that give rise to sperm or eggs.

hemorrhagic stroke: Sudden bleeding into or around the brain.

hormone: A substance that stimulates the function of a gland.

human immunodeficiency virus (HIV): The virus that causes acquired immunodeficiency syndrome (AIDS), which is the most advanced stage of HIV infection.

human papillomavirus (HPV): The virus that causes HPV infection, the most common sexually transmitted infection.

hypertension: Characterized by persistently high arterial blood pressure defined as a measurement greater than or equal to 140 mm/Hg systolic pressure over 90 mm/Hg diastolic pressure.

imaging: In medicine, a process that makes pictures of areas inside the body.

immune system: The complex group of organs and cells that defends the body against infections and other diseases.

immunosuppressant: A drug given to stop the natural responses of the body's immune system.

incontinence: The inability to control urination.

injection drug use: A method of illicit drug use. The drugs are injected directly into the body into a vein, into a muscle, or under the skin with a needle and syringe.

intracerebral hemorrhage: Occurs when a vessel within the brain leaks blood into the brain.

invasive cancer: Cancer that has spread beyond the layer of tissue in which it developed and is growing into surrounding, healthy tissues.

jaundice: A condition in which the skin and the whites of the eyes become yellow, urine darkens, and the color of stool becomes lighter than normal.

lipoprotein: Small globules of cholesterol covered by a layer of protein; produced by the liver.

lobe: A portion of an organ, such as the liver, lung, breast, thyroid, or brain.

lupus: A chronic inflammatory disease that occurs when the body's immune system attacks its own tissues and organs.

lymph nodes: Small glands that help the body fight infection and disease. They filter a fluid called lymph and contain white blood cells.

magnetic resonance imaging (MRI): A type of imaging involving the use of magnetic fields to detect subtle changes in the water content of tissues.

medical test: Tests designed to rule out or avoid disease.

melanoma: A form of cancer that begins in melanocytes (cells that make the pigment melanin).

metabolism: Metabolism refers to all of the processes in the body that make and use energy, such as digesting food and nutrients and removing waste through urine and feces.

monoclonal antibody: A type of protein made in the laboratory that can bind to substances in the body, including tumor cells.

mutation: Any change in the deoxyribonucleic acid (DNA) of a cell. Mutations may be caused by mistakes during cell division, or they may be caused by exposure to DNA-damaging agents in the environment.

neoplasm: An abnormal mass of tissue that results when cells divide more than they should or do not die when they should.

nonseminoma: A group of testicular cancers that begin in the germ cells (cells that give rise to sperm).

obstruction: A clog or blockage that prevents liquid from flowing easily.

oncologist: A doctor who specializes in treating cancer. Some oncologists specialize in a particular type of cancer treatment.

opioid: A natural or synthetic psychoactive chemical that binds to opioid receptors in the brain and body.

opportunistic infection: An infection that occurs more frequently or is more severe in people with weakened immune systems, such as people with HIV or people receiving chemotherapy, than in people with healthy immune systems.

outpatient surgery: A procedure in which the patient is not required to stay overnight in a hospital.

pancreas: A large gland that helps digest food and also makes some important hormones.

Papanicolaou (Pap) test: A procedure in which cells and secretions are collected from inside and around the cervix for examination under a microscope.

positron emission tomography (PET) scan: In a PET scan, the patient is given radioactive glucose (sugar) through a vein. A scanner then tracks the glucose in the body.

plaque: Fatty cholesterol deposits found along the inside of artery walls that lead to atherosclerosis and stenosis of the arteries.

prognosis: A prediction of the probable outcome of a disease.

pubic lice: Also called crab lice or crabs, pubic lice are parasitic insects found primarily in the pubic or genital area of humans.

radiation: The emission of energy in waves or particles. Often used to treat cancer cells.

recurrence: When cancer comes back after a period when no cancer could be found.

relapse: Return of the manifestations of a disease after an interval of improvement.

resection: Surgery to remove tissue, an organ, or part of an organ.

scabies: An infestation of the skin by the human itch mite (Sarcoptes scabiei var. hominis). The most common symptoms of scabies are intense itching and a pimple-like skin rash.

scrotum: The sac of skin that contains the testes.

semen: The fluid, containing sperm, which comes out of the penis during sexual excitement.

serotonin: A neurotransmitter used in widespread parts of the brain, which is involved in sleep, movement, and emotions.

sexually transmitted disease (STD): An infectious disease that spreads from person to person during sexual contact.

spermicide: A topical preparation or substance used during sexual intercourse to kill sperm.

stage: How much cancer is in the body and how far it has spread.

stroke: A stroke occurs when blood flow to your brain stops.

subarachnoid hemorrhage: Bleeding within the meninges, or outer membranes, of the brain into the clear fluid that surrounds the brain.

testes: The male reproductive glands where sperm are produced.

transient ischemic attack (TIA): A short-lived stroke that lasts from a few minutes up to twenty-four hours; often called a mini-stroke.

transmission: The spread of disease from one person to another.

trichomoniasis: A sexually transmitted disease caused by a parasite.

triglycerides: A type of fat in your blood, triglycerides can contribute to the hardening and narrowing of your arteries if levels are too high.

ulcer: An open lesion on the surface of the skin or a mucosal surface, caused by superficial loss of tissue, usually with inflammation.

ultrasound: A type of test in which sound waves too high to hear are aimed at a structure to produce an image of it.

urinalysis: A test of a urine sample that can reveal many problems of the urinary tract and other body systems.

urinary tract: The path that urine takes as it leaves the body. It includes the kidneys, ureters, bladder, and urethra.

vaccine: A substance meant to help the immune system respond to and resist disease.

virus: A microscopic infectious agent that requires a living host cell in order to replicate.

weight control: This refers to achieving and maintaining a healthy weight with healthy eating and physical activity.

X-ray: A type of high-energy radiation. In low doses, X-rays are used to diagnose diseases by making pictures of the inside of the body.

yoga: A mind and body practice with origins in ancient Indian philosophy. The various styles of yoga typically combine physical postures, breathing techniques, and meditation or relaxation.

Chapter 49

Directory of Resources That Provide Information about Men's Health

General

Eunice Kennedy Shriver
National Institute of
Child Health and Human
Development (NICHD)
P.O. Box 3006
Rockville, MD 20847
Toll-Free: 800-370-2943
Toll-Free TTY: 888-320-6942
Toll-Free Fax: 866-760-5947
Website: www.nichd.nih.gov
E-mail: NICHDInformation
ResourceCenter@mail.nih.gov

National Human Genome
Research Institute (NHGRI)
31 Center Dr., 9000 Rockville Pike
Bldg. 31, Rm. 4B09, MSC 2152
Bethesda, MD 20892-2152
Phone: 301-402-0911
Fax: 301-402-2218
Website: www.genome.gov

National Institute of
Diabetes and Digestive and
Kidney Diseases (NIDDK)
31 Center Dr.
Bldg. 31, Rm. 9A06, MSC 2560
Bethesda, MD 20892-2560
Toll-Free: 800-472-0424
Phone: 301-496-3583
Website: www2.niddk.nih.gov
E-mail: niddkinquiries@nih.gov

Resources in this chapter were compiled from several sources deemed reliable; all contact information was verified and updated in June 2019.

Occupational Safety and Health Administration (OSHA)
200 Constitution Ave. N.W.
Washington, DC 20210
Toll-Free: 800-321-6742 (OSHA)
Website: www.OSHA.gov

U.S. Department of Health and Human Services (HHS)
200 Independence Ave. S.W.
Washington, DC 20201
Toll-Free: 877-696-6775
Website: www.hhs.gov

U.S. Food and Drug Administration (FDA)
10903 New Hampshire Ave.
Silver Spring, MD 20993
Toll-Free: 888-INFO-FDA
(888-463-6332)
Website: www.fda.gov

Cancer

American Cancer Society (ACS)
250 Williams St. N.W.
Atlanta, GA 30303
Toll-Free: 800-227-2345
Website: www.cancer.org

American Childhood Cancer Organization (ACCO)
6868 Distribution Dr.
Beltsville, MD 20705
Toll-Free: 855-858-2226
Phone: 301-962-3520
Fax: 301-962-3521
Website: www.acco.org
E-mail: staff@acco.org

Cancer Care
275 Seventh Ave.
22nd Fl.
New York, NY 10001
Toll-Free: 800-813-4673
Phone: 212-712-8400
Fax: 212-712-8495
Website: www.cancercare.org
E-mail: info@cancercare.org

Colorectal Cancer Control Program (CRCCP)
Centers for Disease Control and
Prevention (CDC)
1600 Clifton Rd. N.E.
Atlanta, GA 30329-4027
Toll-Free: 800-232-4636
Toll-Free Fax: 888-232-6348
Website: www.cdc.gov/cancer/
crccp
E-mail: cdcinfo@cdc.gov

National Cancer Institute (NCI)
9609 Medical Center Dr.
BG 9609, MSC 9760
Bethesda, MD 20892-9760
Toll-Free: 800-4-CANCER
(800-422-6237)
Toll-Free TTY: 800-332-8615
Website: www.cancer.gov
E-mail: NCIinfo@nih.gov

Drug Abuse

*National Council on
Alcoholism and Drug
Dependence, Inc. (NCADD)*
217 Bdwy.
Ste. 712
New York, NY 10007
Toll-Free: 800-NCACALL
(800-622-2255)
Phone: 212-269-7797
Fax: 212-269-7510
Website: www.ncadd.org
E-mail: national@ncadd.org

*National Institute on Drug
Abuse (NIDA)*
6001 Executive Blvd.
Rm. 5213, MSC 9561
Bethesda, MD 20892-9561
Phone: 301-443-1124
Website: www.drugabuse.gov
E-mail: media@nida.nih.gov

*Substance Abuse and
Mental Health Services
Administration (SAMHSA)*
5600 Fishers Ln.
Rockville, MD 20857
Toll-Free: 877-SAMHSA-7
(877-726-4727)
Toll-Free TTY: 800-487-4889
Fax: 240-221-4292
Website: www.samhsa.gov
E-mail: SAMHSAInfo@samhsa.
hhs.gov

Eating Disorders

*The Academy for Eating
Disorders (AED)*
11130 Sunrise Valley Dr.
Ste. 350
Reston, VA 20191
Phone: 703-234-4079
Fax: 703-435-4390
Website: www.aedweb.org
E-mail: info@aedweb.org

*The Alliance for Eating
Disorders Awareness ("The
Alliance")*
1649 Forum Pl.
Ste. 2
West Palm Beach, FL 33401
Toll-Free: 866-662-1235
Phone: 561-841-0900
Fax: 561-653-0043
Website: www.
allianceforeatingdisorders.com
E-mail: info@
allianceforeatingdisorders.com

*The British Columbia
Eating Disorders Association
(BCEDA)*
526 Michigan St.
Victoria, BC V8V 1S2
Canada
Phone: 250-383-2755
Website: www.cwhn.ca/en/
node/18300

Center for Eating Disorders (CED)

111 N. First St.
Ste. 2
Ann Arbor, MI 48104
Phone: 734-668-8585
Fax: 734-668-2645
Website: www.center4ed.org
E-mail: info@center4ed.org

Heart Disease

American Association of Cardiovascular and Pulmonary Rehabilitation (AACVPR)

330 N. Wabash Ave.
Ste. 2000
Chicago, IL 60611
Phone: 312-321-5146
Fax: 312-673-6924
Website: www.aacvpr.org
E-mail: aacvpr@aacvpr.org

American Heart Association (AHA)

7272 Greenville Ave.
Dallas, TX 75231
Toll-Free: 800-AHA-USA-1
(800-242-8721)
Phone: 214-570-5978
Fax: 214-706-1551
Website: www.heart.org

Cardiovascular Research Foundation (CRF)

1700 Bdwy.
Ninth Fl.
New York, NY 10019
Phone: 646-434-4500
Website: www.crf.org
E-mail: info@crf.org

Heart Rhythm Society (HRS)

1325 G St. N.W.
Ste. 400
Washington, DC 20005
Phone: 202-464-3400
Fax: 202-464-3401
Website: www.hrsonline.org
E-mail: info@HRSonline.org

National Heart, Lung, and Blood Institute (NHLBI)

NHLBI Health Information
Center
P.O. Box 30105
Ninth Fl.
Bethesda, MD 20824-0105
Phone: 301-592-8573
TTY: 240-629-3255
Fax: 301-592-8563
Website: www.nhlbi.nih.gov
E-mail: nhlbiinfo@nhlbi.nih.gov

Liver Disease

American Liver Foundation (ALF)

39 Bdwy.
Ste. 2700
New York, NY 10006
Toll-Free: 800-GO-LIVER
(800-465-4837)
Phone: 212-668-1000
Fax: 212-483-8179
Website: www.liverfoundation.org

Hepatitis Foundation International (HFI)
8121 Georgia Ave.
Ste. 350
Silver Spring, MD 20910
Toll-Free: 800-891-0707
Phone: 301-565-9410
Website: www.
hepatitisfoundation.org
E-mail: info@
hepatitisfoundation.org

United Network for Organ Sharing (UNOS)
700 N. Fourth St.
Richmond, VA 23219
Toll-Free: 888-894-6361
Phone: 804-782-4800
Website: www.unos.org
E-mail: patientservices@unos.
org

Mental-Health Issues

Depression and Bipolar Support Alliance (DBSA)
55 E. Jackson Blvd.
Ste. 490
Chicago, IL 60604
Toll-Free: 800-826-3632
Fax: 312-642-7243
Website: www.dbsalliance.org

National Institute of Mental Health (NIMH)
6001 Executive Blvd.
Rm. 6200, MSC 9663
Bethesda, MD 20892-9663
Toll-Free: 866-615-6464
Phone: 301-443-4513
TTY: 301-443-8431
Toll-Free TTY: 866-415-8051
Fax: 301-443-4279
Website: www.nimh.nih.gov
E-mail: nimhinfo@nih.gov

Prostate and Urological Disorders

The American Urological Association Foundation
1000 Corporate Blvd.
Linthicum, MD 21090
Toll-Free: 800-828-7866
Phone: 410-689-3700
Fax: 410-689-3998
Website: www.urologyhealth.org
E-mail: info@
UrologyCareFoundation.org

National Kidney and Urologic Diseases Information Clearinghouse (NKUDIC)
National Institute of Diabetes
and Digestive and Kidney
Diseases (NIDDK)
3 Information Way
Bethesda, MD 20892
Toll-Free: 800-891-5390
Toll-Free TTY: 866-569-1162
Fax: 703-738-4929
Website: www.kidney.niddk.nih.
gov
E-mail: nkdep@info.niddk.nih.
gov

Prostatitis Foundation (PF)
1063 30th St.
Smithshire, IL 61478
Phone: 309-325-7184
Fax: 309-325-7189
Website: www.prostatitis.org
E-mail: info@prostatitis.org

Sexually Transmitted Diseases

AIDS Healthcare Foundation (AHF)
6255 W. Sunset Blvd.
21st Fl.
Los Angeles, CA 90028
Toll-Free: 800-263-0067
Phone: 323-860-5200
Website: www.aidshealth.org

Gay Men's Health Crisis (GMHC)
446 W. 33rd St.
New York, NY 10001-2601
Phone: 212-367-1000
Website: www.gmhc.org
E-mail: webmaster@gmhc.org

Sexuality Information and Education Council of the United States (SIECUS)
1012 14th St. N.W.
Ste. 1108
Washington, DC 20005
Phone: 202-265-2405
Fax: 202-462-2340
Website: www.siecus.org
E-mail: info@siecus.org

Suicide

American Association of Suicidology (AAS)
5221 Wisconsin Ave. N.W.
Washington, DC 20015
Toll-Free: 800-273-TALK
(800-273-8255)
Phone: 202-237-2280
Fax: 202-237-2282
Website: www.suicidology.org

Suicide Prevention Resource Center (SPRC)
43 Foundry Ave.
Waltham, MA 02453-8313
Toll-Free: 877-GET-SPRC
(877-438-7772)
TTY: 617-964-5448
Fax: 617-969-9186
Website: www.sprc.org
E-mail: info@sprc.org

Index

Index

Page numbers followed by 'n' indicate a footnote. Page numbers in *italics* indicate a table or illustration.

A

abdominal aortic aneurysm (AAA)
  defined 34
  screening 36
abdominal lymph node dissection *see* lymphadenectomy
abdominal ultrasound
  defined 677
  inguinal hernias tests 426
ablation, defined 677
abnormality, testicular self-examination (TSE) 31
"About Diabetes" (CDC) 181n
"About Stroke" (CDC) 361n
abscess, epididymitis 416
abstinence
  defined 677
  male condoms 489
The Academy for Eating Disorders (AED), contact 687
ACE inhibitors, chronic kidney disease (CKD) 272
acetaminophen (Tylenol), cirrhosis 166

achromatopsia
  color blindness 548
  defined 677
  prostate cancer 347
acquired immunodeficiency syndrome (AIDS)
  gonorrhea 515
  gynecomastia 606
  hemophilia 560
  overview 225–7
  sexually transmitted diseases (STDs) 502
action plan, heart attack 221
active surveillance
  defined 677
  prostate cancer 347
acupuncture
  lung cancer 283
  prostatitis 464
addiction
  defined 677
  eating disorders 663
  gender 5
  violence 656
adjuvant therapy
  defined 677
  described 602
  penile cancer 338
  testicular cancer 358

693

adrenocorticotropic hormone (ACTH),
overweight 101
aerobic activity
adults 135
blood pressure 41
aerobic exercise, high blood
pressure 74
African Americans
chronic kidney disease (CKD) 250
diabetes 183
high blood pressure 40
occupational injuries 321
prostate cancer 57
"Aggressive Driving"
(Omnigraphics) 286n
aggressive driving, overview 286–8
AIDS *see* acquired immunodeficiency
syndrome
AIDS Healthcare Foundation (AHF),
contact 690
Alaska Natives
chronic obstructive pulmonary
disease (COPD) 170
fire injuries 317
prediabetes 182
suicide 370
albumin
chronic liver disease 161
diabetes 253
kidney disease 271
alcohol abuse
eating disorders 663
heart disease 204
osteoporosis 610
premature ejaculation (PE) 470
alcohol poisoning, short-term health
risks 15
alcohol-related deaths
men 647
statistics 16
"Alcohol, Tobacco, and Other Drugs"
(SAMHSA) 646n
alcohol use
eating disorders in men 663
heart disease 201
liver cancer 274
male infertility 478
risks to men's health, overview 14–6
water-related accidents 326

alfuzosin, alpha-blockers 449
allergy
benign prostatic hyperplasia 443
human papillomavirus vaccine
(HPV) 66
scrotum and testicles 417
The Alliance for Eating Disorders
Awareness ("The Alliance"),
contact 687
alopecia, male-pattern baldness 625
alpha-blockers, noncancerous prostate
disorders 448
Alzheimer disease (AD)
causes of death 149
kidney and urological disorders 391
"Alzheimer Disease" (CDC) 153n
American Association of
Cardiovascular and Pulmonary
Rehabilitation (AACVPR),
contact 688
American Association of Suicidology
(AAS), contact 690
American Cancer Society (ACS),
contact 686
American Childhood Cancer
Organization (ACCO), contact 686
American Heart Association (AHA),
contact 688
American Indians
chronic obstructive pulmonary
disease (COPD) 170
diabetes 185
kidney disease 250
American Liver Foundation (ALF),
contact 688
The American Urological Association
Foundation, contact 689
amitriptyline, prostatitis 464
amphetamines
gynecomastia 606
sex differences 18
anabolic steroids, overview 650–2
"Anabolic Steroids" (NIDA) 650n
anal sex
human papillomavirus (HPV) 65
sexually transmitted disease
(STD) 499
"Anatomy of Colon and Rectum"
(NCI) 173n

androgenetic alopecia, described 625
"Androgenetic Alopecia"
(GHR) 625n
anemia
diabetes 197
kidney disease 251
nutrition tips for men 129
sexually transmitted diseases
(STDs) 503
anesthesia
benign prostatic hyperplasia 445
hydrocelectomy 420
kidney stones 380
penile concerns 401
screening tests for men 47
spermatocele 430
vasectomy 484
aneurysm
screening tests 37
stroke 363
angina, heart disease 203
anorexia, eating disorders 662
antiandrogen, defined 678
antibiotic
acute bacterial prostatitis 465
benign prostatic hyperplasia 452
bronchoscopy 244
chronic obstructive pulmonary
disease (COPD) 171
gynecomastia 605
muscular dystrophy (MD) 583
penile concerns 402
pneumonia 236
sexually transmitted diseases
(STDs) 500
spermatocele 430
antibodies
fecal immunochemical test
(FIT) 177
hemophilia 559
hepatitis B 519
targeted therapy 600
antidepressant medications
mental-health concerns 633
muscle dysmorphic disorder
(MDD) 669
premature ejaculation (PE) 471
antimuscarinics, benign prostatic
hyperplasia 450

antipsychotics
healthy weight 95
schizophrenia 642
antiretroviral therapy (ART),
human immunodeficiency virus
(HIV) 246
anus, depicted *431*
apnea *see* sleep apnea
arrhythmia
described 6
heart disease 203
ART *see* antiretroviral therapy
artery
heart attack 218
stroke 362
arthritis
chlamydia 508
chronic obstructive pulmonary
disease (COPD) 171
kidney and urological disorders 389
nutrition tips 127
ascites, cirrhosis 162
Asian Americans, diabetes 185
aspirin
colorectal cancer 175
heart attack 220
male-linked genetic disorders 565
prostatitis 464
screening tests 50
asthma
chronic obstructive pulmonary
disease (COPD) 170
influenza and pneumonia 232
osteoporosis 610
seasonal influenza vaccination 68
smoking 649
atherosclerosis
coronary artery disease (CAD) 215
erectile dysfunction (ED) 468
overweight and obesity 92
sleep apnea 617
atrial flutter, arrhythmia 7
autoimmune disorders
infertility 478
penile concerns 405
sex-specific health differences 6
Avodart (dutasteride)
benign prostatic hyperplasia 449
prostatitis 464

axillary lymph node, breast
concerns 594

B

balanced diet
healthy muscles 129
osteoporosis 611
balanitis, overview 395–7
"Balanitis" (Omnigraphics) 395n
baldness, overview 625–6
bariatric surgery, healthy
weight 119
basal cell
defined 678
skin cancer self-examination 28
"Basic Information about Prostate
Cancer" (CDC) 341n
"Basics about COPD" (CDC) 169n
BDD *see* body dysmorphic disorder
becker muscular dystrophy (BMD),
muscular dystrophy 578
behavioral therapy *see* (CBT)
behavioral weight-loss program,
healthy weight 102
beige fat tissue, healthy weight 94
"Benefits of Exercise" (NIH) 139n
benign prostatic hyperplasia (BPH)
overview 440–59
prostatitis 463
bigorexia, muscle dysmorphic disorder
(MDD) 667
bile, cirrhosis 160
binge drinking, men's health
risks 10, 647
biofeedback
prostatitis 464
urgency incontinence 390
biologic therapy
cancer 151
penile cancer 339
biological clock, sleep 78
biopsy
benign prostatic hyperplasia 447
breast cancer 588
cirrhosis 164
defined 678
penile cancer 333
prostate cancer 60

birth control
vasectomy 482
withdrawal, overview 490–1
bladder
benign prostatic hyperplasia 440
depicted *58*
kidney disease 249, 341
perineal injury 432
prostate cancer 56
urinary incontinence 388
blood alcohol concentration (BAC)
drowsy driving 293
impaired driving 298
blood alcohol levels, men's health
risks 12
blood clot, depicted *362*
blood pressure
chronic kidney disease (CKD) 252
healthy eating for men 126
heart attack 220
men and heart disease 201
screening tests for men 34
sleep apnea 617
stroke 368
blood tests
cholesterol screening 43
cirrhosis 167
genital herpes 511
gynecomastia 607
healthy weight 101
heart attack 224
hemophilia 558
kidney disease 254
kidney stones 380
syphilis 535
blood thinners
falls and injuries 306
BMD *see* Becker muscular dystrophy
BMD *see* bone mineral density
BMI *see* body mass index
body dysmorphic disorder (BDD)
eating disorders in men 662
muscle dysmorphic disorder
(MDD) 667
body image, overview 662–9
body mass index (BMI)
healthy weight 100
screening tests for men 35
weight and health risk 86

bone density test, osteoporosis
  screening 51
bone mineral density (BMD),
  osteoporosis 611
bone-strengthening, physical
  activities 134
BPH *see* benign prostatic hyperplasia
brain
  Alzheimer disease (AD) 154
  cirrhosis 163
  color vision deficiency 545
  endocrine disorders 95
  fall and injuries 306
  hemophilia 557
  perineal injury 432
  schizophrenia 642
  sexual dysfunction 473
  stroke 361
BRCA
  breast self-examination 24
  male breast cancer 587
breast cancer
  men, overview 586–605
  self-examination 24
breast lumps, breast self-
  examination 25
breast self-examination,
  overview 24–6
"Breast Self-Examination"
  (Omnigraphics) 24n
breathing devices, sleep apnea 620
The British Columbia Eating
  Disorders Association (BCEDA),
  contact 687
bronchiole, depicted *236*
brown fat tissue, healthy weight 94
buddy system, water-related
  accidents 328
bulimia, eating disorders in men 662
bump (slang)
  healthy weight loss 111
  human papillomavirus (HPV) 522
  penile intraepithelial neoplasia 398

C

calcium oxalate stones
  kidney stones 385
  see also hypercalciuria

calories
  defined 678
  healthy eating for men 122
  overweight and obesity 93
  physical activity 136
Cambridge Color Test, color
  blindness 548
cancer
  breast self-examination 24
  human papillomavirus (HPV) 65, 522
  men 151
  penile intraepithelial neoplasia 398
  vasectomy 484
"Cancer" (NIH) 151n
"Cancer and Men" (CDC) 151n
Cancer Care, contact 686
candida, balanitis 396
candy (slang)
  healthy weight loss 108
  poisoning 324
carcinoma
  breast cancer in men 586
  cirrhosis 161
  defined 678
  penile intraepithelial neoplasia 398
  skin cancer self-examination 28
cardiomyopathy, heart failure 203
cardiopulmonary resuscitation (CPR),
  water-related accidents 328
cardiovascular disease
  colorectal cancer 175
  screening tests for men 35
  sexual dysfunction 468
Cardiovascular Research Foundation
  (CRF), contact 688
Cardura (doxazosin), benign prostatic
  hyperplasia 449
cataract, vision disorders 10
catheter
  benign prostatic hyperplasia 451
  breast cancer in men 600
  heart attack 224
  heart failure 209
CDC *see* Centers for Disease Control
  and Prevention
Centers for Disease Control and
  Prevention (CDC)
  publications
    alcohol use 13n

Centers for Disease Control and
  Prevention (CDC)
  publications, *continued*
      Alzheimer disease (AD) 153n
      body mass index (BMI) 88n
      cancer and men 151n
      chronic obstructive pulmonary
        disease (COPD) 169n
      colorectal cancer 173n
      coronary artery disease
        (CAD) 215n
      diabetes 181n
      distracted driving 288n
      drowsy driving 291n
      epididymitis 414n
      excessive alcohol use and risks
        to men's health 10n, 647n
      important facts about
        falls 306n
      healthy weight 86n
      heart disease 14n, 200n
      impaired driving 296n
      infertility FAQs 477n
      influenza (flu) 230n
      liver cancer 273n
      losing weight 103n
      lung cancer 277n
      men and heart disease 200n
      mortality in the United
        States 146n
      muscular dystrophy
        (MD) 578n
      older adult drivers 301n
      poisoning 322n
      preventing suicide 369n
      prostate cancer 341n
      scabies FAQs 526n
      stroke 361n
      water-related injuries 325n
cefoxitin, epididymitis 418
ceftriaxone, epididymitis 418
Center for Eating Disorders (CED),
  contact 688
chemotherapy
  breast concerns in men 601
  cancer and men 151
  lung cancer 282
  penile cancer 338
  testicular cancer 358

chest pain
  benign prostatic hyperplasia 455
  chronic kidney disease (CKD) 251
  heart attack 221
  lung cancer 280
children
  body mass index (BMI) 90
  domestic abuse against men 655
  flu vaccine 68
  fragile X syndrome 552
  heart failure 204
  hemophilia 562
  hepatitis B 518
  influenza 231
  overweight and obesity 99
  physical activity 135
  pneumonia 240
  poisoning 322
  sleep apnea 617
chills
  influenza 230
  kidney and urological disorders 379
  noncancerous prostate disorders 444
  prostatitis 463
  seasonal influenza vaccination 67
chlamydia
  defined 678
  epididymitis 416
  gonorrhea 515
  overview 507–9
  pneumonia 245
  sexually transmitted diseases
    (STDs) 500
"Chlamydia Infections" (NIH) 507n
cholesterol
  defined 678
  heart attack 220
  kidney disease 271
  men and heart disease 201
  overweight and obesity 92
  physical activity 139
  screening tests for men 35
  stroke 368
  see also heart disease; high-density
    lipoprotein (HDL) cholesterol;
    low-density lipoprotein (LDL)
    cholesterol
"Choosing a Safe and Successful
  Weight-Loss Program"
  (NIDDK) 112n

chronic bronchitis *see* chronic
  obstructive pulmonary disease
chronic kidney disease (CKD)
  blood pressure 73
  diabetes 195
  overview 249–72
  sleep apnea 617
"Chronic Kidney Disease (CKD)"
  (NIDDK) 249n
chronic obstructive pulmonary disease
  (COPD)
  overview 169–71
  pneumonia 235
Cialis (tadalafil), benign prostatic
  hyperplasia 449
circumcision
  balanitis 396
  described 394
  hemophilia 556
  penile cancer 332
  phimosis 410
"Circumcision" (NIH) 394n
cirrhosis
  breast cancer in men 586
  gynecomastia 606
  hepatitis B 517
  overview 159–68
  sexually transmitted diseases
    (STDs) 505
"Cirrhosis: A Patient's Guide"
  (VA) 159n
cirrhotic, depicted *159*
clinical trials
  breast cancer 604
  penile cancer 337
  testicular cancer 359
clonazepam (Klonopin),
  prostatitis 464
clotrimazole, balanitis 396
clotting
  cirrhosis 161
  hemophilia 554
cocaine
  defined 678
  heart attack 220
  heart failure 204
  sex differences in substance
    abuse 18
  sexual dysfunction 473

cognitive behavioral therapy (CBT)
  depression 634
  muscle dysmorphic disorder 669
cognitive function
  Alzheimer disease (AD) 154
  motor vehicle accidents 302
  schizophrenia 641
colon
  colorectal cancer 173
  colorectal cancer screening 46
  lung cancer 278
colon large intestine, depicted *47*
colonoscopy
  colorectal cancer 178
  colorectal cancer screening 47
color blindness *see* color vision
  deficiency
colorectal cancer
  overview 173–9
  screening tests for men 34
color vision deficiency,
  overview 544–9
Colorectal Cancer Control Program
  (CRCCP), contact 686
computed axial tomography scan
  (CAT; CT)
  breast concerns in men 591
  colorectal cancer 178
  lung cancer 281
  penile cancer 333
  testicular cancer 352
condoms
  defined 678
  genital herpes 510
  hepatitis B 519
  HIV and AIDS 226
  overview 488–9
  safer sex guidelines 494
  trichomoniasis 538
  vasectomy 482
  withdrawal 491
congestive heart failure, influenza 232
constipation
  chronic perineal injury 435
  inguinal hernias 428
  urinary incontinence 388
continuous positive airway pressure
  (CPAP), sleep apnea 622
"Control Your Cholesterol" (NIH) 75n

COPD *see* chronic obstructive pulmonary disease
coronary angioplasty, heart attack 224
coronary artery disease (CAD)
   colorectal cancer 175
   overview 215–6
   physical activities 139
   see also heart disease
"Coronary Artery Disease (CAD)" (CDC) 215n
"Coronary Artery Disease" (NIH) 215n
corpora cavernosa
   penile cancer 331
   Peyronie disease 403
corpus spongiosum, penile cancer 331
Cortisol, endocrine disorders 95
CPAP *see* continuous positive airway pressure
CPR *see* cardiopulmonary resuscitation
crabs *see* pubic lice
Crohn disease, colorectal cancer 174
crusted scabies, scabies 526
cryotherapy *see* cryosurgery
cryosurgery, penile cancer 337
cryptorchidism, testicular self-examination 32
crystal (slang), kidney stones 382
CT scan *see* computed axial tomography scan
Cushing syndrome
   endocrine disorders 95
   male infertility 479
   overweight and obesity 101
cyclobenzaprine, prostatitis 464
cystinuria, kidney stones 377
cystoscopy
   benign prostatic hyperplasia 447
   kidney stones 381

D

dehydration, nutrition 130
dehydroepiandrosterone sulfate (DHEAS) tests
   healthy weight 101
   sleep apnea 619
dementia
   Alzheimer disease (AD) 153
   syphilis 534

depression
   chronic obstructive pulmonary disease (COPD) 171
   defined 679
   erectile dysfunction (ED) 468
   heart disease 214
   kidney disease 263
   Klinefelter syndrome (KS) 570
   overview 629–36
   physical activity 140
   screening tests 34
   sexual assault 657
   sleep apnea 617
   stress 81
   stroke 368
Depression and Bipolar Support Alliance (DBSA), contact 689
desmopressin, hemophilia 561
detrol (Tolterodine), prostatic hyperplasia 455
deuteranomaly, color blindness 546
deuteranopia, color blindness 547
diabetes
   balanitis 395
   benign prostatic hyperplasia 440
   chronic obstructive pulmonary disease (COPD) 171
   defined 679
   erectile dysfunction (ED) 468
   flu 234
   healthy weight 103
   inguinal hernia 421
   kidney disease 253, 389
   liver cancer 274
   nutrition 126
   overview 181–97
   screening tests 34
   sleep apnea 617, 625
   stroke 367
   vaccinations 63
diastolic pressure, blood pressure 72
diet and nutrition, gynecomastia 606
Dietary Guidelines for Americans
   alcohol use 15
   defined 679
   kidney disease 250
dietary supplements
   healthy weight 102
   lung cancer 283

dietary supplements, *continued*
  nutrition 129
  prostatitis 464
digestive system, nutrition 128
digital rectal exam (DRE)
  benign prostatic hyperplasia 445
  prostate cancer 58, 347
digoxin, heart disease 211
dihydrotestosterone (DHT)
  benign prostatic hyperplasia 441
  male-pattern baldness 626
distracted driving, overview 288–91
"Distracted Driving" (CDC) 288n
diuretic
  benign prostatic hyperplasia 448
  decompensated cirrhosis 165
  eating disorders 665
  heart failure 211
  kidney disease 261
DMD *see* Duchenne muscular
  dystrophy
domestic abuse, overview 654–7
dopamine
  addiction 5
  defined 679
  schizophrenia 642
doxazosin, alpha-blockers 449
drowning, water-related accidents 325
drowsy driving
  overview 291–6
  sleep apnea 624
"Drowsy Driving" (CDC) 291n
dry eye, vision disorders 9
dual-energy x-ray absorptiometry (DXA)
  body mass index (BMI) 88
  osteoporosis 612
Duchenne muscular dystrophy
  (DMD), muscular dystrophy 578
ductal carcinoma in situ, breast
  cancer 586
dutasteride
  benign prostatic hyperplasia 449
  prostatitis 464
dysthymia, depression 631

E

EACA *see* epsilon-aminocaproic acid
"Eat Healthy" (ODPHP) 122n

eating disorders
  overview 662–7
  see also body dysmorphic disorder
"Eating Disorders" (HHS) 662n
"Eating Disorders in Men"
  (SAMHSA) 662n
ecstasy, sexual dysfunction 473
edema
  defined 679
  heart failure 206
  kidney disease 251
ejaculation
  benign prostatic hyperplasia 443
  prostate cancer 343
  prostatitis 461
  sexual dysfunction 474
  trichomoniasis 538
  withdrawal 490
electrocardiogram (EKG)
  heart attack 224
  heart disease 207
emphysema
  chronic obstructive pulmonary
    disease (COPD) 169
  defined 679
enablex (darifenacin), noncancerous
  prostate disorders 455
epididymitis
  overview 414–8
  spermatocele 430
"Epididymitis" (CDC) 414n
epididymo-orchitis *see* epididymitis
epsilon-aminocaproic acid (EACA),
  antifibrinolytic medicines 561
erectile dysfunction (ED)
  male menopause 672
  penile cancer 331
  perineal injury 432
  Peyronie disease 403
  physical activity 140
  prostate screening 60
  see also sexual dysfunction
erection
  described 403
  hyperplasia 455
  penile cancer 331
  perineal injury 432
  Peyronie disease 402
  sexual dysfunction 468

erection, *continued*
  vasectomy 484
  see also erectile dysfunction
erythromycin, balanitis 396
erythroplasia of Queyrat *see* penile
  intraepithelial neoplasia
estrogen
  benign prostatic hyperplasia 441
  breast cancer 586
  breast self-examination 24
  hormonal disorders 479
  hormone therapy 600
  hypogonadism 611
Eunice Kennedy Shriver National
  Institute of Child Health and
  Human Development (NICHD)
  contact 685
  publications
      fragile X syndrome 549n
      Klinefelter syndrome (KS) 566n
      sexually transmitted diseases
        (STDs) 498n
      vasectomy 481n
exam
  balanitis 396
  breast concerns 592
  colorectal cancer 179
  depression 632
  erectile dysfunction (ED) 468
  heart disease 207
  inguinal hernias 425
  penile cancer 332
  prostate cancer screening 58
  sleep apnea 618
  testicular cancer 358
  see also self-examinations
excessive drinking, drinking levels
  among men 647
exercise
  alcohol abuse 611
  benign prostatic
  blood pressure 74
  cirrhosis 166
  diabetes 188
  eating disorders 663
  falls 308
  heart disease 14, 210
  hemophilia 564
  hyperplasia 442

exercise, *continued*
  mental health 635
  nutrition 128
  physical activity 141
  prostatitis 464
  smoking 50
  stroke 367
  urinary incontinence 389
  weight-loss program 102
exercise stress tests
  heart disease 15
  tabulated *215*

F

"Fact Sheets—Alcohol Use and Your
  Health" (CDC) 14n
"Fact Sheets—Excessive Alcohol
  Use and Risks to Men's Health"
  (CDC) 10n, 647n
"Facts about Color Blindness"
  (NEI) 544n
fad diets, healthy weight 86
falls
  blood pressure 72
  drowsy driving 292
  inguinal hernia 425
  Klinefelter syndrome (KS) 567
  male infertility 477
  nutrition 127
  occupational injuries 320
  overview 306–8
  physical activity 140
  schizophrenia 641
  screening tests 55
  sleep apnea 622
false-negative test result, prostate
  screening 60
false-positive test result
  lung cancer 281
  prostate cancer 345
  prostate screening 60
familial adenomatous polyposis (FAP),
  colorectal cancer 174
family history
  Alzheimer disease (AD) 154
  blood pressure 74
  body mass index (BMI) 100
  breast self-examination 24

family history, *continued*
  cholesterol 44
  chronic kidney disease (CKD) 250
  depression 632
  diabetes 194
  hemophilia 558
  inguinal hernias 424
  kidney stones 377
  peyronie disease 406
  prostate cancer 342
  sleep apnea 615
Farnsworth Lantern Test, color
  blindness 548
Farnsworth-Munsell 100 Hue Test,
  color blindness 548
fatalities
  drowsy driving 292
  occupational injuries 319
fecal occult blood test (FOBT),
  colorectal cancer 177
fertility
  prostate 440
  sexual dysfunction 474
  spermatocele 428
fight-or-flight, described 21
finasteride (Proscar)
  benign prostatic hyperplasia 449
  prostatitis 464
fire
  overview 309–19
  penile trauma 400
Flomax (tamsulosin), alpha-
  blockers 449
flu *see* influenza
"Flu (Influenza)" (HHS) 67n
flu shots, vaccination 63
flu vaccine, influenza 67, 230
follow-up test
  colonoscopy 178
  epididymitis 417
  healthy weight 105
  lung cancer 281
  penile cancer 340
  penile intraepithelial neoplasia 399
  prostate cancer 60
  syphilis 536
  testicular cancer 353
  viral pneumonia 246

food diary
  healthy weight 105
  nutrition 123
fragile X syndrome, overview 549–54
"Fragile X Syndrome" (NICHD) 549n

G

gallstone
  defined 679
  healthy weight 114
Gay Men's Health Crisis (GMHC),
  contact 690
"Gender Differences in Primary
  Substance of Abuse across Age
  Groups" (SAMHSA) 17n
gene
  breast concerns 587
  cirrhosis 160
  color blindness 544
  defined 679
  diabetes 186
  hemophilia 554
  male-pattern baldness 626
gene therapy
  defined 679
  hemophilia 561
genetic syndromes
  colorectal cancer 174
  healthy weight 95
genetic testing, fragile X
  syndrome 553
Genetics Home Reference (GHR)
  publication
      androgenetic alopecia 625n
genital herpes
  balanitis 396
  overview 509–12
"Genital Herpes" (HHS) 509n
genital warts
  defined 679
  human papillomavirus (HPV) 502
  penile intraepithelial neoplasia 398
germ cell tumor
  defined 679
  testicular cancer 349
"Get a Bone Density Test"
  (ODPHP) 51n
"Get Enough Sleep" (ODPHP) 77n

"Get Tested for Colorectal Cancer"
(ODPHP) 46n
"Get Your Blood Pressure Checked"
(ODPHP) 39n
"Get Your Cholesterol Checked"
(ODPHP) 42n
GFR *see* glomerular filtration rate
Gleason score, prostate cancer 347
glomerular filtration rate (GFR),
kidney disease 254
glucocorticoids
Cushing syndrome 95
male infertility 479
osteoporosis 610
gonorrhea
epididymitis 416
overview 512–5
"Gonorrhea" (HHS) 512n
good cholesterol *see* high-density
lipoprotein (HDL) cholesterol
gynecomastia
breast self-examination 25
overview 605–8
"Gynecomastia" (Omnigraphics) 605n

H

HDL cholesterol *see* high-density
lipoprotein (HDL) cholesterol
head injury, important facts about
falls 306
healthy eating pattern, overview 122–6
healthy muscles, nutrition tips 127
"Healthy Muscles Matter"
(NIAMS) 127n
"Healthy Weight" (CDC) 86n
healthy weight loss, overview 103–11
heart attack
high blood pressure 74
kidney disease 271
overview 217–24
screening tests for men 35
"Heart Attack" (NHLBI) 217n
heart disease
cholesterol screening 43
depression 632
diabetes 181
kidney disease 250
overview 200–24

heart disease, *continued*
preventing high cholesterol 75
stroke 368
"Heart Disease and Men" (CDC) 200n
heart failure
overview 202–14
pneumonia 235
screening tests for men 35
"Heart Failure" (NHLBI) 202n
heart problems
heart failure 209
muscle dysmorphic disorder 668
Heart Rhythm Society (HRS),
contact 688
heavy drinking *see* excessive drinking
hemochromatosis, liver cancer 274
hemophilia, overview 554–66
"Hemophilia" (NHLBI) 554n
hemorrhagic stroke
defined 679
stroke 362
hepatic encephalopathy, cirrhosis 163
hepatitis A
male-linked genetic disorders 560
sexually transmitted diseases
(STDs) 504
viral hepatitis 158
hepatitis B
liver cancer 275
overview 516–20
sexually transmitted diseases 499
vaccinations for men 63
viral hepatitis 158
"Hepatitis B" (HHS) 516n
hepatitis C
liver cancer 275
sexually transmitted diseases
(STDs) 499
viral hepatitis 158
Hepatitis Foundation International
(HFI), contact 689
hepatocellular carcinoma,
cirrhosis 161
heroin
gynecomastia 606
sex differences in substance abuse 18
herpes simplex viruses (HSV)
genital herpes 509
sexually transmitted diseases
(STDs) 499

HHS *see* U.S. Department of Health
and Human Services
high blood pressure *see* hypertension
high-density lipoprotein (HDL)
cholesterol
cholesterol screening 44
kidney disease 271
Hispanics
fire-related injuries 317
healthy weight 98
heart disease 200
kidney disease 250
HIV *see* human immunodeficiency
virus
"HIV/AIDS: The Basics" (HHS) 225n
HIV infection
epididymitis 418
safer sex 494
sexually transmitted diseases
(STDs) 501
hives, noncancerous prostate
disorders 455
homicide
men's health risks 15
occupational injuries 319
hormone
breast cancer 600
defined 679
endocrine disorders 95
male infertility 479
male menopause 671
prostate cancer 348
sex-specific health differences 11
sleep apnea 619
hormone therapy
cancer among men 151
male breast cancer 600
"How the Heart Works" (NHLBI) 200n
"How the Lungs Work" (NHLBI) 277n
"How to Prevent High Blood Pressure"
(NIH) 72n
HPV *see* human papillomavirus
"HPV (Human Papillomavirus)"
(HHS) 65n, 520n
HRR Pseudoisochromatic Color Test,
color blindness 548
human immunodeficiency virus (HIV)
anabolic steroids 650
cancer 152

human immunodeficiency virus (HIV),
continued
condoms 489
defined 679
epididymitis 417
gynecomastia 606
heart disease 204
hemophilia 560
human papillomavirus (HPV) 522
kidney stones 378
overview 225–7
screening tests 35
sexually transmitted diseases
(STDs) 501
human papillomavirus (HPV)
cancer 151
defined 679
oral cancer 26
overview 520–4
penile cancer 332
"Human Papillomavirus (HPV)"
(HHS) 520n
hydrocele, overview 419–20
"Hydrocele" (Omnigraphics) 418n
hydrocelectomy, hydrocele 420
hyoscyamine, noncancerous prostate
disorders 455
hyperarousal, posttraumatic stress
disorder (PTSD) 639
hypercalciuria
kidney stones 377
osteoporosis 610
hyperparathyroidism, kidney
stones 377
hypertension
blood pressure 40
cirrhosis 160
defined 679
male-pattern baldness 625
obesity 92
hypogonadism, gynecomastia 606
hytrin (terazosin), alpha-blockers 449

I

ibuprofen
chronic kidney disease (CKD) 261
cirrhosis 166
hemophilia 565
prostatitis 464

ICD *see* implantable cardioverter
   defibrillator
imaging, defined 680
imipramine (Tofranil)
   benign prostatic hyperplasia 458
   retrograde ejaculation 474
immune function, biological factors 7
immune system
   autoimmune disorders 6
   biologic therapy 339
   cirrhosis 160
   defined 680
   human immunodeficiency virus
      (HIV) 225
   penile intraepithelial neoplasia
      (PEIN) 398
   Peyronie disease 404
   prostate cancer 348
   scabies 526
   targeted therapy 604
immunosuppressant
   defined 680
   muscular dystrophy (MD) 583
impaired driving, overview 296–301
"Impaired Driving: Get the Facts"
   (CDC) 296n
implantable cardioverter defibrillator
   (ICD), heart failure 212
"Important Facts about Falls"
   (CDC) 306n
impotence
   prostate cancer 346
   reproductive health 13, 648
   see also erectile dysfunction
in vitro fertilization (IVF), male
   infertility 480
incontinence, defined 680
indinavir, kidney stones 378
indirect inguinal hernia
   defined 421
   depicted *422*
infertility
   chlamydia 508
   epididymitis 416
   Klinefelter syndrome (KS) 569
   male menopause 672
   overview 477–80
   retrograde ejaculation 475
   sexual function 16

infertility, *continued*
   sexually transmitted diseases
      (STDs) 498
   testicular cancer 352
"Infertility FAQs" (CDC) 477n
influenza (flu)
   described 7
   overview 230–4
inguinal canal, depicted *422*
inguinal hernia, overview 421–8
"Inguinal Hernia" (NIDDK) 421n
injection drug use
   defined 680
   hepatitis B 518
insulin resistance, type 2 diabetes 189
internal penis, depicted *431*
intimate partner violence, excessive
   alcohol use 15
intracerebral hemorrhage
   defined 680
   hemorrhagic stroke 363
invasive cancer
   colorectal cancer 174
   defined 680
ischemic stroke, described 362
Ishihara Color Test, color
   blindness 548
itching
   benign prostatic hyperplasia 455
   chlamydia 508
   penile intraepithelial neoplasia
      (PEIN) 398
   physical activity 136
   scabies 526
   sexually transmitted diseases
      (STDs) 498
   skin cancer 29
   trichomoniasis 538

J

jaundice
   cirrhosis 162
   defined 680
   hepatitis B 517
   liver cancer 274
   syphilis 503
jogging
   healthy muscles 129

jogging, *continued*
  osteoporosis 612
  tabulated *136*

K

Kegel exercises
  prostatitis 464
  urinary incontinence 390
"Key Facts about Influenza (Flu)"
  (CDC) 230n
kidney damage
  benign prostatic hyperplasia 443
  muscle dysmorphic disorder
    (MDD) 668
  smoking 263
kidney disease
  erectile dysfunction (ED) 468
  high blood pressure 73
  overview 249–72
  sleep apnea 617
  type 2 diabetes 189
kidney failure
  chronic kidney disease (CKD) 250
  diabetes 195
  gynecomastia 606
  high blood pressure 40
  kidney stones 382
kidney stones, overview 376–88
"Kidney Stones" (NIDDK) 376n
Klinefelter syndrome (KS),
  overview 566–77
"Klinefelter Syndrome (KS):
  Condition Information"
  (NICHD) 566n
"Know the Facts about Heart Disease"
  (CDC) 14n

L

lactulose, encephalopathy 164
laparoscopic hernia repair,
  described 426
laparoscopy
  hydrocelectomy 420
  inguinal hernia 427
laser surgery
  benign prostatic hyperplasia 453
  penile cancer 337

latex condoms
  balanitis 395
  chlamydia 509
  gonorrhea 514
  syphilis 535
  withdrawal 491
  see also condoms
laxative
  anorexia nervosa 665
  colorectal cancer 47
LDL cholesterol *see* low-density
  lipoprotein cholesterol
Levitra (vardenafil), erectile
  dysfunction (ED)469
lifestyle changes
  benign prostatic hyperplasia 448
  cholesterol 76
  diabetes 182
  erectile dysfunction (ED) 469
  heart attack 220
  heart failure 210
  overweight and obesity 92
  sleep apnea 615
  urinary incontinence 390
lipoprotein
  defined 680
  high cholesterol 76
liver, depicted *159*
liver cancer
  cirrhosis 161
  hepatitis B 520
  overview 273–5
  viral hepatitis 158
"Liver Cancer" (CDC) 273n
liver damage
  hepatitis B 520
  muscle dysmorphic disorder
    (MDD) 668
liver failure
  gynecomastia 606
  hepatitis B 517
  viral hepatitis 158
lobar pneumonia, depicted *236*
lobe
  benign prostatic hyperplasia 440
  breast cancer 586
  defined 680
  pneumonia 237
"Losing Weight" (CDC) 103n

low-density lipoprotein (LDL)
cholesterol
defined 43
heart disease 201
overweight and obesity 92
lung cancer, overview 277–84
lupus
defined 680
described 8
kidney disease 253
lymph nodes
benign prostatic hyperplasia 445
defined 680
human papillomavirus (HPV) 523
lung cancer 277
male breast cancer 590
penile cancer 334
testicular cancer 355
testicular self-examination 31
lymphadenectomy
penile cancer 334
testicular cancer 352

M

magnetic resonance imaging (MRI)
biopsy 447
breast cancer 588
cirrhosis 164
defined 680
gynecomastia 607
heart failure 210
penile cancer 334
perineal injury 436
prostate cancer 347
testicular cancer 352
major depression, described 631
"Male Breast Cancer Treatment
(PDQ®)—Patient Version"
(FDA) 586n
male condom, overview 488–9
"Male Condom" (HHS) 488n
male menopause, overview 671–3
"Male Menopause"
(Omnigraphics) 671n
male-pattern baldness,
overview 625–6
malignant melanoma, potential skin
cancers 28

malnutrition
gynecomastia 606
kidney disease 251
schizophrenia 642
mammogram
breast cancer 588
gynecomastia 607
"Manage Stress" (ODPHP) 81n
marijuana
illegal drugs 646
impaired driving 297
infertility 479
sex differences in substance
abuse 17
MDD *see* muscle dysmorphic disorder
medical test
benign prostatic hyperplasia 446
defined 680
weight-loss program 118
medications
benign prostatic hyperplasia 448
breast self-examination 25
chronic obstructive pulmonary
disease (COPD) 171
cirrhosis 165
colorectal cancer 178
coronary artery disease 216
depression 633
drowsy driving 291
fragile X syndrome 554
gynecomastia 606
human papillomavirus (HPV) 523
inguinal hernia 427
kidney stones 378
liver cancer 273
osteoporosis 610
paraphimosis 411
penile intraepithelial neoplasia
(PEIN) 398
poisoning 322
prostate cancer 344
prostatitis 463
retrograde ejaculation 474
scabies 528
stroke 367
melanoma
defined 680
skin cancer self-examination 29
"Men and Depression" (NIMH) 629n

men and heart disease,
overview 200–2
"Men and Heart Disease Fact Sheet"
(CDC) 14n, 200n
"Men and Mental Health" (NIMH) 628n
"Men: Stay Healthy at Any Age"
(OPM) 34n
men who have sex with men (MSM)
hepatitis B 518
syphilis 534
"Men's Health and Smoking"
(FDA) 648n
mental health
exercises 140
hemophilia 563
kidney disease 263
overview 628–44
mental problems, muscle dysmorphic
disorder (MDD) 668
metabolic syndrome
overweight and obesity 92
physical activity 139
metabolism
defined 680
hypothyroidism 95
physical activity 134
metastasis, cancer 151
methamphetamine *see*
amphetamines
miconazole, balanitis 396
migraine, vision disorders 10
moderate drinking, described 14
moles, skin cancer self-examination 29
monochromacy, described 547
monoclonal antibody
defined 681
hormone therapy 600
mortality
health consequences 92
overview 146–50
"Mortality in the United States, 2017"
(CDC) 146n
mosaicism, fragile X syndrome 551
mouthpieces, described 620
multiple sclerosis (MS)
autoimmune disorders 6
erectile dysfunction (ED) 468
urge incontinence 390
muscle dysmorphic disorder,
overview 667–9

"Muscle Dysmorphic Disorder"
(Omnigraphics) 667n
muscle loss, anabolic steroids 650
muscle strengthening, physical
activities 134
"Muscular Dystrophy Information
Page" (NINDS) 578n
muscular dystrophy (MD),
overview 578–83
mutation
breast self-examination 24
defined 681
fragile X syndrome 549
"Myths and Realities of
Domestic Abuse against Men"
(Omnigraphics) 654n

N

naproxen
hemophilia 565
kidney disease 271
prostatitis 464
National Cancer Institute (NCI)
contact 686
publications
colorectal cancer 173n
male breast cancer 586n
penile cancer 331n
prostate cancer 56n
testicular cancer 349n
National Center for Posttraumatic
Stress Disorder (NCPTSD)
publications
posttraumatic stress disorder
(PTSD) 637n
sexual assault on males 657n
National Eye Institute (NEI)
publication
color blindness 544n
National Heart, Lung, and Blood
Institute (NHLBI)
contact 688
publications
heart attack 217n
heart failure 202n
hemophilia 554n
how the heart works 200n
how the lungs work 277n
overweight and obesity 92n

National Heart, Lung, and Blood
Institute (NHLBI)
publications, *continued*
pneumonia 235n
sleep apnea 615n
National Human Genome Research
Institute (NHGRI), contact 685
National Institute of Arthritis and
Musculoskeletal and Skin Diseases
(NIAMS)
publication
importance of healthy
muscles 127n
National Institute of Dental and
Craniofacial Research (NIDCR)
publication
oral cancer exam 26n
National Institute of Diabetes and
Digestive and Kidney Diseases
(NIDDK)
contact 685
publications
chronic kidney disease
(CKD) 249n
how kidneys work 249n
inguinal hernia 421n
kidney stones 376n
perineal injury in males 430n
Peyronie disease 402n
prostate enlargement (benign
prostatic hyperplasia) 440n
prostatitis 459n
viral hepatitis 158n
weight-loss program 112n
National Institute of Mental Health
(NIMH)
contact 689
publications
depression 629n
men and depression 629n
men and mental health 628n
schizophrenia 640n
National Institute of Neurological
Disorders and Stroke (NINDS)
publication
muscular dystrophy (MD) 578n
National Institute on Aging (NIA)
publication
urinary incontinence in older
adults 388n

National Institute on Drug Abuse
(NIDA)
contact 687
publication
anabolic steroid use 650n
National Institutes of Health (NIH)
publications
benefits of exercise 139n
blood pressure 72n
cancer 151n
chlamydia infections 507n
circumcision 394n
coronary artery disease 215n
oral cancer 26n
pubic lice 524n
sex/gender influence on health
and disease 4n
sleep apnea 615n
National Kidney and Urologic
Diseases Information Clearinghouse
(NKUDIC), contact 689
needle aspiration
hydrocele 420
spermatocele 430
neoplasm
defined 681
hydrocele 418
testicular cancer 30
nerves, depicted *431*
"News Release Bureau of Labor
Statistics" (BLS) 319n
NIA *see* National Institute on Aging
nicotine
osteoporosis in men 611
sleep disorders 79
NIDA *see* National Institute on Drug
Abuse
NIDDK *see* National Institute of
Diabetes and Digestive and Kidney
Diseases
NIH News in Health
publications
controlling cholesterol 75n
sex and gender 4n
NIH Osteoporosis and Related Bone
Diseases—National Resource Center
(NIH ORBD—NRC)
publication
osteoporosis in men 609n

nitroglycerin pill, emergency medical
  care 219
nocturnal erection test, erectile
  dysfunction (ED) 469
nonmelanoma skin cancer, potential
  skin cancers 28
nonseminoma
  defined 681
  testicular cancer 349
nortriptyline, prostatitis 464
Nutrition Facts label
  healthy eating for men 124
  kidney disease 264
  osteoporosis 54

O

obesity
  benign prostatic hyperplasia 442
  colorectal cancer 174
  gynecomastia 606
  healthy eating for men 123
  heart disease 201
  kidney disease 270
  male-pattern baldness 625
  physical activity 139
  sleep apnea 618
  stress 81
  type 2 diabetes 191
  weight-loss program 112
obstruction
  benign prostatic hyperplasia 440
  defined 681
  epididymitis 414
  sleep apnea 621
  spermatocele 429
Occupational Safety and Health
  Administration (OSHA), contact 686
Office of Disease Prevention and
  Health Promotion (ODPHP)
  publications
    abdominal aortic aneurysm 36n
    blood pressure test 39n
    bone density test 51n
    cholesterol test 42n
    colorectal cancer test 46n
    healthy eating 122n
    sleep 77n
    stress management 81n

ofloxacin, epididymitis 416
"Older Adult Drivers" (CDC) 301n
older adults
  older drivers 301
  physical activity 140
  pneumonia 241
  substance abuse 20
  vaccinations for men 63
Omnigraphics
  publications
    balanitis 395n
    breast self-examination 24n
    gynecomastia 605n
    hydrocele 418n
    longer lifespans for
      women 6n
    male menopause 671n
    muscle dysmorphic
      disorder 667n
    myths and realities of
      domestic abuse against
      men 654n
    penile intraepithelial
      neoplasia 398n
    penile trauma 400n
    phimosis and
      paraphimosis 409n
    sexual dysfunction 467n
    skin cancer self-
      examination 28n
    spermatocele 428n
    testicular self-examination 30n
    withdrawal 490n
oncologist
  defined 681
  lung cancer 283
open hernia repair, described 426
opioid
  defined 681
  sleep apnea 619
opportunistic infection
  defined 681
  human immunodeficiency virus
    (HIV) 227
"Oral Cancer" (NIH) 26n
"The Oral Cancer Exam"
  (NIDCR) 26n
oral cancer self-examination,
  overview 26–7

oral sex
  chlamydia 509
  human papillomavirus (HPV) 521
  male condoms 489
  syphilis 533
osteoarthritis
  described 8
  obesity 93
osteoporosis
  Klinefelter syndrome (KS) 573
  male menopause 672
  overview 609–14
  screening 51
"Osteoporosis in Men" (NIH ORBD—
  NRC) 609n
outpatient surgery
  defined 681
  vasectomy 482
overdiagnosis
  lung cancer screening 281
  prostate cancer screening 60
overflow incontinence, described 390
overweight and obesity
  body mass index (BMI) 89
  colorectal cancer 174
  heart disease 201
  overview 92–103
"Overweight and Obesity"
  (NHLBI) 92n
oxybutynin, noncancerous prostate
  disorders 455
oxygen therapy, pneumonia 246

P

pacemaker
  heart failure 212
  muscular dystrophy (MD) 583
Pacific Islanders
  civilian fire injuries 317
  prediabetes 185
Paget disease of the nipple
  male breast cancer 586
  tumor 593
pancreas
  chronic inflammation 617
  defined 681
  diabetes 181
Papanicolaou (Pap) test, defined 681

paraphimosis, described 410
Parkinson disease (PD)
  depression 632
  incontinence 390
paroxetine, antidepressant
  medications 472
PE *see* premature ejaculation
peau d'orange
  inflammatory male breast
    cancer 605
  male breast cancer 587
penectomy, surgery 338
penicillin
  balanitis 396
  epididymitis 417
  syphilis 535
penile cancer
  chronic balanitis 397
  circumcision 394
  overview 331–40
  penile intraepithelial neoplasia
    (PEIN) 398
"Penile Cancer Treatment (PDQ®)—
  Patient Version" National Cancer
  Institute (NCI) 331n
"Penile Curvature (Peyronie Disease)"
  (NIDDK) 402n
penile intraepithelial neoplasia,
  overview 398–9
"Penile Intraepithelial Neoplasia"
  (Omnigraphics) 398n
penile trauma, overview 400–2
"Penile Trauma" (Omnigraphics) 400n
penis
  chlamydia 507
  cystoscopy 447
  depicted *406*
  erectile dysfunction (ED) 469
  gonorrhea 513
  human papillomavirus (HPV) 502
  injury 404
  Klinefelter syndrome (KS) 568
  male condom 488
  paraphimosis 410
  Peyronie disease 402
  premature ejaculation (PE) 470
  priapism 472
  prostatic hyperplasia surgery 452
  prostatitis 461

penis, *continued*
  retrograde ejaculation 474
  scabies 527
  sexual problems 432
  sexually transmitted diseases
    (STDs) 498
  spermatoceles 429
  syphilis sores 536
  trichomoniasis 538
  withdrawal 490
percutaneous nephrolithotomy, kidney
  stones 381
perineal injury, overview 430–7
"Perineal Injury in Males"
  (NIDDK) 430n
perineal urethroplasty, described 433
perineum, depicted *431*
permethrin, pubic lice treatment 525
pertuzumab
  breast cancer treatment 589
  monoclonal antibody therapy 601
  targeted therapy 600
Peyronie disease, overview 402–8
phimosis, described 409
"Phimosis and Paraphimosis"
  (Omnigraphics) 409n
physical activity
  benefits 139, 262
  cholesterol check 39
  colorectal cancer 48
  coronary artery disease (CAD)
    prevention 216
  healthy muscles 128
  healthy weight 86
  healthy weight loss 104
  hemophilia 564
  osteoporosis 52
  overview 132–8
  overweight 96
  sleep apnea 620
  stress relief 188, 263
  trouble sleeping 78
  type 2 diabetes prevention 185
  weight-loss program 116
"Physical Activity Basics"
  (USDA) 132n
physical examination
  erectile dysfunction(ED) 468
  hydrocele 419

physical examination, *continued*
  male menopause 672
  penile trauma 401
  perineal injury 436
  phimosis 409
  premature ejaculation (PE) 471
  priapism 473
  testicular cancer 31
physical inactivity
  coronary artery disease (CAD) 215
  heart disease risk 201
piperonyl butoxide, lice-killing
  lotion 525
plaque
  coronary artery disease (CAD) 215
  defined 681
  depicted *406*
  heart disease 14
  high blood pressure 203
  ischemic heart disease 219
  Peyronie disease 402
pneumonia
  aging 63
  leading causes of death 149
  lung cancer 280
  overview 235–47
  respiratory infections 212
"Pneumonia" (NHLBI) 235n
poisoning, overview 322–4
"Poisoning" (CDC) 322n
polyps, colorectal cancer 48, 173
polyurethane condoms, male
  condom 488
portal vein, depicted *160*
positron emission tomography (PET)
  scan
  defined 681
  described 333
  nuclear heart scan 209
posttraumatic stress disorder (PTSD)
  overview 637–40
  sexual assault 657
potassium permanganate,
  balanitis 396
pregabalin, prostatitis 464
prehypertension, blood pressure 41,
  72
premature ejaculation (PE),
  described 470

prescription pain relievers, primary
substances of abuse 18
presumptive therapy, sexually
transmitted infections (STIs)
treatment 416
"Preventing Suicide" (CDC) 369n
priapism
described 472
male sexual dysfunction 467
prognosis
defined 681
muscular dystrophy (MD) 583
penile cancer 333
described 470
sexual dysfunction 467
propantheline bromide, noncancerous
prostate disorders 455
Propulsid, arrhythmia 7
Proscar (finasteride), 5-alpha
reductase inhibitors 464
prostate, depicted *441*
prostate cancer
overview 341–8
prostatectomy 432
prostate-specific antigen (PSA) blood
test 446
screening 57
testosterone treatment 573
vasectomy 484
prostate cancer gene 3 RNA test,
described 59
prostate cancer screening,
overview 56–60
"Prostate Cancer Screening (PDQ®)—
Patient Version" (NCI) 56n
"Prostate Enlargement (Benign
Prostatic Hyperplasia)"
(NIDDK) 440n
prostate gland, depicted *342*
prostate-specific antigen (PSA) test,
described 59
prostatectomy
perineal injury 432
prostate cancer treatment 60, 347
"Prostatitis: Inflammation of the
Prostate" (NIDDK) 459n
prostatitis
benign prostatic hyperplasia 444
male incontinence 389
overview 459–65

"Prostatitis: Inflammation of the
Prostate" (NIDDK) 459n
Prostatitis Foundation (PF),
contact 690
protanomaly, color blindness
types 546
protanopia, color blindness types 546
protective gear, prevent injuries 130
pruritus, scabies 526
pseudogynecomastia,
gynecomastia 605
psychotherapy, depression 634
PTSD *see* posttraumatic stress
disorder
"PTSD Basics" (NCPTSD) 637n
"PTSD Study: Men versus Women"
(VA) 20n
pubic lice
defined 681
overview 524–5
"Pubic Lice" (NIH) 524n
pulmonary rehabilitation, chronic
obstructive pulmonary disease 171
pulmonologist, lung cancer 283

Q

quality of life (QOL)
Alzheimer disease (AD) 155
benign prostatic hyperplasia 448
chronic obstructive pulmonary
disease (COPD) 171
heart failure 210
hemophilia 563
overweight and obesity 93
sleep apnea 623
quit smoking
abdominal aortic aneurysm 38
chronic obstructive pulmonary
disease (COPD) 171
colorectal cancer 49
lung cancer 278
physical activity 139

R

radiation
breast self-examination 24
defined 682
infertility 479

radical prostatectomy, prostate
cancer 347
raloxifene, gynecomastia 607
rectum
chlamydia 507
colorectal cancer 173
depicted *58*
gonorrhea 512
human papillomavirus (HPV) 65
perineal injury 436
syphilis 533
urinary incontinence 389
recurrence
balanitis 397
defined 682
hydrocele 420
paraphimosis 411
prostatitis 465
relapse
defined 682
psychosocial treatments 643
renal tubular acidosis, kidney
stones 378
resection, defined 682
retrograde ejaculation
overview 474–5
sexual dysfunction 458
risky sexual behavior
men's health risk 15
sex guidelines 494

S

scabies
described 682
overview 526–32
sexually transmitted diseases
(STDs) 499
"Scabies Frequently Asked Questions
(FAQs)" (CDC) 526n
schizophrenia
overview 640–4
sexual dysfunction 473
"Schizophrenia" (NIMH) 640n
sclerotherapy, hydrocele 420
screening tests
cancer 152
colorectal cancer 173
diabetes 190

screening tests, *continued*
lung cancer 280
overview 34–56
scrotum
defined 682
depicted *422*
epididymitis 415
penile cancer 336
prostatitis 461
testicular cancer 354
testicular self-examination 31
vasectomy 582
seasonal flu *see* influenza
secondary syphilis, sexually
transmitted diseases (STDs) 503
secondhand smoke
cancer 152
lung cancer 278
smoking 649
Seldane, sex-specific health
differences 7
self-examinations
breast cancer 24
oral cancer 26
skin cancer 28
testicular cancer 30
semen
benign prostatic hyperplasia 440
defined 678
hepatitis B 516
HIV and AIDS 225
motor vehicle accidents 291
penile trauma 400
premature ejaculation 470
prostate cancer 56, 341
semen analysis, infertility 478
seminal fluid
human immunodeficiency virus
(HIV) 225
vasectomy 481
seminal vesicle, depicted *342*
sentinel lymph node biopsy
described 590
penile cancer 334
serotonin
antidepressant medications 472
defined 682
muscle dysmorphic disorder
(MDD) 669
premature ejaculation (PE) 471

sertraline
  antidepressant medications 472
  posttraumatic stress disorder
    (PTSD) 640
serum tumor marker test,
  described 351
sex and gender, impact on health 4
"Sex and Gender" (NIH) 4n
sex with multiple partners
  excessive alcohol use 648
  genital herpes 511
  HIV screening 35
  human papillomavirus (HPV) 523
  risky sexual behaviors 15
sexual assault
  excessive alcohol use 15
  overview 657–9
  posttraumatic stress disorder
    (PTSD) 637
"Sexual Assault: Males"
  (NCPTSD) 657n
sexual dysfunction
  overview 467–75
  penile trauma 401
  sleep apnea 616
"Sexual Dysfunction"
  (Omnigraphics) 467n
sexual function
  alcohol use 16, 648
  benign prostatic hyperplasia 458
  exercise 140
  perineal surgery 433
Sexuality Information and Education
  Council of the United States
  (SIECUS), contact 690
sexually transmitted diseases
  (STDs)
  circumcision 394
  defined 682
  overview 498–539
  safer sex guidelines 493
  vasectomy 484
"Sexually Transmitted Diseases
  (STDs)" (NICHD) 498n
shingles, vaccinations for men 64
sigmoidoscopy, colorectal cancer 176
sildenafil (Viagra), ED treatment 469
silent killer, hypertension 40
Silodo, prostatitis 464

skin cancers
  overview 28–30
  prostate cancer 341
  sleep apnea 617
  statistics 151
"Skin Cancer Self-Examination"
  (Omnigraphics) 28n
sleep apnea, overview 615–24
"Sleep Apnea" (NHLBI) 615n
"Sleep Apnea" (NIH) 615n
sleep disorders
  drowsy driving 291
  male menopause 672
  overweight and obesity 92
  sleep apnea 615
sleep studies, sleep apnea 618
small intestine rectum, depicted 47
smoking
  abdominal aortic aneurysm 36
  cholesterol screening 44
  chronic obstructive pulmonary
    disease (COPD) 171
  coronary artery disease 216
  exercises 139
  high blood pressure 74
  infertility 479
  inguinal hernias 427
  kidney disease 270
  lung cancer 278
  osteoporosis 610
  osteoporosis screening 52
  overview 648–50
  pneumonia 238
  urinary incontinence 390
smoking cessation
  alcohol abuse 611
  chronic obstructive pulmonary
    disease (COPD) 171
social networks, lifestyle factors 12
solifenacin (VESIcare), noncancerous
  prostate disorders 455
"Some Sleep Drugs Can Impair
  Driving" (FDA) 291n
spermatic cord
  epididymitis 414
  inguinal hernia 421
  testicles 349
spermatocele, overview 428–30
"Spermatocele" (Omnigraphics) 428n

spermicide
  balanitis 396
  defined 682
spleen, depicted *160*
sprain, muscles 128
stage
  AIDS 501
  blood pressure 72
  breast cancer 589
  cirrhosis 162
  colorectal cancer 174
  defined 682
  HIV infection 225, 501
  lung cancer 282
  penile cancer 333
  prediabetes 185
  prostate cancer 56, 347
  syphilis 533
  testicular cancer 31, 351
standard drink, described 13
statin, high blood cholesterol 76
statistics
  accidents and injuries 321
  cancer 151
  death 146
  flu 231
  gynecomastia 606
  sex differences 17
STDs *see* sexually transmitted
  diseases
stem cell transplant
  cancer 151
  pneumonia 235
  testicular cancer 359
steroids
  balanitis 396
  gene therapy 562
  gynecomastia 606
  healthy diet 130
  influenza and pneumonia 239
  muscle dysmorphic disorder 668
  prostatitis 464
  see also anabolic steroids
"Steroids and Other Appearance and
  Performance Enhancing Drugs
  (APEDS)" (NIDA) 650n
strangulated hernia, inguinal
  hernias 424

stress
  chronic kidney disease (CKD) 262
  Cushing syndrome 96
  enlarged breasts 573
  erectile dysfunction (ED) 468
  exercise 140
  fight or flight 21
  gynecomastia 608
  heart failure 214
  male menopause 672
  obesity 96
  Peyronie disease 407
  posttraumatic stress disorder
    (PTSD) 637
  premature ejaculation 471
  sleep 77
  type 1 diabetes 188
  type 2 diabetes 190
  weight-loss program 114
stress management
  blood pressure 75
  overview 81–4
stress test
  described 209
  echocardiography 208
stretching
  nutrition 130
  penile trauma 400
  scar tissue 457
  stress 83
stroke
  blood pressure 73
  cardiovascular risk 7
  defined 682
  described 9
  influenza and pneumonia 237
  kidney disease 271
  overview 361–8
  physical activity 134
  prediabetes 182
  screening tests 35
  sleep apnea 617
subarachnoid hemorrhage
  defined 682
  hemorrhagic strokes types 363
  see also stroke
substance abuse
  adolescence 576
  gender differences 17

substance abuse, *continued*
  mental-health therapists 575
  sexual trauma 658
Substance Abuse and Mental Health
  Services Administration (SAMHSA)
  contact 687
  publications
      alcohol, tobacco, and other
        drugs 646n
      eating disorders 662n
      gender differences in primary
        substance of abuse across age
        groups 17n
suicide
  causes of death 149
  depression 630
  overview 369–71
  sex-specific health differences 15
Suicide Prevention Resource Center
  (SPRC), contact 690
support groups
  schizophrenia 644
  stroke rehabilitation 368
  violence against men 656
surgery
  abdominal aortic aneurysm
    (AAA) 38
  breast concerns in men 601
  cancer among men 151
  erectile dysfunction 470
  heart disease 212
  hemophilia 556
  human papillomavirus (HPV) 523
  hydrocele 420
  influenza and pneumonia 242
  kidney and urological disorders 384
  lung cancer 282
  male breast cancer 590
  male-linked genetic disorders 573
  noncancerous prostate disorders 452
  oral cancer 27
  overweight and obesity 92
  penile cancer 334
  penile trauma 401
  prostate cancer 346
  prostatitis 460
  sleep apnea 621
  stroke 367
  testicular cancer 357
  vasectomy 482

swelling
  balanitis 395
  heart failure 205
  hemophilia 560
  human papillomavirus (HPV) 66
  hydrocele 418
  oral cancer 27
  paraphimosis 410
  Peyronie disease 405
  spermatoceles 429
  testicular cancer 350
  viral hepatitis 158
symptoms of AAA, screening tests 37
syphilis
  overview 533–6
  screening tests 35
  sexually transmitted diseases
    (STDs) 499
"Syphilis" (HHS) 533n
systolic pressure, blood pressure 72

T

tadalafil (Cialis)
  erectile dysfunction 469
  noncancerous prostate disorders 449
tailbone, depicted *431*
"Talk to Your Doctor about Abdominal
  Aortic Aneurysm" (ODPHP) 36n
tamoxifen, breast concerns 600
tamsulosin, benign prostatic
  hyperplasia 449
targeted therapy
  breast concerns 600
  lung cancer 283
tendons, muscles 128
terazosin (Hytrin), benign prostatic
  hyperplasia 449
testes
  defined 682
  see also testicles
testicles
  depicted *342*
  hydrocele 418
  Klinefelter syndrome (KS) 566
  male infertility 478
  male-linked genetic disorders 574
  male menopause 671
  self-examinations 31

testicular asymmetry, testicular self-
examination 31
testicular cancer
epididymitis 417
overview 349–60
testicular self-examination 30
vasectomy 484
"Testicular Cancer Treatment
(PDQ®)—Patient Version" National
Cancer Institute (NCI) 349n
testicular function
alcohol use 648
male infertility 479
sex-specific health differences 16
testicular self-examination,
overview 30–2
"Testicular Self-Examination"
(Omnigraphics) 30n
testicular torsion, epididymitis 415
testosterone
breast concerns 600
healthy weight 101
hyperplasia 441
Klinefelter syndrome (KS) 568
male infertility 479
male menopause 671
sex-specific health differences 11
testicular cancer 349
tetanus, vaccinations 63
thyroid hormone levels, healthy
weight 101
TIA *see* transient ischemic attack
tobacco use
alcohol, tobacco, and other
drugs 646
colorectal cancer 174
tolterodine (Detrol), noncancerous
prostate disorders 455
tonsillectomy, sleep apnea 621
Topiramate, kidney stones 378
total cholesterol, screening tests 43
total testosterone
healthy weight 101
sleep apnea 619
tracheostomy, sleep apnea 622
tranexamic acid, male-linked genetic
disorders 561
transient ischemic attack (TIA),
described 363

transmission
hepatitis B 519
nonsurgical contraception 491
scrotum and testicles 416
syphilis 535
transrectal ultrasound
described 447
prostate cancer 347
trastuzumab, breast concerns 589
Trichomonas vaginalis, sexually
transmitted diseases (STDs) 504
trichomoniasis
overview 537–9
sexually transmitted diseases
(STDs) 502
"Trichomoniasis" (HHS) 537n
triglycerides
cholesterol screening 44
healthy weight 92
kidney disease 271
tritanomaly, male-linked genetic
disorders 547
tritanopia, red-green color
blindness 547
tunica albuginea, penile concerns 401

U

ugly duckling sign, self-
examination 28
ulcer
breast concerns 593
gynecomastia 606
sexual dysfunction 468
ulcerative colitis *see* Crohn disease
ultrasound
breast concerns 588
cirrhosis 164
defined 437
noncancerous prostate disorders 450
penile cancer 334
penile concerns 401
prostate cancer 347
screening tests 37
scrotum and testicles 415
tabulated *215*
undescended testicle, testicular
cancer 350
unemployment, alcohol use 15

Unhealthy Lifestyle Habits,
  overweight and obesity 96
United Network for Organ Sharing
  (UNOS), contact 689
unprotected sex
  alcohol use 648
  chlamydia 507
  human immunodeficiency virus
    (HIV) 35
  male infertility 477
  sex-specific health differences 15
  viral hepatitis 158
ureteroscopy, kidney and urological
  disorders 381
urethra
  chlamydia 507
  kidney and urological disorders 381
  noncancerous prostate disorders 450
  penile cancer 331
  penile trauma 400
  perineal injury 432
  prostate cancer 56
  prostatitis 460
  trichomoniasis 537
  vasectomy 481
urinalysis
  kidney and urological disorders 380
  retrograde ejaculation 474
  spermatocele 429
urinary incontinence
  benign prostatic hyperplasia 442
  kidney stones 382
  prostate cancer 346
"Urinary Incontinence in Older
  Adults" (NIA) 388n
urinary tract
  kidney and urological disorders 376
  kidney disease 249
  noncancerous prostate disorders 451
  perineum 431
urinary tract infections (UTI)
urine flow
  kidney disease 249
  kidney stones 382
  noncancerous prostate
    disorders 447
  prostate cancer 341
  prostatitis 465

uroflowmetry, noncancerous prostate
  disorders 447
U.S. Bureau of Labor Statistics (BLS)
  publication
    occupational injuries 319n
U.S. Department of Agriculture
  (USDA)
  publication
    physical activity 132n
U.S. Department of Health and
  Human Services (HHS)
  contact 686
  publications
    flu (influenza) 67n
    genital herpes 509n
    gonorrhea 512n
    hepatitis B 516n
    HIV/AIDS 225n
    human papillomavirus
      (HPV) 65n, 520n
    male condom 488n
    syphilis 533n
    trichomoniasis 537n
    vaccines for adults 62n
U.S. Department of Veterans Affairs (VA)
  publications
    cirrhosis 159n
    PTSD study: men versus
      women 20n
    safer sex 493n
U.S. Fire Administration (USFA)
  publication
    fire-related injuries 309n
U.S. Food and Drug Administration
  (FDA)
  contact 686
  publications
    sleep drugs and impaired
      driving 291n
    smoking 648n
U.S. Office of Personnel Management
  (OPM)
  publication
    screening tests 34n

V

vaccines
  defined 683

vaccines, *continued*
  overview 62–4
Vaccines for Adults, overview 62–4
"Vaccines for Adults" (HHS) 62n
vardenafil (Levitra), erectile
  dysfunction (ED) 469
varicocele, male infertility 478
vas deferens
  testicular cancer 349
  vasectomy 481
vasectomy, overview 481–5
"Vasectomy: Condition Information"
  (NICHD) 481n
ventricular fibrillation, heart
  attack 218
veterans crisis line, mental health
  concerns 637
Viagra, erectile dysfunction (ED) 469
vigorous physical activities
  physical activity 132
  tabulated *136*
virus
  childhood vaccines 64
  hemophilia 560
  hepatitis B 520
  liver cancer 274
  Peyronie disease 404
  pneumonia 235
  schizophrenia 642
  sexually transmitted diseases
    (STDs) 498
  type 1 diabetes 186
  viral hepatitis 158
vision disorders, described 9
vitamin D supplement,
  osteoporosis 613
vomiting
  abdominal aortic aneurysm
    (AAA) 37
  bulimia 666
  chronic liver disease 167
  diabetes 184
  heart attack 218
  influenza 230
  inguinal hernia 424
  kidney and urological disorders 379
  kidney disease 251
  liver cancer 274

vomiting, *continued*
  prostatitis 462
  sex-specific health differences 5
  viral hepatitis 504

W

waist circumference
  overweight and obesity 100
  weight and health risk 86
walking pneumonia, bacteria 236
warm-up exercises, nutrition
  tips 130
"Water-Related Injuries"
  (CDC) 325n
weight loss
  liver cancer 274
  overview 103–11
  sleep apnea 623
  syphilis 534
"What Is BMI?" (CDC) 88n
"What Is Colorectal Cancer?"
  (CDC) 173n
"What Is Lung Cancer?"
  (CDC) 277n
"What Is Muscular Dystrophy?"
  (CDC) 578n
"What Is 'Safer Sex'?" (VA) 493n
"What Is Viral Hepatitis?"
  (NIDDK) 158n
white fat tissue, overweight and
  obesity 94
whooping cough, vaccines for
  adults 62
"Why Women Live Longer than Men"
  (Omnigraphics) 10n
withdrawal, overview 490–1
"Withdrawal" (Omnigraphics) 490n

X

X-linked disorder, color blindness 546
X-ray
  defined 683
  inguinal hernia 425
  male breast cancer 590
  osteoporosis 612
  Peyronie disease 408

Y

yawning, drowsy driving 292
yeast infection, balanitis 396
yoga
  defined 683
  kidney disease 270
  physical activity 137

"Your Kidneys and How They Work"
  (NIDDK) 249n

Z

zero tolerance laws, impaired
  driving 298